PRINCIPLES AND APPLICATIONS OF

RADIOLOGICAL
PHYSICS

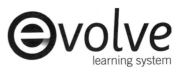

learning system

Evolve Learning Resources for Students and Lecturers.
See the instructions on the inside cover for access to the website.

Think outside the book...evolve

Commissioning Editor: Claire Wilson
Development Editor: Veronika Watkins
Project Manager: Mahalakshmi Nithyanand
Designer: Charles Gray
Illustration Manager: Merlyn Harvey
Illustrator: Jennifer Rose

PRINCIPLES AND APPLICATIONS OF
RADIOLOGICAL
SIXTH EDITION
PHYSICS

Edited by

Donald T. Graham MED TDCR
Former Director, Radiography,
School of Health Sciences,
Robert Gordon University, Aberdeen, UK

Paul Cloke MSc TDCR
Former Lecturer in Diagnostic Imaging,
Centre for Radiographic and Medical Studies,
Department of Materials and Medical Science,
Cranfield University, Shrivenham Campus, Swindon, Wiltshire, UK

Martin Vosper MSc PgDip HDCR
Senior Lecturer,
School of Health and Human Sciences,
University of Hertfordshire, Hatfield, Hertfordshire, UK

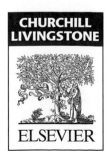

CHURCHILL
LIVINGSTONE

ELSEVIER

EDINBURGH   LONDON   NEW YORK   OXFORD   PHILADELPHIA   ST LOUIS   SYDNEY   TORONTO   2011

CHURCHILL
LIVINGSTONE
ELSEVIER

© 2012 Elsevier Ltd. All rights reserved.

First edition 1981
Second edition 1987
Third edition 1996
Fourth edition 2003
Fifth edition 2007
Sixth edition 2012

Formerly 978-0-7020-4309-3
ISBN: 978-0-7020-5215-6

British Library Cataloguing in Publication Data
A catalogue record for this book is available from the British Library

Library of Congress Cataloging in Publication Data
A catalog record for this book is available from the Library of Congress

Notices
Knowledge and best practice in this field are constantly changing. As new research and experience broaden our understanding, changes in research methods, professional practices, or medical treatment may become necessary.

Practitioners and researchers must always rely on their own experience and knowledge in evaluating and using any information, methods, compounds, or experiments described herein. In using such information or methods they should be mindful of their own safety and the safety of others, including parties for whom they have a professional responsibility.

With respect to any drug or pharmaceutical products identified, readers are advised to check the most current information provided (i) on procedures featured or (ii) by the manufacturer of each product to be administered, to verify the recommended dose or formula, the method and duration of administration, and contraindications. It is the responsibility of practitioners, relying on their own experience and knowledge of their patients, to make diagnoses, to determine dosages and the best treatment for each individual patient, and to take all appropriate safety precautions.

To the fullest extent of the law, neither the Publisher nor the authors, contributors, or editors, assume any liability for any injury and/or damage to persons or property as a matter of products liability, negligence or otherwise, or from any use or operation of any methods, products, instructions, or ideas contained in the material herein.

ELSEVIER your source for books,
journals and multimedia
in the health sciences
www.elsevierhealth.com

Printed in China

Contents

Contents

Preface

Since the publication of the fifth edition of *Principles of Radiological Physics* in 2006, radiography education has continued to evolve. The four-tier nature of the radiography profession is now well established and radiography courses appropriate to all grades from Assistant Practitioner to Consultant Radiographer have been established. Much of the 'pure physics' is no longer taught and many courses concentrate more on the basic principles and the application of these principles to radiographic science. Before commencing the sixth edition we surveyed university staff and students and received many useful comments on what they would like to see in the new edition.

We have tried to reflect these comments as a result have changed the title of the text to *'Principles and Applications of Radiological Physics.'* This has resulted in expansion of the text, and some sections which were previously appendices are now full chapters. Also, six new chapters considering the applications of radiological physics have been written. We have rearranged some of the sections so that the text follows a more logical order. The sixth edition now consists of the following sections:

- Basic Physics
- Atomic Physics
- X-rays and Matter
- Dosimetry
- Equipment for X-ray production
- The radiographic Image
- Applications of radiological Physics
- Radiation Protection
- Appendices
- Tables

There has been significant updating of many sections, especially the section dealing with the radiographic image, where the change from film/screen imaging to digital imaging has been acknowledged. Colour has also been used to clarify some of the diagrams and photographic images have been included where appropriate.

Sections which students and staff felt were valuable have been retained. These include 'insight boxes' to allow consideration of some topics at greater depth – and self-assessment questions have been added to the accompanying Evolve website.

In writing this new edition we would like to acknowledge the help we have received from Academic and clinical staff, students and the manufacturers of radiographic equipment who have kindly allowed us to use some of their published material. We also acknowledge with gratitude the help and encouragement we have received from the publication team at Elsevier all of whom have made a significant contribution to this publication.

Despite the changes in the education of radiographers, the principal role of the radiographer remains unchanged, namely the selection of appropriate imaging techniques and the production of high quality images or treatments. These should be performed with the minimum of radiation hazard to the patient, staff and others whose presence is a necessary part of the examination or treatment. An understanding of physics and its application to radiographic technology is essential to enable us to do this effectively.

Donald T Graham
Paul Cloke
Martin Vosper

Aberdeen, Bicester and Hatfield
2011

Part | 1 |

Introduction

Chapter | 1 |

Principles of radiography

1.1 AIM

This chapter considers the basic principles of diagnostic radiography, therapeutic radiography and radiation protection. This should allow the reader to appreciate how the individual chapters within the text form part of a whole study.

1.2 DIAGNOSTIC AND THERAPEUTIC RADIOGRAPHY

X-rays (and other forms of radiation) can have two main uses in medicine. They can be used to investigate the patient's illness or physical state through the production of an image – this forms the basis of *diagnostic radiography*; or they can be used to eliminate unwanted abnormal cells in certain body tissues – the basis of *therapeutic radiography*.

1.2.1 Diagnostic radiography

In diagnostic radiography, an image of structures within the patient's body is produced on an image receptor or a monitor screen. Normally, of course, we cannot see inside each other's bodies because light photons, to which our eyes are sensitive, are absorbed and reflected very close to the surface of body tissues.

> **Insight**
>
> To examine internal body structures using light, an instrument called an endoscope must be inserted into the body. This consists of fibre optic bundles which transmit the light to and from the region of interest and so allows the operator to view the organ. Such techniques are used in 'keyhole surgery'. This type of imaging does carry some risk, or it may be uncomfortable for the patient, and so radiography will often be considered as an alternative.

Figure 1.1 shows a radiographer preparing the equipment for a common X-ray diagnostic examination.

As light is a form of *electromagnetic radiation* (see Ch. 17) and it seems logical to suggest that if we can take photons of electromagnetic radiation which have higher energies than light photons, then these may have sufficient energy to penetrate body tissues and allow us to visualize internal organs. X-rays are in this part of the electromagnetic spectrum and so will penetrate body tissues and allow us to image internal organs. Unfortunately the retina of the eye cannot detect X-rays and so we cannot see an image of a structure just by directing an X-ray beam on it. This means that the X-rays, which have passed through the body, must be made to strike an image receptor that will produce a visible image, for example an imaging plate.

3

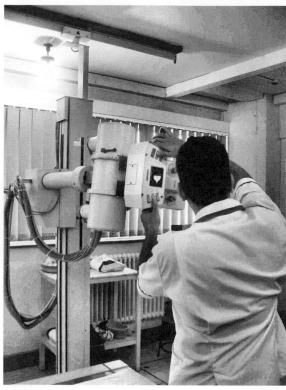

Figure 1.1 A radiographer preparing to examine a patient's chest.

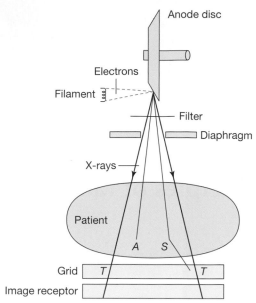

Figure 1.2 The principal interactions involved in the production of a radiographic image. *A* represents absorbed photons, *S* represents scattered photons and *T* represents transmitted photons.

The principal interactions involved in the basic requirements for the formation of a radiographic image are shown in Figure 1.2.

X-rays are produced in the X-ray tube by accelerating electrons and causing these to collide with the target of the X-ray tube. To understand how this works we need to know about *energy* (see Ch. 4) and *electricity* (see Chs 7 and 11) as well as the construction of the X-ray transformer and X-ray tube (see Chs 14 and 30). The X-rays so produced are over a wide band of energies. Most of the photons that have insufficient energy to be of diagnostic value are removed from the beam using *filtration* (see Ch. 22) and the area of the patient irradiated is restricted using a *diaphragm* (see Ch. 25). The beam now interacts with the patient and a number of things may happen to the X-ray photons. These may be:

- *transmitted* (*T* in Fig. 1.2): these photons pass through the patient without interacting with the patient's tissues. They are thus unaffected by their passage through the patient
- *absorbed* (*A* in Fig. 1.2): these photons interact with the patient's tissues and as a result lose all of their energy. As the photon consists only of energy, then these photons disappear from the spectrum of radiation transmitted through the patient

- *scattered* (*S* in Fig. 1.2): these photons interact with the patient's tissues and are then deflected from their original path. Such a deflection may or may not result in a loss of some of the photons' energy.

Different tissues will absorb different amounts of radiation (see Ch. 25) and so a differentiated radiation pattern leaves the patient. The scattered radiation is not helpful to the image, so when the scatter production is significant, as much as possible of this is removed using a *secondary radiation grid* (see Ch. 25). Finally, the radiation interacts with the image receptor, where it is 'captured' and passed into a digital imaging system (see Ch. 34).

Radiographers employ other radiations in the course of their clinical work. Magnetic resonance imaging (MRI; see Ch. 39) makes use of powerful magnetic fields as well as radiofrequency waves. Both of these are examples of *non-ionizing radiations*, which are not thought to cause cancers but can have other biological effects on the human body. Radiofrequency waves are a form of electromagnetic radiation, just like X-rays, but have a much lower frequency. As a result they are much less energetic and fit lower down the electromagnetic spectrum. Ultrasound (see Ch. 42) is another example of a non-ionizing radiation used in radiography. But unlike X-rays and radiofrequency waves, ultrasound needs a medium like fluid or body tissue to pass through. This is because it consists of a series of vibrations passing through molecules and is not a form of electromagnetic radiation. Sound cannot be heard in a vacuum. But X-rays, radio waves and light, which are all electromagnetic, can pass freely through outer space.

Sound waves travel at different speeds in different body tissues, whereas X-rays always travel at the same extremely high speed, which is termed the 'speed of light' – about 300 000 kilometers per second!

1.2.2 Therapeutic radiography

In therapeutic radiography, we are not trying to produce images but are using the *biological effects* of radiation to kill tumour cells. At the same time, we try to cause as little damage as possible to the healthy cells in the body.

Insight

There are four main methods of cancer treatment: surgery, chemotherapy, alteration of the hormone balance and radiotherapy. They may be used in isolation or together to give the optimum treatment regime for a given cancer in a given patient. The treatment may be *radical* or *palliative*. The former is an all-out effort to achieve a cure and the latter is used to relieve pain and other distressing symptoms when no cure for the disease is possible. This is normally in the terminal stages of the disease.

The relative success of radiotherapy in the management of cancer lies in the fact that malignant cells are more sensitive to radiation than healthy cells in the same organ. In spite of this, a number of healthy cells are affected by radiation and so must be given time to recover. Thus the radiation dose is delivered as a number of treatments rather than as a single dose. This technique is known as fractionation and may mean that a patient has 15–30 treatments over a period of 3–6 weeks.

1.3 METHODS OF RADIATION TREATMENT

A detailed description of the different methods of radiation treatment is beyond the scope of this introductory chapter and the reader is directed to some of the more specialized texts on the subject. In considering the overview of radiation treatment methods, we can, however, identify some distinct types, which we will discuss further. These are:

* teletherapy
* brachytherapy
* nuclear medicine.

1.3.1 Teletherapy

Here an external source of radiation (normally X-rays or gamma rays) is directed at the tumour. The aim is to give the maximum dose to the tumour and the minimum dose to the healthy tissue. This is often achieved by treating the tumour with a number of fields (see Fig. 1.3). The areas in the patient that receive doses of equal value are joined by lines called *isodose lines*. The shape and the position of these lines may be altered by the use of absorbing wedges and compensators and also by altering the energy and shape of the treatment beam. Once the treatment plan has been produced, the positions of the treatment fields on the patient are checked in a *simulator* where the treatment angles can be set up and the fields marked. In areas of the patient around the head and the neck, accurate positioning and immobilization are achieved by placing this part in a specially prepared clear plastic shell.

1.3.2 Brachytherapy

When we use external radiation beams, the radiation must travel through healthy tissue to reach the tumour. There are some situations where tumours are relatively accessible from the body surface or are in body cavities where sealed *radioactive sources* (see Ch. 19) may be inserted. This technique is known as brachytherapy. The technique can often mean that a large dose can be delivered to the tumour while a much smaller dose strikes the surrounding tissues because of the effects of the inverse square law (see Ch. 26). If the sources were implanted directly by the radiotherapist, the dose to the hands of the operator could be quite large. This is overcome by inserting a number of guides into the correct position and mechanically inserting the sources over the guides for the required treatment. This technique is called *afterloading* and is often used in the treatment of pelvic cancers.

1.3.3 Nuclear medicine

A third possibility is that the radiation can be delivered to the tissue by allowing the tissue to absorb a certain *radionuclide* (see Ch. 19). This is probably best illustrated by considering the treatment of an overactive thyroid gland. The activity of the gland can be reduced by surgical removal of part of the gland, or some of its tissue may be destroyed using radiation. To allow the thyroid to produce the required hormones, it must absorb iodine. The patient may be given sodium iodide (where the iodine is in the form of ^{131}I) as a capsule or in an oral solution. Some of this *isotope* (see Ch. 19) is taken up by the gland and the rest is secreted in the urine. ^{131}I is a *beta particle* emitter (see Ch. 19) and this results in a radiation dose to the thyroid tissue, which reduces its metabolic rate to normal. Because of the limited range of the beta particles produced, there is less radiation dose to structures around the thyroid than there would be if we used an external radiation beam. ^{131}I also has a relatively short *half-life*

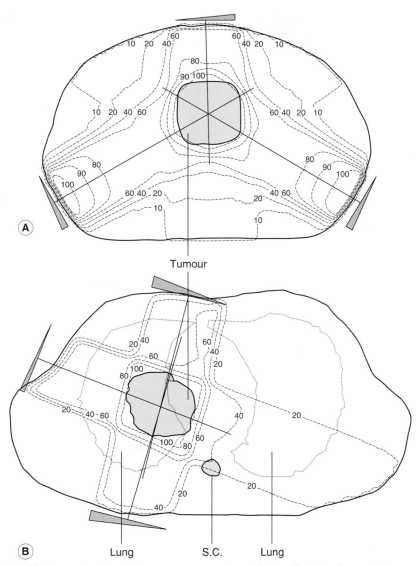

Figure 1.3 Grossly simplified examples of radiotherapy treatment plans. (A) Three-field plan for a pelvic tumour. (B) Three-field plan for a mediastinal tumour (note how the fields minimize dose to the spinal cord (SC) on the plan).

(8 days) (see Ch. 19) and so the radiation hazard posed by the patient to others can be minimized.

1.4 RADIATION PROTECTION

All ionizing radiation of the cells which make up our bodies carries a risk of damage to those cells. It is also true that some tissues are more sensitive to radiation than others. The use of ionizing radiation in medicine is of great value to humans, but it is the largest single factor which contributes to the *artificial radiation dose* received

by the human race. The contribution of the various radiation sources is shown in Figure 1.4.

Because of this, we have a duty to minimize the dose to our patients and colleagues and so minimize the risk of radiation damage. The radiation dose is composed of *primary radiation* and *secondary radiation*, and so we need to look at the ways in which these are produced and absorbed. This will be considered in Chapter 44. Because of the known hazards of radiation, there are certain statutory requirements for *radiation protection* and *monitoring* in diagnostic and therapy departments (see Ch. 44). In terms of assessing the risk, it is important to know the dose received by both patients and radiation workers and this will be discussed in Chapter 27, which deals with the topic of *radiation dosimetry*.

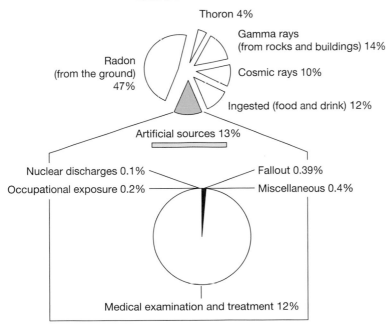

Figure 1.4 Sources of radiation exposure to humans.
(Based on data from the radiation section of the Health Protection Agency (formerly the National Radiological Protection Board.)

Summary

This brief overview should enable the reader to understand certain physical principles which underpin diagnostic and therapy radiography. Patients and staff should be exposed to the minimum risk from the radiation and the principles governing this have been outlined.

FURTHER READING

This overview covers a very large subject area and so only the principal texts are identified. Further reading in specialized topics will be covered in the chapter bibliographies.

Diagnostic radiography

Moores, B.M., Wall, B.F., Stieve, S.E., et al., 1989. Optimisation of Image Quality and Patient Exposure in Diagnostic Imaging. British Institute of Radiology Report 18. British Institute of Radiology, London.

Therapeutic radiography

Bomford, C.K., 1993. Walter's and Miller's textbook of radiotherapy. Churchill Livingstone, Edinburgh.

Souhami, R., Tobias, J., 1987. Cancer and its Management. Blackwell Scientific, Oxford.

Wang, C.C., 2000. Clinical Radiation Oncology: Indications, Techniques and Results, Second edn. Wiley, New York.

Radiation protection

Dowd, S.B., Tildon, E.R., 1999. Practical Radiation Protection and Applied Radiobiology, Second edn. WB Saunders, Philadelphia.

Statutory Instrument 1999/3232 The ionising radiation regulations, 1999. HMSO, London.

UK National Radiation Protection Division. (http://www.hpa.org.uk/radiation).

Part | 2 |

Basic physics

Chapter | 2 |

Power sources for radiation production

2.1 AIM

This chapter explains how energy is obtained to produce radiations in diagnostic and therapeutic radiography. There are a range of devices to be considered, including X-ray generators, linear accelerators, ultrasound machines and magnetic resonance imaging (MRI) scanners. This variety of equipment contributes to making modern radiography an exciting and powerful tool for diagnosis and treatment.

2.2 OBTAINING ENERGY FOR RADIATION PRODUCTION

As will be seen in Chapter 3, energy cannot be created out of nothing, but may be converted from one form to another. This principle is called the law of conservation of energy. It is a bit like saying that we must have cash in our bank account before we can make a purchase, with no borrowing permitted! So we must have energy available before we can produce the range of radiations that are used in diagnostic and therapeutic radiography. Normally the production of radiations in radiography involves a conversion of electrical energy into wave energy, via various stages. These waves are either electromagnetic (see Ch. 17) or sound (see Ch. 42). At this point it would be useful to identify the types of radiations that we will encounter. These include X-rays, sound waves and radio waves.

Most of the radiations used in radiography can be regarded as 'waves' (this topic is covered in Ch. 17) and may be divided into two major types – ionizing and non-ionizing:

- Ionizing radiations have sufficient energy to remove electrons from atoms, in a process which is of course termed ionization. You will probably already know that electrons are small negatively charged particles which orbit the nuclei of atoms. Atoms are the fundamental building blocks of matter and can group together to form molecules and extended structures in living and non-living things. More can be learnt about atoms in Chapter 18. The process of ionization can break chemical bonds in the DNA of living cells, resulting in damage. X-rays are a type of ionizing radiation.
- Non-ionizing radiations include the sound waves used in ultrasound, and radio waves used in MRI. These radiations are less energetic than X-rays, but can agitate body tissues to some extent, generating heat. The biological effects of these radiations are not thought to result in long-term harm. Sound has a special place among the radiations used in radiography, as it is not electromagnetic (see Ch. 17) and is transmitted via vibrations passing through atoms and molecules.

All of the above mentioned radiations – X-rays, sound waves and radio waves, are 'generated' by man-made devices. These devices have to be powered in order to produce the radiations. Table 2.1 summarizes the commonly used power sources found in radiography.

Table 2.1 Sources of power for the radiations found in radiography

RADIATION	POWER SOURCE	RESULT AND APPLICATIONS
X-rays – diagnostic imaging and radiotherapy	An X-ray generator – this takes electrical power from the mains and provides a high voltage, typically up to 150 000 volts for diagnostic use and 300 000 volts for radiotherapy, across the two electrodes of an X-ray tube Found in fixed ('static') units in X-ray or low-energy radiotherapy treatment rooms and high-output mobile X-ray machines	Electrons in an X-ray tube are promoted to a high electrical potential This potential energy, when released and converted to kinetic energy, results in X-rays at the target of the X-ray tube Applications include conventional diagnostic X-ray procedures, computed tomography (CT) scanning and superficial radiotherapy for skin cancers
X-rays – mobile and portable radiography	Batteries or capacitors Charged up from the mains Found in low-output mobile and portable X-ray machines, used in hospital wards, casualty, operating theatres and sometimes people's homes	An X-ray tube is used as above, but applications are limited to diagnostic X-ray procedures which only require low X-ray tube outputs, such as conventional chest and abdominal radiography
X-rays – radiotherapy linear accelerators	A linear accelerator (LINAC) This takes electrical power from the mains in order to produce a high voltage and also to power acceleration of electrons in a wave guide Found in fixed ('static') units in radiotherapy treatment rooms	Electrons in the LINAC are promoted to a high electrical potential and then accelerated to an enormous speed by microwaves in a wave guide This results in very high kinetic energy (including some increase in electron mass) which in turn produces very high-energy X-rays at the target of the LINAC The rays are used to kill cancer cells in radiotherapy
Sound waves	Electrical power is taken from the mains and a voltage is applied across a piezoelectric crystal in the probe of an ultrasound machine Ultrasound machines are compact and portable	The applied alternating voltage waveform causes the crystal to vibrate The resultant mechanical oscillations of the crystal produce high-frequency sound waves which are termed 'ultrasound'
Radio waves	Electrical power is taken from the mains and applied to a radiofrequency (RF) transmitter coil Additionally, electrical power is used to generate very strong magnetic fields in an MRI magnet, normally involving the process of 'superconductivity', which requires refrigeration of coils of wire to extremely low temperatures	Radio waves emitted from the transmitter coil are used to excite the magnetic spins of atomic nuclei in a human body Subsequent 'relaxation' of this spin energy results in a returning radio wave signal. Used in MRI

It will be seen that all of the above sources obtain electrical power from the mains (National Grid). There are two voltages available in the United Kingdom – a single-phase 240-volt supply for low-powered hospital devices such as dental X-ray tubes (as shown in Fig. 2.1) and domestic use, and a three-phase 415-volt supply where more power is needed, as in conventional static X-ray sets. The number of phases refers to how many voltage waveforms are combined within the electrical output. This subject is covered in more detail in Chapter 11.

2.3 A SPECIAL CASE – RADIOACTIVE SOURCES

Radioactive materials, many of which are found 'naturally' on Earth, are rather different from the above mentioned sources of radiation, in that they do not require man-made electrical power in order to emit radiation. They emit radiation spontaneously, in some cases over many years. Radioactive materials may emit gamma rays (often written as γ rays, using the Greek letter gamma) which are waves, as well as alpha and beta particles (often written as α and β) which have mass. These are all examples of ionizing radiations. Radioactive materials consist of atoms which are unstable due to having an excess of neutrons or protons in their atomic nuclei. Chemical elements always have a fixed number of protons in their atomic nuclei (uranium, for example, always has 92 protons), but isotopes of elements have different numbers of neutrons. Two isotopes of uranium are uranium-235 (with 235 − 92 = 143 neutrons) and uranium-238 (with 238 − 92 = 146 neutrons). Radioactive materials are covered in more detail in Chapters 19 and 37. They have diagnostic applications in radionuclide imaging (RNI) and therapeutic applications in teletherapy, brachytherapy and nuclear medicine, as mentioned in Chapter 1.

There is just one more added complication with regard to radioactive materials – some radioactive isotopes used in radiography in the imaging technique called positron emission tomography (PET) are man made and do not occur naturally on Earth. These isotopes are unstable due to having too few neutrons in their nuclei and require power for their artificial synthesis, using a device called a cyclotron. This topic is explored in Chapter 40.

2.4 X-RAY GENERATORS

In the world at large, the term 'generator' means a device for producing electricity. This might range from a huge apparatus at a power station to a mobile unit at a camp site! But in radiography, the term 'generator' normally refers to a device that increases (or 'steps-up') the mains voltage to values sufficient to produce X-rays. At one time the generator tank in an X-ray room would be a bulky affair, containing a large transformer and various switches, surrounded by insulating oil. More will be said about transformers in Chapter 14. But modern generator tanks tend to be much more compact, due to the advent of more efficient 'medium-frequency' voltage converters. An example of a modern generator tank can be seen in Figure 2.2.

As mentioned previously, the 'driving force' for X-ray production at X-ray energies up to 300 keV (300 kilo electron volts, or 300 000 electron volts) is a source of current electricity from the mains. This mains electricity is alternating current (AC) which means that the electrons in the circuit flow first in one direction and then another. Electricity is a flow of small negatively charged electrons drifting through a conducting material, as explained in more detail in Chapter 7.

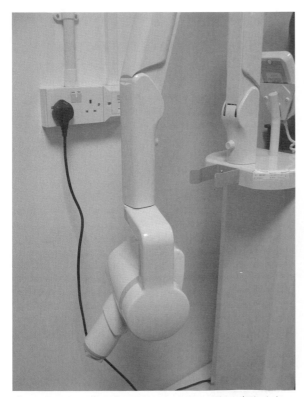

Figure 2.1 A modern dental X-ray machine. This relatively low-powered device can be operated from a 240-volt mains supply.

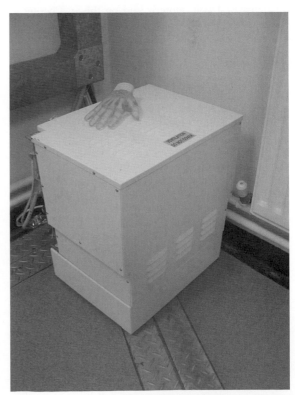

Figure 2.2 A modern medium-frequency generator tank in an X-ray room. The compact size of the unit can be seen with reference to the hand phantom.

Why are X-ray energies (and also the energies of gamma rays and particle radiations) expressed in electron volts (eV)? Well the electron volt is a unit of energy. It equals the kinetic energy (energy of movement) gained by an electron when it is accelerated by an electrical potential difference of 1 volt. More is said on this in Chapter 4. This has real practical relevance in X-ray tubes, in which electrons are accelerated by large voltages. The transfer of energy from a fast-moving electron to produce an X-ray photon (a little packet of wave energy) occurs in the target of an X-ray tube. To be of practical use in diagnostic radiography, X-ray photons are typically produced with energies ranging from 30 000 to 150 000 eV (30 keV to 150 keV). In radiotherapy, X-rays with energies of about 50–150 keV may be used for the treatment of superficial (shallow) cancers. Orthovoltage radiotherapy operates at about 200–300 keV. These techniques all use X-ray tubes. Radiotherapy linear accelerators (LINACs) use more exotic technology (not X-ray tubes) and typically operate at 6 or 16 MeV (mega electron volts). These radiotherapy topics are followed up in Chapter 32.

The voltage across the X-ray tube in kilovolts corresponds to the maximum possible X-ray energy in kilo electron volts, as will be explained in Chapter 21. Another term which needs explaining is the 'kVp' or 'peak kilovoltage' applied to an X-ray tube. There is a peak value since there may be slight voltage fluctuations in the AC output of an X-ray generator.

Traditional X-ray generators included large 'step-up' transformers, designed to increase the mains voltage of 415 volts to the kilovoltage levels needed for X-ray production. The transformer, as will be detailed in Chapter 14, consists of two coils of conducting wire, termed primary and secondary coils, mounted on an iron core.

Alternating (AC) electrical current in the primary coil produces a time-varying magnetic field which in turn induces an alternating electrical current in the secondary coil. The relative size of the primary and secondary voltages depends on the relative number of loops of wire on the primary and secondary coils. Alternating current is especially good at this process of electromagnetic induction, which is covered further in Chapter 10, as it produces a lot of magnetic flux change.

Modern X-ray generators make use of 'medium-frequency' devices, which are not only more compact and more efficient but also offer more precise control of electrical output. The term medium frequency means a frequency higher than the 50 Hz (Hertz or cycles per second) supply obtained from the mains and is typically about 5000 Hz in radiographic generators. A key principle of working with voltages that vary with a high frequency is that they are very efficient at producing electromagnetic induction in a transformer. The transformer can be more compact as a result of this. The frequency of a wave is the number of wave cycles which will fit into a second, as explained further in Chapter 17. The modern generator assembly additionally first converts mains alternating current to direct current. This direct current is fed to a voltage inverter, which in turn provides a high-frequency alternating current supply for the primary coil of a step-up transformer.

2.5 THE LINEAR ACCELERATOR

A linear accelerator (LINAC) is a complex apparatus used in radiotherapy to deliver very high-energy X-rays to destroy tumours. This topic is covered in more detail in Chapter 32. The advantage of very high-energy X-rays is that they can deliver lethal radiation doses to unwanted tumour cells deep in the human body, but deliver low doses to the skin. This is termed 'skin sparing'. Conventional X-ray tubes have real problems in trying to work with voltages much above 300 kVp (including the problem that electrical insulation is likely to break down, resulting in a violent spark!). Thus different approaches have to be used for generating X-rays in the MeV range.

The LINAC is quite exotic, in that it not only features a high-voltage supply to generate a stream of electrons which bombard a target, but also uses microwaves passing down a tube (called a waveguide) to accelerate those electrons. The electrons 'hitch a lift' on the travelling microwaves and end up travelling at incredibly high speeds, which approach (but can never reach) the speed of light. As a result they have incredibly high energies when they reach the LINAC target material and can transfer large amounts of energy to X-rays.

Insight

As particles (such as electrons) approach the speed of light, their mass increases. Thus their kinetic energy, which is expressed as $\frac{1}{2}mv^2$ (m is mass, v is velocity) is very high. The increase in mass is a consequence of Einstein's theory of relativity. This would be a problem for fictional space ships like the starship Enterprise, as a ship travelling at the speed of light would have an infinite mass. But is faster than light travel (warp speed) possible? We just don't know!

2.6 ULTRASOUND GENERATION

Ultrasound machines produce very high-frequency sound waves at 2–20 MHz, above the audible range for humans. These waves, unlike the other waves found in radiography, consist of alternating compressions and rarefactions passing through atoms and molecules and are *not* electromagnetic. More will be said about ultrasound in Chapter 42. The probes of ultrasound machines contain special crystals which have piezoelectric properties. This means that if a varying electrical voltage is applied to them, the material of the crystals vibrates at a frequency which can be varied by altering the applied electrical frequency. The mechanical vibration produces sound waves which can be transmitted into human tissues.

2.7 MAGNETIC RESONANCE IMAGING

Magnetic resonance imaging (MRI) scanners draw electrical power from the mains in order to generate radiofrequency (RF) waves. These RF waves are produced by transmitter coils at the Larmor or resonance frequency for hydrogen nuclei placed in a powerful magnetic field. This frequency is 42.6 MHz for a scanner operating at a 1-Tesla field strength. More will be said about MRI in Chapter 39. An RF transmitter uses an oscillating electrical current, with power being provided by an AC supply. The varying current in the oscillator causes charges to oscillate in an antenna. This induces an electromagnetic field which radiates out from the antenna. The radiofrequency wave energy is applied to a patient in the MRI scanner and increases the energy of the magnetic 'spins' of atomic nuclei (especially hydrogen nuclei) present in the human body. The subsequent 'relaxation' of these spins, in which energy is lost, produces a returning radio wave signal.

MRI scanners (with the exception of permanent magnet systems) also require electrical current in the main magnet coils to generate very powerful magnetic fields. This works on the principle of electromagnetic induction (see Ch. 10). In resistive systems (which are electromagnets), large amounts of electrical current are required. Superconducting magnet systems operate in conditions where there is zero electrical resistance in the magnet coils, at just a few Kelvin (K) above absolute zero temperature. But, as was mentioned at the start of this chapter, it is never possible to get energy from nothing! In this case, electrical power must be put into the system to refrigerate the coils and maintain liquid helium coolant at extremely low temperature.

Summary

In this chapter you should have learnt that:
- Electrical energy is used to generate radiations in diagnostic and therapeutic radiography.
- Natural radioactive sources are a special case, as they produce radiations by spontaneous decay.
- The majority of radiations used in radiography are waves, either electromagnetic or sound. However, particle radiations may be emitted from radioactive sources and may also be used to treat some tumours in radiotherapy.

Many of the topics included in this chapter are followed up in more detail later in the book.

Chapter | 3 |

Laws of classical physics

3.1 AIM

The chapter introduces the reader to some of the laws of classical physics. An understanding of these laws will aid in understanding some of the later chapters of the book. (Some of the physics in the later chapters of this book (e.g. pair production as an absorption mechanism) cannot be explained in terms of the laws of classical physics.) Before these concepts are considered (Ch. 20 onwards), the laws of modern physics will be considered (in Ch. 16).

3.2 LAW OF CONSERVATION OF MATTER (MASS)

3.2.1 Statement of the law

Matter is neither created nor destroyed, but it may change its chemical form as the result of a chemical reaction.

This law tells us that the total mass of the ingredients after a chemical reaction is equal to their mass before the reaction.

Insight
Consider the reaction: $H_2O \rightarrow OH^- + H^+$ Here a molecule of water has been ionized by radiation. Matter has neither been created nor destroyed by the reaction.

3.3 LAW OF CONSERVATION OF ENERGY

3.3.1 Statement of the law

Energy can neither be created nor destroyed but can be changed from one form to another. The amount of energy in a system is constant.

This law tells us that energy is never used up but changes from one form to another.

Insight
When an electron is released from the filament of an X-ray tube, it has potential energy. As it is accelerated across the tube, this potential energy is converted to kinetic energy. When it makes contact with the target of the tube, this kinetic energy is converted to heat and X-ray energy. At any time, the sum of all the energies remains constant.

Some of the common forms of energy are:

- chemical
- potential
- electrical
- kinetic
- heat
- radiation.

These two laws of conservation of mass and energy are combined into one law by modern physics (see Ch. 16).

3.4 LAW OF CONSERVATION OF MOMENTUM

3.4.1 Statement of the law

The total linear or rotational momentum in a given system is constant.

This law is important when we consider collisions between two bodies.

Insight

There are two types of collision that occur, elastic and inelastic. An elastic collision is one where all kinetic energy is conserved, as in the case of a 'perfect' billiard ball colliding with a similar but stationary billiard ball; the moving ball stops, while the ball which was previously stationary moves with the same velocity as the first ball had before collision. In an *inelastic* collision, the total kinetic energy is not conserved, as in the case of two billiard balls colliding with a glancing blow, so that both continue to move after the collision. In both cases, the *momentum* is conserved, although the *velocities* of the bodies in each case will be different.

In radiographic science, conservation of momentum is mainly concerned with the interactions of X-rays with matter; these will be dealt with in Chapter 23.

3.5 NEWTON'S LAWS OF MOTION

Newton's laws of motion can be derived from the above laws, but they are so useful that they merit a separate section. They are defined as follows:

3.5.1 Law 1

A body will remain at rest or will travel with a constant velocity unless acted upon by a net external force.

3.5.2 Law 2

The rate of change of momentum of a body is proportional to the applied force.

3.5.3 Law 3

The action of one body on a second body is always accompanied by an equal and opposite action of the second body on the first.

Note: The terms *velocity* and *momentum* in the first two laws imply direction, as both are vector quantities (see Ch. 4).

A body of mass m and velocity u has a force F applied to it. After a time t, its velocity has changed to v. Then the second law of motion can be stated as:

$$\frac{(mv - mu)}{t} \propto F$$

$$\frac{m(v - u)}{t} \propto F$$

Now $(v - u)/t$ is the rate of change of velocity or the acceleration, a, of the body (see Ch. 4). So, we can say that:

$$ma \propto F \text{ or } F = kma$$

where k is the constant of proportionality (see Appendix A).

If we choose suitable units, it can be arranged that k is equal to 1 and we finally have:

Equation 3.1

$$F = m \times a$$

In the International System of Units (SI; see Ch. 4), F is measured in newtons, m is measured in kilograms and a is measured in m.s^{-2}. This makes Equation 3.1 the familiar mathematical statement of Newton's second law and can also be used as the basis for the definition of the newton ($1\,\text{N} = 1\,\text{kg} \times 1\,\text{m.s}^{-2}$).

Insight

As an illustration of the use of this law, we are now in a position to calculate the kinetic energy of a body of mass, m, travelling with a velocity, v. If we apply a steady force, F, in the opposite direction to that of v, the body will slow down and eventually come to rest. The work done in bringing the body to rest must be equal to its kinetic energy. We can state this mathematically as:

Equation 3.2

$$E = -F \times s$$

where s is the distance taken for the body to come to rest. (The force, F, and its associated acceleration, a, are regarded as negative as they are applied in the opposite direction to v.)

From Equation 3.1 we can now change Equation 3.2 as follows:

Equation 3.3

$$E = -m \times a \times s$$

The acceleration, a, is the change in velocity per unit time. Stated mathematically, this is:

$$-a = \frac{(v - 0)}{t}$$

$$a = \frac{-v}{t}$$

As the action of the force is consistent throughout the deceleration, the time taken for the body to stop can be calculated by dividing the distance travelled by the average velocity ($v/2$). So:

$$t = \frac{s}{\frac{1}{2}v} = \frac{2s}{v}$$

Thus we get:

$$a = \frac{-v}{t}$$

$$= \frac{-v}{(2s/v)}$$

$$= \frac{-v^2}{2s}$$

If we now consider Equation 3.3, this can be rewritten:

Equation 3.4

$$E = \frac{-m(as)}{\frac{1}{2}}$$

$$= -m(-\tfrac{1}{2}v^2)$$

$$E = \tfrac{1}{2}mv^2$$

Newton's third law is usually paraphrased as: 'To every action there is an equal and opposite reaction'. There are many examples of this in everyday life, such as a hammer hitting a nail, but it is important to realize that there need not necessarily be physical contact between the two bodies for one to act on the other. If we take two charged bodies and bring these close together (but not actually touching), the forces between the two bodies will be equal and opposite. The significance of this in the design of the cathode of the X-ray tube will be considered in Chapter 30.

3.6 AVOGADRO'S HYPOTHESIS, THE MOLE AND AVOGADRO'S NUMBER

As we will see in Chapter 18, all substances consist of atoms or molecules. These may react chemically with the atoms or molecules of other substances. These reactions occur with fixed proportions in order to produce a given chemical compound and it is possible to predict the number of molecules of the compound from knowledge of the number of molecules of the original elements or compounds, for example:

$$2H_2 + O_2 = 2H_2O$$

In the case of gases, Avogadro's hypothesis postulated that *equal volumes of gases at the same temperature and pressure contain equal numbers of molecules*. This hypothesis was first postulated in the early nineteenth century and has been verified by a number of experiments since then.

This is taken one stage further within the SI system in the more general statement that *the number of molecules per mole is the same for any substance*. The mole is the SI unit of the amount of substance and is defined as:

Definition
The *mole* is the amount of substance which contains as many elementary particles as there are atoms in 0.012 kg of carbon-12.

Carbon-12 is used as the standard for technical experimental reasons. From this, we can predict the number of atoms or molecules in a substance by knowing its atomic mass number and comparing this with carbon-12. For example, if we consider cobalt-60, then there will be the same number of atoms in 0.6 kg of cobalt-60 as there will be in 0.012 kg of carbon-12, as each constitutes one mole of substance. The number of molecules in a mole is given by Avogadro's number (or constant) and is 6×10^{23} molecules.

Insight
If we consider X-ray photons being attenuated by matter, this is a reaction between the photons and the electrons of atoms of the material through which they pass. If we know the number of atoms per mole of the material, we can calculate the number of atoms per unit mass. By knowing the atomic number of the material, it is then possible to establish the electron density and so predict the likelihood of an X-ray photon interacting with an electron. This will be discussed further in Chapter 23.

Summary

In this chapter you should have learnt:

- the law of conservation of matter (see Sect 3.2)
- the law of conservation of energy (see Sect 3.3)
- the law of conservation of momentum (see Sect 3.4)
- Newton's laws of motion (see Sect 3.5)
- Avogadro's hypothesis, the mole and Avogadro's number (see Sect 3.6).

FURTHER READING

Further reading on the laws of classical physics can be found in most textbooks which are used in schools for study of AS level or A2 level physics. In addition, the following may prove useful:

Allan, E., Harris, J., 1999. New Higher Chemistry. Hodder Gibson, London (Chapter 3).

Ball, J.L., Moore, A.D., Turner, S., 2008. Ball and Moore's Essential Physics for Radiographers, fourth edn. Blackwell Scientific, London (Chapter 1).

Chapter | 4 |

Units of measurement

4.1 AIM

This chapter introduces the reader to the main units that are used in measurement in radiographic science.

4.2 UNITS OF MEASUREMENT

Science has three fundamental tools that are used in its attempts to understand the external world:

1. theory
2. logic
3. experimental measurements.

Problems arise when making experimental measurements as to what quantities to measure and how to measure them. In particular, the *units* in which these quantities are expressed must be defined so that when two people make the same measurement they get the same results. Also, there are obvious advantages if one set of units is universally adopted as the basis for all measurements.

Each of the *base* units discussed in the next section relies on the appropriate *standard* to which each measurement is compared. Thus, there are units of standard length, standard mass, standard time interval and so on. Without such standards, no accurate measurements can be made. This in turn retards the development of adequate theories, or models, of the world.

4.3 SI BASE UNITS

There are a plethora of units of measurement used throughout the world. The International System of Units (SI) attempts to replace this with seven standard units. These standards are termed *SI units* (see Table 4.1) and represent the fundamental measurements that we might wish to make of a body:

- What is its size? (unit of *length – metre*)
- How massive is it? (unit of *mass – kilogram*)
- How bright is it? (unit of *luminous intensity – candela*)
- How much electrical current flows through it? (unit of *electrical current – ampere*)
- How many elementary particles does it contain? (unit of *amount of substance – mole*)
- How hot is it? (unit of *temperature – Kelvin*)
- How do all the quantities vary with time? (unit of *time – second*)

The very precise definitions of the units are not required for the rest of this text, but if you wish to see them, they are given in Appendix C.

The base units of mass, length and time are termed *fundamental or base units* since one or more of them is always involved in the measurement of any other quantity.

These seven SI base units may be combined to give *derived units,* as described in the next section.

4.3.1 Derived SI units

A number of derived SI units can be formed by the combination of the seven base units. Some of these are sufficiently important to be given their own names and they are listed in Table 4.2 and discussed in the rest of this chapter.

Further derived units are of a more specialized nature (e.g. absorbed radiation dose) and will be discussed in the specific chapters which require such measurement.

Table 4.1 SI base units

QUANTITY	UNIT OF MEASUREMENT	SYMBOL
Length	Metre	m
Mass	Kilogram	kg
Luminous intensity	Candela	cd
Electric current	Ampere	A
Amount of a substance	Mole	mol
Temperature	Kelvin	K
Time	Second	s

Insight

For some quantities, we can consider a body moving between two points. For certain measurements, it is important to know how far the body has travelled between the two points. In other cases, we wish to know not only how far it has travelled but also the direction it has travelled. Measurements where the direction is important are termed *vector* quantities whereas those where the direction is not important are known as *scalar* quantities.

Table 4.2 Derived SI units and their definitions

QUANTITY	DEFINITION	SI UNIT	SCALAR/VECTOR
Speed	Distance travelled in unit time	Metre per second ($m.s^{-1}$)	Scalar
Velocity	Distance travelled in unit time in a given direction	Metre per second ($m.s^{-1}$)	Vector
Acceleration	Change of velocity in unit time	Metre per second ($m.s^{-2}$)	Vector
Force	The application of unit force to unit mass produces unit acceleration	Newton (N) ($kg.m.s^{-2}$)	Vector
Pressure	Force applied per unit area	Pascal (Pa) ($N.m^{-2}$)	Vector
Weight	Force acting on a body due to gravity	Newton (N) ($kg.m.s^{-2}$)	Scalar
Work	Product of the force acting on a body times the distance the body moves	Joule (J) (n.m)	Scalar
Energy	Kinetic energy: work which can be done by a system because of its velocity	Joule (J)	Scalar
	Potential energy: work which can be performed because of the position or state of a system	Joule (J)	
Power	Rate of doing work	Watt (W) ($J.s^{-1}$)	Scalar
Momentum	Product of mass and the velocity of the body	($kg.m.s^{-1}$)	Vector

4.3.2 Speed and velocity

The speedometer in a car is calibrated in terms of kilometres per hour (kph) or miles per hour (mph). Either of these shows that *speed* means distance travelled in unit time.

In SI units, speed (S), distance (d) and time (t) are related by the equation:

Equation 4.1

$$S = \frac{d}{t}$$

where d is in metres, t is in seconds and S, therefore, is in metres per second ($m.s^{-1}$). The speedometer in a car gives no indication of the *direction* in which the car is moving so we can see that speed is a scalar quantity. *Velocity is* measured in the same units as speed ($m.s^{-1}$) but this time the *direction* of movement is also measured. Thus, a car travelling at a constant speed around a roundabout is continuously changing its velocity.

4.3.3 Acceleration

Acceleration implies a change in velocity and is defined as the *change in velocity per unit time* (a vector quantity).

For example, the acceleration due to gravity is approximately 9.8 meters per second per second ($9.8\,m.s^{-2}$). This means that for a free-falling body, the velocity increases by $9.8\,m.s^{-1}$ after each second. Thus, if a body is dropped, its downward velocity is $9.8\,m.s^{-1}$ after the first second, $19.6\,m.s^{-1}$ after the next second and so on.

The acceleration due to gravity causes a free-falling body to increase its velocity, but if the accelerating force is in the opposite direction to the direction of movement of the body, then it will cause it to lose velocity. This force causes a negative acceleration or a *deceleration*.

Also, notice that acceleration is a vector quantity as the acceleration has direction (a vector measurement).

4.3.4 Force

Newton's second law of motion (see Ch. 3) shows that the net force acting on a body is proportional to the mass of the body multiplied by the acceleration produced on the body. The units of force are therefore $kg.m.s^{-2}$ in SI units. However, this quantity is sufficiently important to be given its own special name and is known as the *newton*. This can be defined as follows:

Definition
A net force of 1 *newton* acting on a body of mass 1 kg causes it to have an acceleration of $1\,m.s^{-2}$.

Force is a vector quantity as it has direction. The acceleration produced by the action of the force (also a vector quantity) is in the same direction as the force.

4.3.5 Pressure

Pressure is defined as the *force exerted per unit area*. The units of pressure would therefore be $N.m^{-2}$ Again, it is sufficiently important to merit its own unit, known as the *pascal*, and is defined as follows:

Definition
The pressure acting on a body is 1 *pascal* if 1 newton of force is applied per square metre of body surface.

Insight
The difference between force and pressure can be readily appreciated if one considers crossing some snow wearing either shoes or skis. In both cases, the force is the same but this force is applied to a smaller area in the case of shoes (the pressure on the snow is greater) so they tend to sink into the snow.

4.3.6 Weight and mass

As we have already seen, mass is a base SI unit, is defined as the amount of matter in a body and is defined against the standard kilogram. This is sometimes confused with the mole (the amount of substance in a body) and so it is possibly easier to understand the concept of mass if we consider it in terms of inertia. We know that a force acting on a body will produce an acceleration and that the force, the mass and the acceleration are linked by the equation $F = m \times a$ (see Equation 3.1) so that inertia can be defined as the body's resistance to acceleration. From the equation, it can be seen that as the mass of the body increases, so the force required to produce a given acceleration also increases, i.e. *the inertia of the body increases with mass*.

The *weight* of a body is the downward force on the body due to the gravitational attraction of Earth. Hence, the weight of a body is expressed in newtons, not in kilograms. An equation similar to Equation 3.1 links weight (w), mass (m) and gravity (g):

Equation 4.2

$$w = m \times g$$

From the above discussion and equation, we can see that a body always has mass but it only has weight in the presence of a gravitational field. Hence, a body in deep space has no weight (because of the zero gravitational field) but it has mass as it still requires a force to cause it to change its velocity (i.e. it has inertia).

4.3.7 Work and energy

Both *work* and *energy* are measured using the same units. A force is said to do work if it moves its point of application in the same direction as the applied force. This can be expressed as:

Equation 4.3

$$W = F \times d$$

where W is work, F is force and d is distance.

Thus, the units of work are newtons and meters (N.m). Again, the concept of work is sufficiently important to merit its own unit, which is the *joule*.

Definition

1 joule of work is performed when a force of 1 newton moves its point of application through a distance of 1 metre.

Energy can be considered as the capacity of a body to do work. There are two types of energy that we need to consider separately:

1. Kinetic energy.
2. Potential energy.

4.3.7.1 Kinetic energy

Kinetic energy is energy that a body possesses by virtue of its motion. This motion may be translational (movement along a path) or rotational, or a combination of both types. The kinetic energy is simply the work that must be done in the process of bringing the body to rest. We have already looked at this when we considered Newton's laws of motion and established an equation (Equation 3.4) for the kinetic energy of a body of mass m having a velocity of v.

Equation 4.4

$$E = \frac{1}{2}mv^2$$

Insight

Consider an electron, which has been accelerated across the X-ray tube and is travelling with a velocity v at the point when it starts to collide with the atoms of the target.

It has a kinetic energy ($= \frac{1}{2}mv^2$) and then starts to liberate some of that energy in the form of X-ray photons. The energy of X-ray photons is measured in electron-volts (eV).

4.3.7.2 Potential energy

Potential energy is energy possessed by a body (or a system) by virtue of its condition or state. Thus, a stationary body has potential energy if it is in a condition that allows it to release its stored energy. The potential energy of the system can be thought of as the work that the system will perform in bringing its potential energy to zero. If we consider a body of mass m, which is at a height h above the ground, then we can apply Equation 4.3 to this situation.

$$W = F \times d$$

The force at work here is the weight of the body (mg) and the distance it can move its height above the ground (h), so we now have the equation for the potential energy (PE):

Equation 4.5

$$PE = mg \times h$$

Insight

Consider the case of a hospital lift sitting at the ground floor. Attached to this lift, over a pulley system, is a counterweight. This counterweight has potential energy because of its position. If the brakes on the lift are released, it will assist in moving the lift up to the top floor (i.e. the counterweight performs work).

Work and energy are both scalar quantities, as they do not have direction.

4.3.8 Power

A particular car may reach a speed of 60 mph in 6 s while another car of the same mass does the same speed in 20 s. The first car is said to be more *powerful* than the second. Assuming that the cars are travelling in the same direction, then their velocity is the same and so their kinetic energy ($= \frac{1}{2}mv^2$) is the same, but the first car reached that energy more quickly. Hence, *power* can be expressed as the *rate at which energy is expended* and, since energy and work are basically the same thing, we can say that:

Definition

Power is the rate at which work is done.

Thus, power is measured in joules per second ($J.s^{-1}$) but is again an important enough concept to merit its own unit, the *watt*. Thus:

$$watts = \frac{joules}{seconds}$$

or 1 watt is 1 joule of work per second.

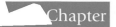

4.3.9 Momentum

In everyday speech, *momentum* expresses the ability of a moving body to 'keep going'. This depends on the mass of the body and its velocity and so momentum is defined:

> **Definition**
>
> The *momentum* of a body is the product of its mass and its velocity.

We have already, briefly, come across the concept of momentum in the law of conservation of momentum (Ch. 3).

> **Insight**
>
> Consider the situation where a projectile (e.g. a bullet) strikes a barrier. The depth to which it penetrates the barrier is dependent on the mass of the projectile and its *velocity* at the point of impact. This fits in with our concept of *momentum* as the ability of a body to keep going.

4.4 UNITS USED IN RADIOGRAPHY

Many derived SI units (such as the joule, coulomb, etc.) are used in radiographic science. However, other units that do not strictly adhere to the SI system are especially useful to radiography and are unlikely to be discontinued, because of their practical convenience. These are shown and defined in Table 4.3.

4.4.1 mA and mAs

X-rays are produced in an X-ray tube when electrons from the cathode, with high kinetic energy, strike the anode (see Chs 21 and 30). If we assume that each electron has a chance of producing X-rays, then the intensity of X-ray production is proportional to the number of electrons striking the anode per second. The number of electrons flowing per second is related to the *current* flowing through the tube (see Ch. 8). The SI unit of current is the ampere (A), as we saw earlier in this chapter, and it is equivalent to a current of 6×10^{18} electrons per second. This unit of current is too large a unit for radiography so current is measured in milliamperes ($1\,mA = 10^{-3}\,A$).

We only wish the tube to produce X-rays in sufficient quantity to produce the image on the recording medium (e.g. film) and so an exposure time is selected by the operator. It can be seen that, all other factors remaining constant,

Table 4.3 Units used in radiography

UNIT	DEFINITION
mA	The average electrical current passing through an X-ray tube during an exposure (measured in milliamperes)
mAs	The average current passing through the tube during an exposure multiplied by the exposure time in seconds (1 mAs = 1 millicoulomb)
keV	The energy imparted to an electron when passing through a potential difference of 1 kV in a vacuum

Table 4.4 Different combinations of mA and time to produce a given mAs

CURRENT (mA)	EXPOSURE TIME (S)	mAs
10	6.0	60
20	3.0	60
100	0.6	60
200	0.3	60
300	0.2	60
600	0.1	60

the amount of blackening (or optical density) of the film will be determined by the number of X-rays leaving the tube. From the above arguments, this is determined by the total number of electrons striking the anode of the tube. The total number of electrons striking the target (and hence the X-ray output) is determined by the number of electrons flowing in unit time (related to the mA) and the length of time for which the current flows (the exposure time in seconds, s). The X-ray output from a tube (if all other factors remain unaltered) is determined by the mAs.

Any combination of mA and time which produces a given mAs will result in the same quantity of X-rays being emitted by the tube. If 60 mAs was required to produce an acceptable image, this could be delivered in the ways listed in Table 4.4.

The reasons why we might wish to use the different combinations of mA and time will be discussed in Chapter 25.

As we shall see in Chapter 7, the mAs is equivalent to the *millicoulomb* ($10^{-3}\,C$), which is the unit of electrical charge. The mAs is, however, used in preference to the millicoulomb as it makes it more obvious that this can be altered by altering the tube current (mA) or the exposure time (s).

4.4.2 keV

As we have already seen in this chapter, energy is measured in joules. When we come to consider the energies involved in the atom or the energies of the photons of the X-ray beam, the coulomb is an extremely large unit. The electron-volt (eV) and the kiloelectron-volt (keV = 10^3 eV) are much more convenient units of measurement for such energies.

Definition

If an electron is accelerated from rest across a potential difference of 1 volt in a vacuum, it gains a kinetic energy of 1 *electron-volt*.

Similarly, an electron accelerated from rest across a potential difference of 1 kilovolt in a vacuum gains a kinetic energy of 1 kiloelectron-volt. The energy (E) in joules can be calculated from the equation:

Equation 4.6

$$E = e \times V$$

In this equation, e is the charge on the electron $(1.6 \times 10^{-19}\,C)$ and V is the potential difference measured in volts. Thus:

$$1\,ev = 1.6 \times 10^{-19}\,J$$

$$1\,keV = 1.6 \times 10^{-16}\,J$$

Insight

If 75 kVp is selected by an operator for a specific exposure, then some of the electrons travelling across the X-ray tube will have a kinetic energy of 75 keV when they strike the anode. If we assume that some of these electrons give up all their energy as a single X-ray photon, then the energy of this photon will be 75 keV and it will represent the maximum photon energy in this beam. Thus, by altering the kVp, the operator can alter the maximum photon energy of the beam.

Summary

In this chapter, we considered the following factors related to units of measurement:
- The SI base units for length, mass, luminous intensity, electric current, amount of substance, temperature and time.
- The SI derived units for speed, velocity, acceleration, force, pressure, weight, work, energy, power and momentum.
- Units of measurement used in radiography in the form of mA, mAs and keV.

FURTHER READING

Ball, J.L., Moore, A.D., Turner, S., 2008. Ball and Moore's Essential Physics for Radiographers, forth ed. Blackwell Scientific, London (chapter 1).

Chapter | 5 |

Heat

Insight

In fact, we are better at noticing 'hotter' or 'colder' than we are at determining an absolute value of 'hot' or 'cold'. This can easily be shown from a simple experiment for which you require a bowl of hot water, a bowl of cold water and two bowls of tepid water. Place the right hand in the bowl of hot water and the left hand in the bowl of cold water and leave them in position for about 2 minutes. Now transfer both hands to the bowls of tepid water. You will note that this water feels cold to the right hand and warm to the left hand. This shows that we are better at detecting changes in temperature than we are at detecting absolute values of temperature.

5.1 AIM

This chapter considers heat as a transfer of energy. Links between heat and temperature are established. The mechanisms of transferring heat are also established.

5.2 INTRODUCTION

We are familiar with the feelings of *hot* and *cold*; indeed, we are crucially dependent on our bodily temperature staying within a very limited range in order to survive. Compared to the vast ranges of temperature which exist across the universe, our experience of 'hot' and 'cold' is very limited indeed.

In order to investigate heat further, we must use objective measures of heat and cold, as described in the following sections.

5.3 HEAT ENERGY AND TEMPERATURE

When heat is given to a body, its atoms or molecules are given increased kinetic energy in the form of increased lattice vibration (this is the reason why substances expand when heated). A body whose atoms have a higher kinetic energy than those of another body is said to be hotter or at a higher temperature. If two bodies are placed in contact, then heat will be transferred from the hotter body to the cooler body by collisions between the molecules at the point of contact. The molecules of the cooler body receive

27

a net increase in kinetic energy and so its temperature rises. The molecules of the hotter body have lost kinetic energy and so its temperature falls. This process continues until the two bodies are at the same temperature when no further exchange of *energy* takes place. The bodies are now in a state of *thermal equilibrium*. Notice that the thermal energy is always transferred from the body at the higher temperature to the body at the lower temperature, irrespective of the size of the bodies. Also note that the temperature existing at thermal equilibrium will always lie somewhere between the initial temperatures of the two bodies.

Insight

If a body is made to give *away* thermal energy, then the lattice (the bound framework of a solid or semisolid) vibrations of its atoms or molecules will decrease. It is logical to assume that there must be a temperature at which no lattice vibration exists. As all movement of molecules ceases to exist at this temperature, this is the lowest temperature that we can attain. This temperature is known as absolute zero and will be further discussed in the next section.

5.3.1 Temperature scales

There are two temperature scales used in modern physics: Celsius (also called centigrade) and kelvin. The Celsius scale is defined as $0°C$ at the temperature of melting ice, and $100°C$ at the temperature of boiling water at an atmospheric pressure of 1.01×10^5 newtons per square metre (76 mm of mercury). On this scale, the temperature of absolute zero (see previous Insight) is approximately $-273.15°C$. This temperature is zero on the kelvin scale ($0\,K$) while the temperature of melting ice is $273.15\,K$. From this, we can see that the units of temperature are the same on both scales but the scales have different starting points, i.e. one unit on the Celsius scale is equivalent to one unit on the kelvin scale. Note that temperature on the kelvin scale does not have the degree symbol in front of the K. It is a convenient approximation to assume that $0°C = 273\,K$, so that the simple conversion formula may be used:

Equation 5.1

$$T°C = (T + 273)K$$

where T is temperature.

5.3.2 Units of heat energy, specific heat capacity and thermal capacity

If heat is given to a body, then its molecules will have a higher kinetic energy and its temperature will rise.

Hence, it is convenient to express a quantity of heat in terms of the temperature change it produces in a given body. Consider the situation where we wish to apply an amount of energy, Q, which will raise the temperature of a body by 1 kelvin unit (for simplicity, assume that this does not change the state of the body, i.e. it does not change from a solid to a liquid). This will be affected by the mass and the type of material of the body. It also seems logical to assume that we would need twice the amount of heat to raise the temperature of the body by 2 kelvin units. If we take all these factors together, we can write the equation:

Equation 5.2

$$Q = mc(T_2 - T_1)$$

where Q is the heat energy required to raise the temperature of a body of mass m from T_1 to a temperature T_2. The factor c is approximately constant for a particular material and is known as the specific heat capacity of the material. We can rearrange Equation 5.2 to get:

Equation 5.3

$$c = \frac{Q}{m(T_2 - T_1)}$$

so that c, the specific heat capacity, is in units of c joules per kilogram per kelvin ($J.kg^{-1}.K^{-1}$). Specific heat capacity can be defined thus:

Definition

The specific heat capacity of a body is the energy in joules required to raise the temperature of 1 kilogram of the body by 1 kelvin unit.

The specific heat capacity of a substance is thus unique to that substance and it allows us to predict the behaviour of different masses of the same substance.

Example

The specific heat capacity of water is about it 4.2 ($J.kg^{-1}$. K^{-1}). How much heat energy is required to raise a mass of 10 g of water from 280 K to 285 K? (Remember that the unit of energy is the joule and the unit of mass is the kilogram.)

Using Equation 5.2, we have:

$$Q = mc(T_2 - T_1)$$
$$= 10^{-2} \times 4.2 \times 10^3 \times (285 - 280)$$
$$= 210\,J$$

In the situations considered so far, we have considered the amount of heat required to raise the temperature of 1 kg of the material. Another unit of heat energy, which is useful in practice, is the thermal capacity.

Definition

The thermal capacity of a body is the heat energy in joules which is required to raise the temperature of the body by 1 kelvin unit.

Note that this definition differs from the previous one for specific heat capacity in that no mention is made of unit mass. Thus, the thermal capacity refers to the whole of the body and not just 1 kg of it. It should also be noted that the thermal capacity of a body is the specific heat capacity of the body multiplied by the mass of the body. The units of thermal capacity are joules per kelvin.

Example

The anode discs of two X-ray tubes are made of the same material but one has twice the mass of the other. If the same amount of heat is applied to each anode, which will have the higher temperature rise at the end of the exposure?

The thermal capacity is the product of the mass and the specific heat. Thus, the larger anode will have twice the thermal capacity of the smaller one. If the same amount of heat is applied to each, the smaller one will experience twice the temperature rise of the larger one. The importance of this will be considered when we consider the rating of the X-ray tube (see Ch. 31).

5.4 TRANSFER OF HEAT

As mentioned at the beginning of this chapter, heat can be given to a body from some other structure with greater thermal energy than the body. Similarly, if a body can be isolated from its environment or is in a state of thermal equilibrium with its surroundings, there is no net gain or loss of heat from the body.

The mechanisms of heat transfer form an important part of the study of radiography because of the large amounts of heat energy produced at the target of the X-ray tube. The mechanical and thermal stresses associated with this make it possible to damage the X-ray tube unless adequate precautions are taken. The anodes of all X-ray tubes must therefore be designed to transfer heat away from the focal spot area as quickly as possible in order to minimize the temperature rise in this region. The practical application of this knowledge to the design of X-ray tubes will be considered in Chapter 31. However, we must first understand the different mechanisms of heat transfer: these are *conduction, convection* and *radiation*.

5.4.1 Conduction

Conduction is the transfer of heat between bodies by physical contact of those bodies and results in a transfer of kinetic energy by interatomic collision, thus forming the main process by which heat is transferred through a solid. If heat is applied to one end of a metal bar, the atoms at this end of the bar receive copious supplies of kinetic energy. These atoms, because of their increased vibrational energy, collide with neighbouring atoms and so kinetic energy is gradually transferred along the bar. This method of heat flow along the bar is known as *conduction* of heat.

We can find by experiment that the rate of flow of heat, q (joules per second), by conduction is controlled by a number of things:

- $q \propto A$ (the cross-sectional area of the rod)
- $q \propto (T_1 - T_2)$ (the temperature difference between the ends of the rod; this is known as the temperature gradient)
- $q \propto (1/l)$ (where l is the length of the rod)
- q depends on the material of the rod.

Combining all these factors, we have:

Equation 5.4

$$q \propto \frac{A(T_1 - T_2)}{l}$$
$$q = \frac{kA(T_1 - T_2)}{l}$$

Here k is the constant of proportionality and this is a constant for any given material. It is known as the thermal conductivity of the material. Materials are classed as 'good' or 'bad' conductors depending on the value of k. Typical values of k are shown in Table 5.1 (See page 30).

Note that the rate of flow of heat along a bar can be changed by altering the length, the cross-sectional area and the temperature gradient as well as by altering the material.

5.4.2 Convection

Convection is the main process by which heat is transferred in fluids (i.e. liquids and gases). Consider heat being applied to a liquid in a beaker (Fig. 5.1). The liquid near the source of heat has thermal energy transferred to it by conduction. This increase in thermal energy causes the liquid to expand and become less dense than the surrounding liquid. The heated liquid rises (because of hydrostatic pressure) and, as it rises, it transfers heat to the surrounding molecules by conduction. The temperature

Table 5.1 Thermal conductivity of materials

MATERIAL	THERMAL CONDUCTIVITY $(\text{W.m}^{-1}.\text{K}^{-1})$	COMMENTS
Copper	386	Excellent conductor – used as the anode material in the stationary anode tube
Tungsten	202	Fairly good conductor – used as the target material in stationary X-ray tubes
Molybdenum	147	Relatively poor conductor – used as the anode stem in the rotating anode tube
Glass	1.0	Poor conductor – involved in the transfer of heat to the oil in the tube housing
Rubber	0.05	Very poor conductor
Air	0.02	Very poor conductor – removes heat from the housing of the X-ray tube by convection

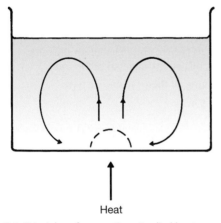

Heat

Figure 5.1 Principles of convection. Applied heat causes the broken-line region of fluid to expand, become less dense and rise, being replaced by cooler parts of the fluid. This sets up convection currents.

of the small section of heated liquid returns to the same temperature as the surrounding liquid and so sinks back into the beaker, to be heated a second time. Thus, convection currents are established, as shown in Figure 5.1. The overall effect is that the whole volume of fluid is heated and not just the region where the heat is applied.

Some interesting points emerge from this:

- Convection can only occur where the molecules are free to move through the medium, i.e. in liquids and gases.
- It is not possible to have convection currents without some conduction.

- It is necessary to have a gravitational field in order for the convection currents to be initiated as the warm fluid moves in the opposite direction to the gravitational force, by hydrostatic pressure.

5.4.3 Radiation

In this process, heat is lost from a body with high thermal energy in the form of electromagnetic radiations. Radiation is the only heat transfer process that will take place through a *vacuum*. The most obvious and striking example is the heat we can feel from our sun where the radiation must pass through a near-perfect vacuum for 93 million miles (approximately 150 million km) to reach us. Light and heat also reach us from other stars but we are only able to discern the light, as we are not sufficiently sensitive to small amounts of heat (although the latter can be detected with infrared sensors).

We are able to feel heat by radiation because it imparts kinetic energy to molecules of our tissues, which we discern as an increase in temperature. Heat radiations occur in a band of energies just beyond the red part of the visible spectrum (see Ch. 17 for further detail of the electromagnetic spectrum). This band of energies is known as infrared radiations. All bodies radiate electromagnetic energies if their temperature is above absolute zero. This does not necessarily mean that we can discern the radiations, as we perceive only a narrow band of energies extending from violet light to infrared. Bodies of different colours and different surface compositions radiate somewhat differently and so it is conventional to consider *black-body radiation*. This we will do next.

5.4.3.1 Black-body radiation

A body looks black because very little of the light incident upon it is reflected or transmitted. A black body is defined as one that will absorb 100% of all radiations at all frequencies incident upon it. If such a black body is in a state of thermal equilibrium with its surroundings, equal amounts of radiation must be absorbed and emitted per second. From this it can be deduced that the black body must radiate more energy than any other type of body since no other body absorbs 100% of the energy incident upon it. The foregoing statements can be summarized thus:

- All bodies are capable of emitting radiation.
- A black body absorbs 100% of all radiations incident upon it.
- A black body is the most efficient emitter of radiation of any body.

We now need to know in more detail the spectrum of radiations emitted by a black body. Figure 5.2 shows such a spectrum for a black body at different temperatures. The following should be noted from the graph:

- The wavelength corresponding to the peak radiation progressively decreases as the temperature of the body increases.
- The height of the graph (intensity of radiation) is very sensitive to changes in temperature.
- The spectrum of the radiation is a smooth curve, of which we perceive only a small part (violet to infrared).
- The total intensity of the radiation emitted by a body at a given temperature is the sum of the intensities at each wavelength. This is related to the area under the curve in each case. *Stefan's law* states that the total intensity of the emitted radiation is proportional to the *fourth power* of the *kelvin temperature*. Thus:

Equation 5.5

$$I \propto T^4$$
$$\text{or } I = \sigma T^4$$

where σ is Stefan's constant.

Doubling of the kelvin temperature results in the amount of heat radiation emitted being increased by a factor of $2^4 = 16$ times. As this shows, the intensity of the radiation emitted varies greatly with the temperature of the body. This has important consequences in the design of the rotating anode X-ray tube disc, as we shall see in Chapter 30.

A curve of emitted radiation at about 1000 K is equivalent to a metal rod which has been heated until it is glowing cherry-red. As the temperature increases, the colour changes through light red to white since an increasing amount of the violet end of the spectrum is emitted along with the red (see 2000 K and 2500 K lines in Fig. 5.2). At higher temperatures, objects emit white light. This is true of the filament of an electric light bulb or the anode disc of the rotating anode tube after a large exposure.

The interactions of energetic atoms produce a broad band of emitted quanta wavelengths because of the range of interactions that are possible. All of these radiations form part of the electromagnetic spectrum. A narrow range of frequencies (in the infrared part) is capable of being absorbed by the whole atom (as opposed to the electron shells or the nucleus) and so these atoms gain kinetic energy. This increase in the kinetic energy of the atoms is in the form of heat. Higher frequencies of radiation interact with the electrons in the orbitals and even higher frequencies will interact with the atomic nuclei.

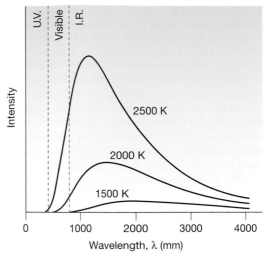

Figure 5.2 The spectrum of electromagnetic radiation emitted by a black body at different temperatures. The total intensity (I) is a function of the kelvin temperature ($I \propto T^4$). IR, infrared; UV, ultraviolet.

Insight

The mechanism that causes the emission of radiation is the acceleration and deceleration of the charged particles, which make up the atoms or molecules of the body involved. An example particularly relevant to radiography is the sudden deceleration of electrons when they strike the anode of the X-ray tube – the *Bremsstrahlung* or braking radiation. Here, some (or all) of the kinetic energy of the electron is transformed into an X-ray photon (see Ch. 21). Another example is the production of radio waves, where electrons are forced to oscillate at high frequencies in a radio-transmitting aerial.

5.5 THERMAL EXPANSION

Most substances expand when heated, owing to the increased kinetic energy of the atoms. The *linear expansivity* is a measure of this thermal expansion, defined as the *fractional change in unit length per unit change in kelvin temperature*. The thermal expansion of different parts of the X-ray tube is an important design consideration as the tube is subject to large temperature variations during its working life. If materials of very different thermal expansivity are used, this can cause mechanical stress that could result in fracture of one of the components. A particularly weak point in this respect is the seal between the glass and the copper anode in a stationary anode tube. A special type of glass with a thermal expansivity very similar to copper is chosen. This reduces the mechanical stress and thus the chances of fracture of the glass envelope and loss of vacuum in the tube.

5.6 EVAPORATION AND VAPORIZATION

We are all familiar with the evaporation of liquids that occurs when heat is applied to them, e.g. boiling kettles. Evaporation is caused by the loss of *whole atoms* from the surface of the liquid. Some of the atoms are given sufficient kinetic energy to escape from the forces of attraction of their neighbours near the surface of the liquid and produce a vapour in the free space above this surface.

Whole atoms may also be liberated from the surfaces of solid materials under the action of heat. There is a stronger force of attraction between the atoms in a solid compared to a liquid and so liberation of the atoms is more difficult to accomplish. This means that in a solid the atoms require higher kinetic energy for liberation, i.e. solids need to be subjected to a higher temperature. The tungsten at the target and in the filament of the X-ray tube is subjected to such high temperatures that a certain amount of *vaporization* takes place. The tungsten vapour can condense to form a thin layer of tungsten on the inside of the glass of the envelope. A major effect of this is to reduce the electrical insulation provided by the glass, as tungsten is a reasonable conductor of electricity. This can produce an effect called a 'gassy tube', which renders the X-ray tube inoperable. Fortunately, this does not occur readily as tungsten has a low *vapour pressure so* does not readily vaporize at its normal working temperatures.

Summary

In this chapter, you should have learnt:
- That heat is a form of energy produced by the kinetic energy of atoms in a body (see Sect. 5.3).
- The greater the kinetic energy of the atoms, the higher the temperature and vice versa (see Sect. 5.3).
- That bodies which are in thermal equilibrium with their surroundings lose heat as fast as they gain heat and so experience no change in temperature (see Sect. 5.3).
- Absolute zero temperature corresponds to zero atomic kinetic energy and has a temperature of 0 K (see Sect. 5.3.1).
- On the kelvin scale, the temperature at which ice melts is approximately 273 K (see Sect. 5.3.1).
- The link between heat and temperature provided by specific heat capacity and thermal capacity (see Sect. 5.3.2).
- Heat may be transferred from one point to another by conduction (mainly in solids), convection (in fluids) and radiation (may travel through a vacuum) (see Sects 5.4.1–5.4.3).

FURTHER READING

Further information on X-ray tube design and rating is available in Chapters 30 and 31 of this text. The following may also prove useful:

Heat and heat transfer processes
Ball, J.L,, Moore, A.D., Turner, S., 2008. Ball and Moore's Essential Physics for Radiographers, fourth ed. Blackwell D Scientific, London (Chapter 2).

Chapter | 6 |

Electrostatics

CHAPTER CONTENTS

6.1 AIM

This chapter introduces the reader to the concepts involved in understanding the electrostatics which is relevant to radiographic science. This involves the consideration of electrical charge, charge distribution and electrical potential and potential difference.

6.2 INTRODUCTION

Electrostatics, as the name implies, is the study of static electrical charges. We are familiar with many examples of electrostatics from our ordinary lives, from sparks which may occur from our clothes when undressing, to the large discharges of electricity which occur during lightning strikes. Much of the early experimentation with electricity involved electrostatics. It was discovered at an early stage that there were two types of electrical charge, one called negative and the other positive. While it is mathematically convenient to regard charge in this way, it does not explain what electrical charge actually is and how it behaves. This will be the subject of this chapter.

6.3 PROPERTIES OF ELECTRICAL CHARGES

The general properties of electrical charges are as follows:

- Charges can be considered as being of two types: positive and negative.
- The smallest unit of negative charge which can exist in isolation is that possessed by an electron, and the smallest unit of positive charge which can exist in isolation is that possessed by a proton.
- Electrical charges exert forces on each other even when they are separated by a vacuum. The forces are mutual, equal and opposite, as expected by Newton's third law (see Sect. 3.5).
- Like charges (i.e. charges of the same sign) repel each other while unlike charges (of opposite signs) attract each other.

- The magnitude of the mutual forces between the charges is influenced by:
  - the magnitude of the individual charges
  - the medium in which they are embedded, being greatest when the medium is a vacuum
  - the inverse square of the distance between the charged bodies – this is another application of the inverse square law (see Ch. 26).
- Electrical charges may be induced in a body by the proximity of a charged body, leading to a force of attraction between the two bodies.
- Electrical charges may flow easily in some materials (called *electrical conductors*) and with difficulty in other materials (called *electrical insulators*). Both types of material are capable of having charges induced in them.
- When electrical charges move, they produce a magnetic field.

6.4 FORCE BETWEEN TWO ELECTRICAL CHARGES IN A VACUUM

Consider two charges, q_1 and q_2, separated by a distance, d, in a vacuum, as shown in Figure 6.1.

If we assume that both charges are of the same sign, then q_1 will exert a force of repulsion (F) on q_2 and q_2 will exert the same force of repulsion on q_1. As we have already stated above, it can be shown that:

1. $F \propto q_1$
2. $F \propto q_2$
3. $F \propto \dfrac{1}{d_2}$

Thus, F is proportional to the magnitude of each charge and to the inverse square of the distance separating them.

If we combine the factors in 1, 2 and 3 above, we can produce the equation:

Equation 6.1

$$F \propto \frac{q_1 q_2}{d^2}$$

If q_1 and q_2 both have the same sign, then F will be positive and will represent a force of repulsion. If the charges have opposite signs, then F will be negative and will represent a force of attraction.

If we wish to replace the proportionality sign in Equation 6.1 by an equals sign then we need to introduce a constant of proportionality (see Appendix A). This equation now reads:

Equation 6.2

$$F = \frac{q_1 q_2}{4\pi\varepsilon_0 d^2}$$

This equation is often referred to as *Coulomb's law of force* between two charges and has particular relevance when we consider the charges between subatomic particles (see Chs 18 and 19).

The constant of proportionality is $\frac{1}{4}\pi\varepsilon_0$, where ε_0 is the *permittivity of a vacuum* and has a value of $6.85 \times 10^{-12}\,\mathrm{F.m^{-1}}$. The charges q_1, and q_2 are expressed in coulombs, the separation d is in meters and the force F is in newtons.

The coulomb corresponds to the charge carried by 6×10^{18} electrons or protons. An alternative (and more practical) definition of the coulomb is:

Definition
A charge of 1 coulomb is possessed by a point if an equal charge placed 1 metre away from it in a vacuum experiences a force of repulsion of $\frac{1}{4}\pi\varepsilon_0$ newton.

Insight
The influence of the inverse square law on the force between charged bodies may be grasped if we assume that charged bodies emanate lines of force in all direction similar to the light emission from a point source of light obeying the inverse square law. The number of such lines is proportional to the magnitude of the charge (analogous to the brightness of the light source). This is shown diagrammatically in Figure 6.2, where the arrows point in the direction of force experienced by a positive charge if placed at that point. There will be further discussion of lines of force in the section of this chapter dealing with electrical field strength (see Sect. 6.6).

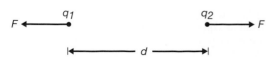

Figure 6.1 The forces (F) between two electrical charges, q_1 and q_2, separated by a distance (d) are equal and opposite.

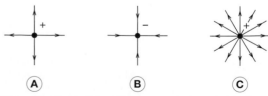

Figure 6.2 Electric 'lines of force' associated with (A) a weak positive charge, (B) a weak negative charge and (C) a strong positive charge.

6.5 PERMITTIVITY AND RELATIVE PERMITTIVITY (DIELECTRIC CONSTANT)

Equation 6.2 only holds true when the charges are in a vacuum, as ε_0 is the permittivity of a vacuum. In any other medium, the equation requires to be modified to:

Equation 6.3

$$F = \frac{q_1 q_2}{4\pi\varepsilon d^2}$$

where ε is the permittivity of the medium.

It is, however, often convenient to compare the permittivity of the medium relative to that of a vacuum, e.g. if the permittivity of the medium is twice that of a vacuum, then the *relative permittivity* (K) *is* 2. This can be obtained from the simple formula:

$$K = \frac{\varepsilon}{\varepsilon_0}$$

or by cross-multiplying:

Equation 6.4

$$\varepsilon = \varepsilon_0 K$$

so Equation 6.3 may be rewritten as:

Equation 6.5

$$F = \frac{q_1 q_2}{4\pi\varepsilon_0 K d^2}$$

K is known as the *dielectric constant* of the medium and so we can see that the relative permittivity and the dielectric constant are the same. Note that as the dielectric constant is a comparative number, it does not have any units. (The dielectric constant is further discussed in Ch. 13 where we consider its importance in capacitors.)

6.6 ELECTRICAL FIELD STRENGTH

We have already seen that an electrical charge is capable of influencing other charges placed at a distance from it. This influence on other charges at a distance is known as a field and, for the purpose of comparing electrical charges, E is measured in units of newton/coulomb. Consider the electrical field around a point charge. If we wish to know the field strength at a point, we simply place a unit of positive charge at that point and measure the magnitude and direction of the force exerted upon it. If we consider Equation 6.5 and have $q_2 = 1$ (unit charge), then we can say:

Equation 6.6

$$E = \frac{q_1 \times 1}{4\pi\varepsilon_0 K d^2}$$

$$E = \frac{q_1}{4\pi\varepsilon_0 K d^2}$$

We have already considered a diagrammatic representation of a field around a point charge (Fig. 6.2). The arrows represent the direction of the force acting on a unit positive charge (if placed at that point) and the line density represents the intensity of the electrical field.

6.7 ELECTROSTATIC INDUCTION OF CHARGE

As mentioned earlier (Sect 6.3), a charge may be induced on an electrical conductor or on an insulator. Each will now be considered.

6.7.1 Induction of a conductor

The situation that exists if an electrically charged body (B) is placed close to a conductor (A) is shown in Figure 6.3. A conductor is a body which will allow a flow of electrons. The positive charge on B attracts electrons to it and leaves equal numbers of positive charges on the opposite surface of A. Notice that the opposite charge is induced on the surface of the conductor closest to the inducing charge and that equal numbers of positive and negative charges are induced. Eventually a state of equilibrium is reached where the electrons on the surface of A experience an equal force of attraction from the two sets of positive charge. When this happens, no further electron flow takes place.

The charge distribution results in a net force of attraction as the unlike charges are closer to the charged body than the like charges.

Withdrawal of the charged body results in uniform distribution of the charges in A.

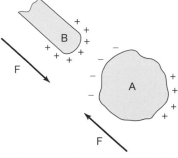

Figure 6.3 Induction of a charge on a conducting body, *A*, results in a force of attraction, *F*, with the inducing body, *B*.

6.7.2 Induction of an insulator (dielectric)

If we bring a charged body close to an insulator, a similar force of attraction occurs – this can be demonstrated by running a comb through your hair and holding it close to a small piece of paper, which will be attracted to it. This result is somewhat surprising, as electrons cannot move as freely through an insulator as a conductor. Some insulators are more efficient at producing induced charges than others and it is found that this varies with the dielectric constant (see Sect. 6.5) of the material. There are two explanations of the induced charge in an insulator, *molecular distortion* and *polar molecules*.

6.7.2.1 Molecular distortion

A body is composed of atoms or molecules. These contain equal numbers of protons (+ve) and electrons (−ve), thus making the body electrically neutral. As can be seen in Figure 6.4A, the electrons normally form symmetrical orbits around the nucleus so that the average position of the electron is over the nucleus, and the two sets of charges cancel each other out. If a charged body is placed close to the atom (Fig. 6.4B), the electron orbits are distorted relative to the atomic nucleus. The average position of the electrons is now displaced to one side of the atom, and so the atom has been *polarized* into an *electrical dipole*.

6.7.2.2 Polar molecules

Some molecules exist in which the atoms are so arranged that the average position of the electrons is not coincident with that of the nuclei, even when the atoms are not

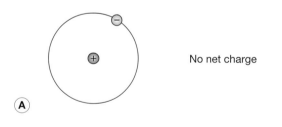

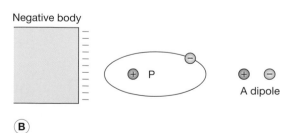

Figure 6.4 The effect of an external field on an atom. (A) The atom with no external field applied; (B) the polarization of the atom to form a dipole caused by the proximity of a negatively charged body.

subject to an electrical field. These molecules are polarized even when not subject to an electrical field.

The effect of an external electric field is to rotate these molecules such that they tend to become aligned with the field. This means that the structure now has definite positive and negative ends. Adjacent dipoles cancel each other's effects. Practical dielectrics use such materials as they produce a much stronger effect than molecular distortion alone.

6.8 ELECTRICAL POTENTIAL

There are a number of similarities between electrical potential and potential energy. In the case of potential energy, this represents the work done raising a body to a height from a zero level. Similar concepts will now be discussed for electrical potential.

6.8.1 Zero electrical potential

The most convenient point to choose as having zero potential is the point at which the force exerted by the charged body on unit charge would be zero. This point is *infinity* and all work performed on a unit charge is measured from there. Obviously, infinity is chosen for its mathematical convenience rather than its practicality!

Insight

It is often stated that 'the Earth is at zero potential'. The Earth is assumed to be electrically neutral in that it contains equal numbers of positive and negative charges. Thus, there is no force between the neutral Earth and a unit positive charge and so no effort is needed to move the latter towards Earth. Hence, no work is done and the electrical potential of Earth or any other neutral body is zero.

6.8.2 Absolute potential and potential difference

From the discussion so far, we may define the *absolute electrical potential* at a point as follows:

Definition

The absolute electrical potential at a point is the work done moving a unit positive charge from infinity to that point.
In practice, it is more convenient to compare the potential at one point relative to another than to know its absolute potential. If the potential at point A is V_A and the potential at point B is V_B then the potential difference (PD) between

---

A and B is $V_A - V_B$ and represents the difference in the work done moving unit positive charge from infinity to point A and from infinity to point B. It can be seen that this is the same as the work which would be required to move a unit positive charge to point B. This leads to the definition of potential difference.

Definition

The potential difference between two points is the work done on a unit positive charge in moving it from one point to the other.

6.8.3 The volt

The volt is the International System of Units (SI) unit of potential and is defined as:

Definition

1 volt of potential exists at a point if *1 joule of work* is performed in moving *1 coulomb of positive charge* from infinity to that point.

Similarly, for potential difference we have:

Definition

1 volt of potential difference exists between two points if *1 joule of work* is performed in moving *1 coulomb of positive charge* from one point to the other.

These definitions can be shown in the form of an equation:

Equation 6.7

$$\text{volts} = \frac{\text{joules}}{\text{coulombs}}$$

6.8.4 Electrical potential due to a point charge

Consider a point charge, Q, as shown in Figure 6.5. A unit of positive charge has been moved from infinity to a distance r from Q. The nearer the charge comes to Q, the greater the force of repulsion (if Q is positive) or attraction (if Q is negative). Thus the potential is positive if Q is positive and negative if Q is negative since the potential is the work done on the unit positive charge. If we consider that the work done on all unit positive charges which are equidistant

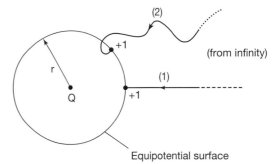

Figure 6.5 The electrical potential energy of a point charge, Q.

from Q will be the same, then it is logical to assume that equipotential surfaces will be concentric spheres with Q as the centre. It is also worth noting that the particular path chosen to bring a unit positive charge from infinity to the point r is of no importance and so paths (1) and (2) give exactly the same electrical potential.

Electrical potential is usually given the symbol V and so we can produce the equation:

Equation 6.8

$$\text{work} = \text{force} \times \text{distance}$$
$$V = \frac{Q \times r}{4\pi\varepsilon_0 r^2}$$
$$V = \frac{Q}{4\pi\varepsilon_0 r}$$

where V is in volts, Q is in coulombs and r is in metres.

The electrical potential due to a point charge is given the term *coulomb potential* and the force between two charges is the *coulomb force* (see Sect. 6.4).

6.8.5 Electrical potential due to a conducting sphere

If we place a charge Q on a conducting sphere, then the charged particles will mutually repel each other and the charges will be evenly distributed on the outer surface of the sphere as shown in Figure 6.5. This is true whether the sphere is hollow or solid. No potential difference exists between any points either on the surface or within the sphere (if a potential difference did exist, the charge would redistribute in such a way that the whole body was at a constant potential). When the potential exists outside the sphere, it may be shown mathematically that the sphere behaves as though all the charge Q is placed at its centre. This is shown in the graph in Figure 6.6 (See page 38). Thus Equation 6.8 can be used to calculate the potential of points outside the sphere where r is the distance from the centre of the sphere. This is important from a practical viewpoint in radiography in the design of components such as the X-ray tube shield where we wish to have the charge distributed evenly over the internal surfaces of the tube shield.

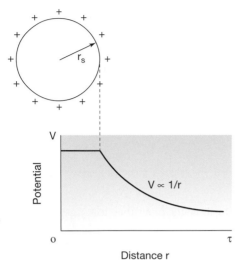

Figure 6.6 Distribution of electrical potential on a conducting sphere of radius *r*. The potential is constant within the sphere and reduces outside it (*V* ∝ 1/*r*).

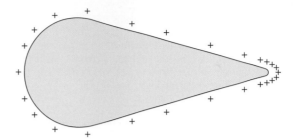

Figure 6.7 Distribution of positive charge on an irregularly shaped conductor. Note the high intensity of charge at the area of low radius of curvature.

6.9 DISTRIBUTION OF ELECTRICAL CHARGE ON AN IRREGULARY SHAPED CONDUCTOR

Having considered the charge distribution on a sphere, it is now useful to consider the distribution of charge on a conducting body of irregular shape. Such a body is shown in Figure 6.7. Again the charge is distributed so that no potential difference exists between any points *within the body*. This gives the charge distribution shown in Figure 6.7. Note that there are large collections of charge at parts of the body that have a small radius of curvature. This is important in the design of the X-ray tube both in the prevention of coronal discharge (where electrons are forcibly removed from their orbits to create an electrical spark) from sharp corners and also the use of a sharp-edged focusing cup for electron focusing (see Ch. 30).

Summary

In this chapter you should have learnt:
- The properties of electrical charges (see Sect. 6.3).
- The force between two electrical charges in a vacuum (see Sect. 6.4).
- The meaning of permittivity and relative permittivity (dielectric constant) (see Sect. 6.5).
- The concept of electrical field strength (see Sect. 6.6).
- The meaning of electrostatic induction (see Sect. 6.7).
- Electrostatic induction of a conductor (see Sect. 6.7.1).
- Electrostatic induction of an insulator or dielectric (see Sect. 6.7.2).
- The concept of electrical potential (see Sect. 6.8).
- The meaning of zero electrical potential (see Sect. 6.8.1).
- The meaning of absolute potential and potential difference (see Sect. 6.8.2).
- The definition of the volt (see Sect. 6.8.3).
- Electric potential due to a point charge (see Sect. 6.8.4).
- Electric potential due to a conducting sphere (see Sect. 6.8.5).
- Electrical charge distribution on an irregularly shaped conductor (see Sect. 6.9).

FURTHER READING

Ball, J.L., Moore, A.D., Turner, S., 2008. Ball and Moore's Essential physics for radiographers, Fourth edn. Blackwell Scientific, London (Chapter 3).

Chapter | 7 |

Electricity (DC)

7.1 AIM

The aim of this chapter is to introduce the reader to the concept of electron flow as a means of conducting electricity. Factors affecting the resistance to this flow will be explored and Ohm's law will be discussed. The consequences of resistance in terms of electrical 'power loss' will be discussed and the practical implications of this in the design of X-ray-generating apparatus will be considered.

7.2 INTRODUCTION

In Chapter 6 we considered the behaviour of static electrical charges. This chapter considers the behaviour of electrical charges which are *unidirectional* in their movement – *direct current* or *DC electricity*. Batteries produce a DC current and it is also found in the form of a rectified supply (see Ch. 28). In a vacuum, liquid or gas (e.g. in an air ionization chamber; see Ch. 27), both positive and negative charges move with relative freedom. These charges are called *ions*. In a solid, however, the atomic nuclei are relatively tightly bound to other atoms and so take no part in the flow of charge. The electrical properties of a given solid are determined by the way in which the orbiting electrons behave.

7.3 SIMPLE ELECTRON THEORY OF CONDUCTION

To explain why some materials readily allow a flow of electrons (i.e. are good electrical conductors) and other materials will only allow electron flow in extreme conditions (i.e. are good insulators), we need to look more closely at the structure of the atom. This chapter will only look at atomic structure in terms of explaining the electrical properties of the material and there will be a fuller description of the atom in Chapter 18.

The nucleus of the atom contains protons (+ve charge) and around this in orbitals are electrons (−ve charge). We can appreciate that electrons near the nucleus experience a high level of attraction (unlike charges attract) and are thus said to be *tightly bound*. Electrons in the more remote orbitals experience less force of attraction from the nucleus (remember $F \propto 1/d^2$) and are also repelled by other electrons which lie between them and the nucleus and so are said to be more *loosely bound*. Because the electrons in a given single atom are influenced by only that atom, the electrons lie at discrete energy levels, as shown in Figure 7.1A.

When electrons are brought closer together, as in a solid, the orbitals of the electrons are strongly influenced by the proximity of neighbouring atoms. This means that electrons are no longer at discrete energy levels but that they are now within a band of energies. This situation is shown in Figure 7.1B.

For the purpose of this discussion, only the outer two energy bands are of interest to us: the *valence band* and the *conduction band*. The valence band is that band which contains the outermost electrons of the atom and may be partially or completely full of its permitted maximum number of electrons. The configuration of electrons in the valence band determines the *chemical properties* of the atom, i.e. its ability to form *chemical bonds* with other atoms. If electrons exist further away from the nucleus than the valence band, then their energies lie in the conduction band. This band is populated with electrons that have, for some reason, become free from their original atoms. Because of this, once an electron is in the conduction band of a solid, it is able to move relatively freely and may take part in electrical conduction through the material. A material with a large number of electrons in the conduction band is a *good electrical conductor* whereas a material with no electrons in the conduction band is a *perfect electrical insulator*. Whether or not a material is a conductor, an insulator or a semiconductor is determined by the number of electrons in the conduction band. This number is in turn determined by the size of the *forbidden energy gap* (E) which exists between the top energy of the valence band and the bottom energy of the conduction band. The arrangement of the valence and conduction bands for conductors, semiconductors and insulators is shown in Figure 7.2. Each of the above will now be considered individually.

7.3.1 Electron arrangements in a conductor

As can be seen from Figure 7.2A, the conduction band and the valence band of energies overlap in a conductor. As a result, a large number of electrons always exist in the conduction band and because of this there is a ready exchange of electrons between the valence and conduction bands. This means that these electrons can be moved through the solid with *little resistance* to their flow. The main opposition to their flow arises from collisions with other electrons or atoms. If the temperature of the conductor is increased, there is an increase in the vibration of the atoms and a corresponding increase in the likelihood of collision with moving electrons. From this we can see that *the opposition (or resistance) to the flow of electrons in a conductor will increase with an increase in its temperature.*

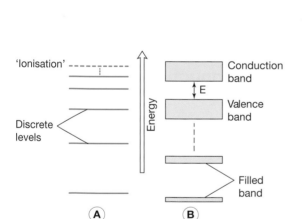

Figure 7.1 (A) Electron energy levels in a solitary atom. (B) Electron energy bands in an atom of a solid.

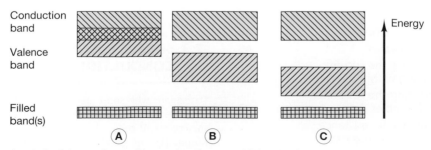

Figure 7.2 Energy bands for (A) a conductor, (B) a semiconductor and (C) an insulator.

Insight

As mentioned in Section 7.3.1, the main cause of resistance to the flow of electrons in a conductor is collisions with other atoms. It would seem logical to suggest that if the vibration of the atoms could be reduced, or even stopped, then the resistance of the conductor could be reduced. This is done by cooling the conductor to temperatures close to absolute zero. At these temperatures, atomic vibration ceases to exist and so flow of electrons through the conduction band is virtually unimpeded. Materials operating in this mode are known as superconductors and this technique is used to produce the large magnetic field required for magnetic resonance imaging (MRI).

In order to produce a current, the following conditions must be satisfied:

- There must be a source of electric *potential difference* (see Sect. 6.8.2).
- There must be a *complete circuit* around which the electrons are able to travel.

These two points are illustrated in Figure 7.4. The battery (B) is a source of potential difference, but if the switch (S) is open (as in Fig. 7.4A), no electric current flows and the bulb does not light up. When the switch is closed (Fig. 7.4B), a complete circuit exists around which electrons are able to flow and so the bulb lights up. The *potential difference* may be thought of as the *driving force* that causes electrons to flow, while the *current is* the rate of flow of electrons, i.e. the number of electrons passing a given point in unit time.

7.3.2 Electron arrangements in a semiconductor

In a semiconductor, there is a gap between the maximum energy of the valence band and the minimum energy of the conduction band (Fig. 7.2B) and so electrons need to be given energy to bridge this gap and flow through the material (this will be discussed in more detail in Ch. 15, which deals with semiconductors). Thus, *semiconductors have a greater resistance to the flow of electrons than conductors.* If we increase the temperature of the semiconductor, we will increase the energy of the electrons in the valence band and so make it easier for them to transfer to the conduction band and move through the solid. Thus, *increasing the temperature of a semiconductor will reduce its resistance to the flow of electrons.*

7.3.3 Electron arrangements in an insulator

In an insulator, there is a significant gap between the maximum energy of the valence band and the minimum energy of the conduction band (Fig. 7.2C). This means that electrons cannot readily bridge this energy gap, and so the conduction band contains no electrons, making conduction impossible. If the material is heated, then the electrons in the valence band gain energy, and so the gap between the valence and the conduction bands is narrowed, making it more likely that electrons can jump the gap. *Thus, increasing the temperature of an insulator reduces its resistance.*

The effect on the resistance to the flow of electrons of increasing the temperature is shown in Figure 7.3.

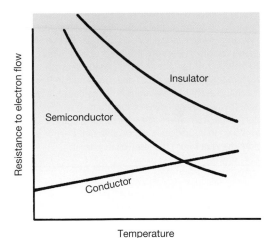

Figure 7.3 Effect of temperature on the electrical resistance of a conductor, a semiconductor and an insulator.

7.4 ELECTRIC CURRENT

Electricity is the flow of electrons in a material. The rate of flow of electrons is a measure of the *electric current.*

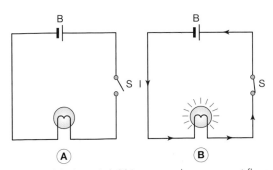

Figure 7.4 (A) The switch (S) is open and so no current flows through the circuit. (B) When the switch is closed, current will flow through the circuit and the bulb will light. This shows that a continuous circuit is necessary for electrical current to flow.

Definition

An *electric current of 1 ampere* (A) flows at a point if a charge of 1 *coulomb* (C) flows past that point *per second*.

Thus, we can say mathematically:

Equation 7.1

$$\text{ampers} = \frac{\text{coulombs}}{\text{seconds}}$$

From Section 6.4, we know that a charge of 1 coulomb is equivalent to approximately 6×10^{18} electrons so 1 ampere is simply this number of electrons passing a point in 1 second.

Insight

We are accustomed to an instant response when we close an electrical switch and so it is surprising to discover that the average velocity of electrons in a circuit is only in the order of $0.5\,\text{mm.s}^{-1}$. When the switch is closed, electrons start to flow through the whole circuit and so the bulb in Figure 7.4 will light up even if the electrons from the battery have not yet reached it – this is similar to the situation where water enters a pipe from a reservoir when a tap is opened; water leaves the tap immediately, although it might be some time before the water from the reservoir reaches it.

7.5 mA, mAs AND MILLICOULOMBS

The electric current through an X-ray tube is a small one and so it is measured in *milliamperes* (mA) rather than in amps: $1\,\text{mA} = 10^{-3}\,\text{A}$. This measures the rate of flow of electrons through the X-ray tube. If we wish to measure the number of electrons that have travelled across the tube during a given radiographic exposure, then we need to multiply the rate of flow by the time of the exposure. This unit is in *milliampere-seconds* (mAs) where:

Equation 7.2

$$\text{mAs} = \text{mA} \times \text{seconds}$$

Now the total number of electrons, which have crossed the X-ray tube, is just a measure of the charge, measured in *coulombs*. From Equation 7.1:

$$\text{amps} = \frac{\text{coulombs}}{\text{seconds}}$$

By cross-multiplying (see Appendix A):

$$\text{coulombs} = \text{amps} \times \text{seconds}$$

so:

Equation 7.3

$$\text{millicoulombs} = \text{milliamps} \times \text{seconds}$$

So we can say that:

Equation 7.4

$$1\,\text{mAs} = 1\,\text{millicoulomb}$$

7.6 POTENTIAL DIFFERENCE AND ELECTROMOTIVE FORCE

We have already considered potential difference in Section 6.8.2 and defined the potential difference in volts:

Definition

The potential difference in volts is the work done in moving 1 coulomb of positive charge from one point to another.

Thus:

Equation 7.5

$$\text{volts} = \frac{\text{joules}}{\text{coulombs}}$$

In electricity, we are concerned with moving charges and, as mentioned previously, we can regard the potential difference as the 'driving force', which moves the electron along a conductor.

Electromotive force (EMF) is also expressed in *volts* and is a measure of electrical potential energy developed across *a source* of electricity (e.g. a battery or a generator). The EMF is the 'driving force' behind the electron flow in the circuit.

It is therefore possible to speak about the potential difference (PD) across any part of the circuit including the source of electricity, whereas the term EMF is reserved solely for the latter. It would not be correct to use the term 'EMF across a resistor' as a resistor is not a source of electricity – the appropriate terminology would be 'the PD across a resistor'.

Insight

It is interesting to note that the PD across the terminals of a battery is less than the EMF when a current flows. This is due to the internal resistance of the battery. The effect is known as *regulation*. Similar effects are observed with transformers and will be discussed more fully in Chapter 14.

7.7 RESISTANCE

The elementary theory of conduction discussed earlier in this chapter refers to two mechanisms that impede electron flow:

1. Lack of 'free' electrons in the conduction band – as in an insulator.
2. Collisions between flowing electrons with other vibrating electrons in the material.

This impedance to the flow of electrons is given the term *electrical resistance* or simply *resistance* and is measured in *ohms*. Obviously, from the earlier discussion, insulators have much higher resistance than conductors of the same shape and size. The resistance of a conductor can vary depending on a number of factors, which will be discussed below.

7.7.1 Factors affecting resistance

The resistance of a substance will be affected by:

* the *shape* of the substance
* the *type* of the substance
* the *temperature* of the substance.

Note that the resistance of the substance is not affected by either the potential difference across it or by the current flowing through it.

7.7.1.1 Shape

The shape of a body is capable of infinite variation, so for simplicity we shall consider circular conductors of constant cross-sectional area.

Figure 7.5 illustrates such a body and the effect on the resistance R of altering its length l and its cross-sectional area A.

The resistance is proportional to the length of the conductor ($R \propto l$). If we consider a situation where the length of the conductor is doubled, then electrons travelling along the conductor have twice as many vibrating atoms to get past, so the resistance to their flow will be doubled.

The resistance is inversely proportional to the cross-sectional area ($R \propto l/A$). If the area is doubled, there are twice as many electrons capable of conducting charge. The number of atoms each electron must get past for the length of the conductor remains the same and so doubling the area will halve the resistance.

7.7.1.2 Type of substance

By definition, good electrical conductors will have a lower resistance than insulators. Different metals also have different values of resistance. As we have just seen, the shape of the substance also affects its resistance, so that a standard shape and size must be used when comparing

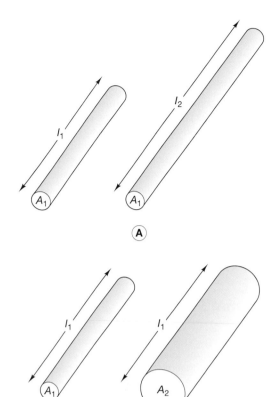

Figure 7.5 Factors affecting resistance of a conductor. In (A) the conductors are of different lengths and the resistance increases with the length. In (B) the conductors have differing cross-sectional areas and the resistance is inversely proportional to the cross-sectional area.

the resistance of different materials. The standard used is a cube of side 1 metre and the resistance is measured when a current is passed between opposing faces of the cube. The value of the resistance so obtained is called the *resistivity* or the *specific resistance* of the material and is measured in ohm-metres. Resistivity is given the symbol ρ (Greek rho) and it is clear that the resistance of the material will be directly proportional to its resistivity: $R \propto \rho$.

If we now consider all the factors discussed above, we have:

Equation 7.6

$$R \propto \frac{\sigma l}{A}$$

In the International System of Units (SI) system, ρ is defined so that the constant of proportionality in the above equation is unity and we can say:

Equation 7.7

$$R = \frac{\sigma l}{A}$$

The resistivity of insulators is about 1 million times greater than those of semiconductors, which in turn are about 1 million times greater than those of metallic conductors.

7.7.1.3 Temperature

As described at the beginning of this chapter, a change in temperature affects the resistance of a body. This effect is different for conductors, semiconductors and insulators, as shown in Figure 7.3. Because of these variations, resistance is usually quoted at a particular temperature (e.g. 20 °C). The *temperature coefficient* of resistance, α, is defined as the fractional change in resistance (or resistivity) per unit temperature change:

$$\alpha = \frac{\text{change in resistivity}}{\text{original resistivity}} / \text{temperature change}$$

Note: α is different for different conductors.

7.8 OHM'S LAW

Ohm's law applies to metallic conductors and combines, in a simple way, the relationship between *current, potential difference* and *resistance.* It is found experimentally that the current flowing through a conductor is proportional to the potential difference applied across it – *as the driving force on the electrons is increased, so the number of electrons passing a point in unit time increases by a proportional amount.* If a potential difference of 2 volts causes a current of 1 amp to flow through a conductor, then a potential difference of 4 volts will cause a current of 2 amps to flow. Ohm's law may be formally stated as follows:

> **The** current flowing through a **metallic conductor is proportional to the** potential difference **which exists across it provided that all** physical conditions **remain constant.**

The main *physical condition,* which must remain *constant,* is the temperature of the conductor, as an alteration in the temperature will cause an alteration in the resistance (see Sect. 7.7.1).

Ohm's law may be stated mathematically thus:

Equation 7.8

$$I \propto V$$

where I and V are the magnitude of the current and the potential difference respectively.

Note that Ohm's law does not mention the word *resistance.* The resistance of the body (R) is introduced into Equation 7.8 as a constant of proportionality (see Appendix A) and so the equation may now be rewritten:

Equation 7.9

$$V \propto I$$
$$\therefore V = R \times I$$
$$\therefore V = I \times R$$

As we have already established, R is a *constant* for a given conductor at a given temperature and *does not* depend on V or I.

R is measured in ohm (Ω) and we can see from Equation 7.9 that when $V = 1$ volt and $I = 1$ amp, then R will be 1 ohm. The ohm may be defined as follows:

Definition

A body is said to have an electrical resistance of *1 ohm* if a potential difference of *1 volt* across it produces an electrical current through it of *1 ampere.*

(Note that a potential difference always occurs *across* a body, never *through* it. Likewise, an electrical current always flows *through* a body and does not exist *across* it.)

Although Ohm's law is simple in its formulation, it has far-reaching implications which can be applied to radiological physics. The most important of these will now be discussed.

7.8.1 Resistors in series

If we join resistors *in series* (end-to-end) and apply a potential difference of V volts across the unit, then a current of I amp flows through it. This is shown in Figure 7.6. Note that the same current flows through each resistor since the whole unit may be regarded as a continuous circuit and so electrons are neither lost nor gained throughout the circuit. Also note that the potential difference across the ends of the unit is simply the sum of the potential differences across each resistor ($V = V_1 + V_2 + V_3$). We wish to calculate the effective resistance of the unit (R), i.e. *what would be the value of a single resistor which would behave in exactly the same way as the whole unit?*

If we apply Ohm's law to each resistor in turn then we get:

$$V_1 = IR_1; \ V_2 = IR_2; \ V_3 = IR_3$$

We already know that:

Equation 7.10A

$$V = V_1 + V_2 + V_3$$
$$V = IR_1 + IR_2 + IR_3$$
$$V = I(R_1 + R_2 + R_3)$$

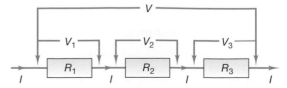

Figure 7.6 Combining resistors in series to produce a total resistance, R.

If we apply Ohm's law to the total unit then:

$$V = I \times R$$
$$R = \frac{V}{I}$$

By substituting this value of V/I into Equation 7.10A, we get:

Equation 7.10

$$R = R_1 + R_2 + R_3$$

Thus, when resistors are connected in series, the total resistance may be obtained simply by adding together the values of each separate resistor.

7.8.2 Resistors in parallel

A potential difference of V exists across points A and B in Figure 7.7 and, since each resistor is connected to A and B, the potential difference across each resistor is also V volts. Electrons flow into the circuit at point A and then some will pass through each resistor to meet again at point B. Since electrons are neither gained nor lost in the circuit:

Equation 7.11A

$$I = I_1 + I_2 + I_3$$

If we apply Ohm's law to each of the resistors, we get:

$$V = I_1 R_1; V = I_2 R_2; V = I_3 R_3$$

By substituting these values in Equation 7.11A:

$$I = \frac{V}{R_1} + \frac{V}{R_2} + \frac{V}{R_3}$$

$$\text{or } I = V\left(\frac{1}{R_1} + \frac{1}{R_2} + \frac{1}{R_3}\right)$$

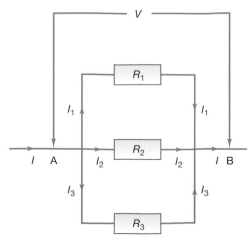

Figure 7.7 Combining resistors in parallel to produce a total resistance, R.

so:

Equation 7.11B

$$\frac{1}{V} = \frac{1}{R_1} + \frac{1}{R_2} + \frac{1}{R_3}$$

If we apply Ohm's law to the whole unit (assuming it has a resistance R), then we get:

$$V = IR$$

or

$$\frac{I}{V} = \frac{1}{R}$$

If we now substitute this value in Equation 7.11B, we get:

Equation 7.11

$$\frac{1}{R} = \frac{1}{R_1} + \frac{1}{R_2} + \frac{1}{R_3}$$

7.9 ELECTRICAL ENERGY AND POWER

To get an electric current to flow through a conductor, the electrons must be driven by a potential difference. As the electrons move through the conductor they are involved in collisions with the atoms of the conductor and so *work* must be done to keep all the electrons moving in the same direction. The electrons dissipate energy to the atoms of the material, which they pass through, and so heat is produced in the material – this is the mechanism by which the filament of the X-ray tube is heated to produce electrons by thermionic emission (see Chapter 30).

7.9.1 The joule

As already discussed (Sect. 4.3), the joule is the SI unit of energy. The key to the method of calculating electrical energy lies in the definition of potential difference. As we discovered in Section 6.8.3, *the potential difference between two points is 1 volt when 1 joule of work is done in moving 1 coulomb of positive charge from one point to the other.* Thus, we can say:

Equation 7.12

$$\text{volts} = \frac{\text{joules}}{\text{coulombs}}$$

or:

Equation 7.13

$$\text{joules} = \text{volts} \times \text{coulombs}$$

45

Since the ampere is a rate of flow of charge of 1 coulomb per second, then we can say:

Equation 7.14

$$\text{joules} = \text{volts} \times \text{amperes} \times \text{seconds}$$

7.9.2 The watt

We also saw in Section 4.3 that the SI unit of power is the watt, where 1 watt = 1 joule per second. Thus, we can say that:

$$\frac{\text{joules}}{\text{seconds}} = \frac{\text{volts} \times \text{amperes} \times \text{seconds}}{\text{seconds}}$$

or:

Equation 7.15

$$\text{watts} = \text{volts} \times \text{amperes}$$

This is a general equation used in the calculation of electrical power, which applies to any electrical system. It is, however, particularly useful to apply this formula to a metallic conductor which obeys Ohm's law.

7.9.3 Power in a resistor

Consider a current I passing through a metallic resistor of resistance R when a potential difference V is applied across its ends. As previously discussed:

$$W = V \times I$$

However, we can apply Ohm's law to the resistor:

$$V = I \times R$$

so

$$W = I \times R \times R$$

or

$$W = I^2R$$

By similar manipulations of Ohm's law, we can get two possible equations for the electrical power in a resistor:

Equation 7.16

$$W = VI$$
$$W = I^2R$$

The second equation is probably the most useful one in radiography.

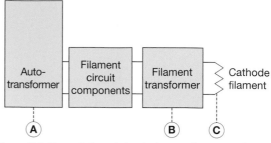

Figure 7.8 Transmission of electrical power from the voltage selector to the X-ray tube filament. Between points A and B power is in the optimum form for transmission with minimum power loss – high voltage and low current. Thus 100 watts of power would be transmitted in the form of 100 volts and 1 ampere. Between points B and C power is in the optimum form for heat generation at the filament. Thus 100 watts of power would be transmitted in the form of 10 volts and 10 amperes.

7.10 POWER LOSS IN CABLES

If we consider electricity in the form of a current I passing through a cable with a resistance R, it becomes apparent that some of the available electrical power will be 'lost' in the cable. The term 'lost' does not imply that there is a breach of the law of conservation of energy but that the power is not available for the user at the far end of the cable – the 'lost' energy is in fact converted into heat.

It is obviously desirable that the power which is lost in the cables be kept to a minimum as this is not available to the user. If we consider that the power loss is given by the equation $P = I^2R$, then it can be seen that the power loss can be kept to a minimum in one of two ways:

1. Reducing the current flowing within the cable.
2. Reducing the resistance of the cables.

7.10.1 Reducing the current flowing within the cable

Electrical power (P) is a combination of the potential difference (V) across the cables and the current (I) flowing through them, i.e. $P = VI$. If we wish to transmit a given amount of electrical power with the minimum loss in the cables, this can be done by using a high voltage and a low current. This is shown in Figure 7.8 where a power of approximately 100 watts is required to heat the filament of the X-ray tube. This power is transmitted from the voltage selector to the filament transformer (see Ch. 14) in the form of a relatively high voltage and low current. At the filament we wish to use this power to generate heat, so it is converted to a relatively low voltage and high current at the filament transformer. Similar techniques are used in transmitting power from the generating stations to our homes.

7.10.2 Reducing the resistance of the cables

This is achieved in two ways: making the cables of a material with a low resistivity (usually copper) and making the cables as thick (large cross-sectional area) as possible. Because the cables are required to transmit power from one point to another, there is little scope for the third possibility – reducing the length of the cables.

7.10.3 Mains cable resistance and X-ray exposures

As we have previously discussed, there is a potential difference across any resistor which is related to the current through the resistor ($V = IR$). This volt drop is removed from the EMF available when a current flows to an X-ray unit. This can be seen in Equation 7.17:

Equation 7.17

$$V = \text{EMF} - IR_c$$

where R_c is the resistance of the mains cables and V is the PD available at the mains supply when the unit is 'on load'. It is also worth noting that this volt drop is related to the resistance of the cables and the current to the X-ray unit.

In practice, with static X-ray units, the resistance of the mains cables is fairly constant so it is possible to compensate for this volt drop using a *static mains resistance compensator*. For mains-dependent mobile units the volt drop can vary for different parts of the hospital – obviously, the mains cables that reach the tenth floor are longer than the cables to the ground floor. This means that *this type of mobile unit has an adjustable mains resistance compensator*. Usually, the plug for the unit in the ward is coded in some way so that we know the correct setting for the compensator.

Insight

Many modern mobile X-ray units overcome this problem by being 'mains independent'. Such units remove power from the mains in small amounts between exposures (they require to be plugged into the mains when not in use) and then release this power through the X-ray tube during the exposure. The electrical power may be stored in special batteries or in capacitors (see Chapter 13).

Summary

In this chapter you should have learnt the following:

- Simple electron theory of conduction (see Sect. 7.3).
- The requirements for a flow of electric current (see Sect. 7.4).
- The relationships between mA, mAs and millicoulombs (see Sect. 7.5).
- The meaning of potential difference and EMF (see Sect. 7.6).
- The meaning of electrical resistance (see Sect. 7.7).
- The factors affecting electrical resistance (see Sect. 7.7.1).
- Ohm's law (see Sect. 7.8).
- The effect of connecting resistors in series (see Sect. 7.8.1).
- The effect of connecting resistors in parallel (see Sect. 7.8.2).
- The meaning of electrical energy and power (see Sect. 7.9).
- The meaning of the joule (see Sect. 7.9.1).
- The meaning of the watt (see Sect. 7.9.2).
- Power in a resistor (see Sect. 7.9.3).
- Power loss in cables (see Sect. 7.10.1 and Sect 7.10.2).
- Mains cable resistance and X-ray exposures (see Sect. 7.10.3).

FURTHER READING

Ball, J.L., Moore, A.D., Turner, S., 2008. Ball and Moore's Essential Physics for Radiographers, fourth ed. Blackwell Scientific, London (Chapter 7).

Dowsett, D.J., Kennedy, P.A., Johnson, R.E., 1998. The Physics of Diagnostic Imaging. Chapman & Hall Medical, London (Chapter 2).

Chapter | 8 |

Magnetism

8.1 AIM

In this chapter the key principles of magnetism are considered. Magnetism plays a vital role in the scanning technique called magnetic resonance imaging (MRI), which uses powerful magnetic fields to portray human tissues.

8.2 MAGNETIC FIELDS

As long ago as the 11th century, the Chinese were employing magnetic compasses. These consisted of a length of permanently magnetized iron which will tend to align itself in the direction of the Earth's magnetic field when free to pivot. The phenomenon that two like magnetic poles (such as two north poles) repel and two unlike magnetic poles (such as a north and a south pole) attract was demonstrated by Peter Peregrinus in the 13th century.

Whenever an electrical charge is in motion, a magnetic field is produced. This takes place when electrons flow in a conductor such as a metal wire. There are also electron orbital motions and spins in atoms, which produce tiny magnetic fields.

Whenever a field is produced in a volume of space, an energy gradient exists. In other words there is a change of energy within that volume. The energy gradient means that force may be exerted on a charge present within the field. For example, force may be exerted on a current-carrying wire, on a compass needle which experiences a twisting force, or on the magnetic spins of nuclei within the field of an MRI magnet. Materials which are capable of being temporarily magnetized experience a force when placed in a magnetic field. A vivid demonstration of this effect (not to be attempted!) is the sight of an object such as a pair of scissors accelerating through the air towards the bore of an MRI magnet. This is an example of the 'projectile effect' in which a magnetic field exerts a 'torque' (or twisting force) on a ferromagnetic object such as iron, tending to align it with the field and bring it closer to the strongest point in the field.

A magnetic north and magnetic south pole separated by a distance is known as a *magnetic dipole*. A dipole can comprise the two poles of a permanent magnet or the two ends of a current-carrying loop of conductor. If two magnetic poles of strength p are separated by a distance l, then the *magnetic dipole moment* of the system, $m = p \times l$.

The force F between two magnetic poles is equal to the product of their individual strengths divided by the square of the distance between them.

F is proportional to $(p_1 \times p_2)$ divided by d^2, where p_1 and p_2 are the individual magnetic pole strengths and d^2 is the square of the distance between them. Thus it can be seen that the force on an object entering a magnetic scanner room increases greatly as the distance to the scanner decreases. This is an example of an 'inverse square law'. Further examples of the law, which is particularly important in radiography, are provided in Chapter 26.

The direction of a magnetic field is taken as the direction in which a hypothetical isolated magnetic north pole would move if placed in the field. Hence lines of magnetic field pass from the north to the south pole of a permanent magnet, as shown in Figure 8.1 (see page 50).

49

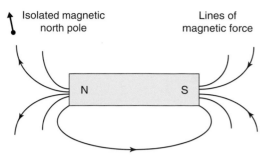

Figure 8.1 Lines of magnetic field surrounding a permanent bar magnet.

Insight

It isn't correct to talk about the north and south poles of an MRI scanner. Such scanners produce a very powerful magnetic field in the z-axis (or long axis) of a patient lying within the scanner, and we can talk about a 'spin-up' orientation parallel to the field and a 'spin-down' orientation antiparallel to it. But the concept of an MRI scanner as a large bar magnet is misleading.

The field around a bar magnet is non-uniform, that is it varies in strength and direction with location. In contrast, the Earth's magnetic field is relatively uniform and the magnetic field lines run fairly parallel to each other. Although this is generally true, there may be small local variations due to the presence of iron-containing rock. The Earth's magnetic flux density is typically about 0.5 gauss (G) or 0.5×10^{-4} tesla. A tesla equals 10 000 gauss. The gauss is an old centimetre gram second (cgs) unit but is still in common use as it is sometimes easier to use. For example, it is easier to talk about a '5-gauss exclusion zone' surrounding an MRI scanner than a 0.0005 tesla zone! The larger and more current SI unit of tesla (T) for magnetic flux density and magnetic inductance is used a lot to describe the 'field strength' of MRI scanners, where 0.2 T would be regarded as a 'low field' magnet and 3 T as a 'high field' magnet. A 3-T magnet provides a magnetic field about 60 000 times more powerful than that of the Earth.

Note: although the tesla is commonly used to describe the 'strength' of the magnetic field B in radiography, strictly the tesla is a unit of magnetic flux density or inductance.

The static (or constant) magnetic field produced by an MRI magnet needs to be as uniform as possible within the bore itself, in order to maximize image quality. Magnetic field homogeneity needs to be achieved, with a maximum permissible variation of 1 part in 100,000 for clinical MR imaging and to about 1 part in 10 million for in-vivo (living) magnetic resonance spectroscopy, which produces spectral signatures of chemicals present in the body. In practice, small inhomogeneities (non-uniformities) arise when an object such as a patient is present within the magnetic field.

Insight

There are two contributions to the magnetic moment of an electron, namely an *orbital magnetic moment* due to angular momentum around the nucleus, and a *spin magnetic moment* due to spin about the electron's own axis. The permitted spins of an electron are +1/2 and −1/2. Paired electrons within full orbitals have opposing spins and cancel out each other's magnetic moments. Likewise, the net magnetic moment of a filled electron shell is zero, since all the orbitals within it are full. Only the unfilled electron shell needs to be considered when examining magnetic properties. Contributions to the spin and angular momentum for each individual outer shell electron need to be added vectorially.

Paramagnetic materials have a small positive *magnetic susceptibility*, symbol χ, of the order of $+10^{-3}$ to $+10^{-5}$. The magnetic susceptibility of a material refers to the extent to which it can become temporarily magnetized in a magnetic field. Materials with positive susceptibility reinforce the effect of a magnetic field. The magnetization of paramagnets is weak but parallel to the direction of the applied magnetic field. These materials usually have unpaired electrons. They include atoms and ions of transition elements, rare Earth elements, some metals, oxygen and free radicals. Examples are aluminium, platinum, manganese and the ion Gd^{3+}, which is used within MRI contrast agents to reduce MRI T1 relaxation times and hence brighten the signal. Fe^{2+} ions in the liver, bound to organic molecules, also reduce T1 times. See Chapter 39 for an explanation of the T1 process.

Diamagnetic materials have a small negative magnetic susceptibility, of the order of 10^{-5}. Their magnetic response is in opposition to the applied magnetic field. These materials, such as copper, silver, gold, bismuth and beryllium, have filled electron shells and no net magnetic moment. Their induced magnetization opposes the magnetic field, in a manner predicted by Lenz's law. The applications of Lenz's law are covered in Chapter 10.

Ferromagnetic materials have a very high positive magnetic susceptibility of the order of +50 to +10 000. Ferromagnetic materials retain their magnetization once exposed to a magnetic field. They are used within permanent MRI magnets. The disadvantage of such magnets is their low maximum field strength. The property of ferromagnetism is due to the bulk effects of many electrons within the material, rather than to the magnetic effects of the electrons within individual atoms. Examples are iron, cobalt and nickel.

Superparamagnetic materials exhibit a large positive magnetic susceptibility. They differ from ferromagnetic materials in consisting of small size particles which do not display the bulk properties of ferromagnetic materials. They become transiently magnetized within a magnetic field. An example is coated particles of iron oxide, used as a negative contrast agent which reduces MRI T2 times and reduces signal intensity.

Insight

The magnetic susceptibility properties of body tissues can be used in MRI to provide useful signal information. For example, the magnetic susceptibility of liver and haemorrhage is altered by their iron content. Metallic implants often produce a large magnetic susceptibility artefact in MRI, by distorting the local magnetic field. The magnetic susceptibilities of oxygenated and deoxygenated blood differ and this can be used in functional MRI of tissue blood supply

So far we have only considered the magnetic effects due to electrons. However, there is a small contribution to the total angular momentum of the atom from the nucleus, due to its spin. This contribution is about one-thousandth of that of an electron, but is a very important property in MRI.

Insight

Nuclei, like electrons, possess ground energy levels and excited energy levels. Protons and neutrons, the constituents of nuclei, have a spin quantum number of +1/2 or −1/2. They also have orbital angular momentum by virtue of their motion in the nucleus. Both the proton and the neutron possess a magnetic moment (the latter despite not having an overall electrical charge, for reasons which need not concern us here). The sum total of the spin and orbital angular moments of the nucleons in the nucleus is referred to as the *nuclear spin*. Since an odd number of spin 1/2 particles always combine to give a half integer total spin, it follows that nuclei with an odd mass number have nuclear spins of values 1/2, 3/2, 5/2, etc. It is these nuclei that concern us in MRI and have useful magnetic spins. The most important one is the hydrogen-1 nucleus, which is just a single proton and has a 1/2 spin. Phosphorus-31 is used in MR spectroscopy. Note that the individual nucleon spins are cancelled out in nuclei with even mass numbers and thus these nuclei are of no use to us in MRI.

MRI used to be termed *nuclear magnetic resonance*, because it depends upon the magnetization of the atomic nucleus. The name was changed because the public tended to confuse it with the nuclear reactions, involving the fission of atomic nuclei, that occur in power stations and atom bombs.

We commented earlier that the magnetic moment of an electron is much greater than that of a nucleus. Indeed, electron spin resonance has been studied to examine its potential for imaging. However, electron spin resonance occurs on the gigahertz or GHz frequency range, and leads to considerable heating of tissues. In addition, these frequencies are absorbed superficially in the body, leading to poor deep imaging.

8.3 BULK MAGNETIC PROPERTIES AND PERMANENT MAGNETS

We saw above that some elements and materials like iron are highly magnetic (ferromagnetic) while others like gold, plastics and most body tissues have almost no magnetization. A ferromagnetic material like a block of iron in fact consists of many tiny crystals, not just one slab of homogeneous material. These small crystals can be considered as individual domains, each with an overall magnetization in a particular direction. If the domains are aligned randomly, very little overall magnetization will result, although the domains may become more aligned in the presence of a strong magnetic field, producing temporary magnetization. This is the case when a pair of scissors hurtles into an MRI magnet!

In permanent magnets, the domains tend to align in a particular direction and are fixed in this direction, giving a permanent overall magnetization, as shown in Figure 8.2.

A small number of MRI scanners employ permanent magnets to produce a magnetic field. These magnets have the disadvantages of being bulky and producing a relatively low magnetic field strength. More will be said about the types of available MRI scanners in Chapter 39. There have been improvements in the technology of permanent magnets and a range of materials, such as neodymium iron, ceramics, ferrites and rare Earth elements can be employed in their construction.

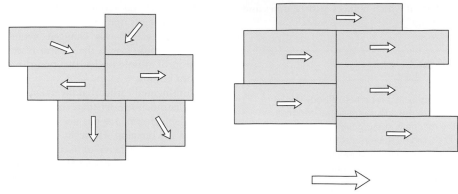

Figure 8.2 Individual magnetic domains are randomly aligned (but can be influenced) in non-permanent magnetic materials (left) while permanent magnets (right) have their domains in fixed alignment, giving an overall magnetization.

Summary

In this chapter you should have learnt the following:
- Magnetic properties exist in nuclei and electrons at the atomic level (see Sect. 8.3) and also in whole materials at the macroscopic level (see Sect. 8.4).
- Magnetism may be temporary or permanent and many materials become magnetized within a magnetic field (see Sect. 8.4).
- There are many applications of these principles in magnetic resonance imaging and general radiography.

FURTHER READING

Bushong, S.C., 2008. Radiologic Science for Technologists, ninth ed. Mosby, St Louis.

Halliday, D., Resnick, R., Walker, J., 2007. Fundamentals of Physics, eigth ed. John Wiley, New York.

Chapter | 9 |

Electromagnetism

9.1 AIM

The aim of this chapter is to consider the basic properties of magnetism discussed in Chapter 8 and show how these can be applied to a current-carrying conductor, giving an electromagnet.

9.2 INTRODUCTION

In Chapter 8, it was shown that magnetism is a phenomenon associated with atoms, and is due to the spinning and orbiting of electrons around those atoms. Electrons are negatively-charged particles so we may conclude that magnetism is caused by moving electric charges. It is reasonable to ask whether an electric current in a wire (for example) can also produce a magnetic field, since an electric current is just the flow of electrons in a conductor (Sects 7.3 and 7.4). This is found to be so in practice and the term *electromagnetism is* used to describe this effect (i.e. *electricity* producing *magnetism*).

9.3 ELECTRON FLOW AND 'CONVENTIONAL' CURRENT

When electricity was first discovered, it was assumed that it was the *positive* charges that flow in a conductor, and not the negative charges. This concept is now known as the 'conventional' current. It is now known that the positive charges in a solid material do *not have any net movement* (although they vibrate with heat energy; Ch. 5), since they form the protons in the nuclei of atoms (Ch. 18). Thus, it is the electrons that move in a solid, as explained by the elementary electron theory of conduction.

In gas or liquid, any positive and negative charges present may take part in current flow, since the positive charges are free to move, unlike in a solid. In radiography and many other subjects, it is the electron flow in conductors which is most frequently under consideration, and herein lies a difficulty, for many rules (or conventions) in electromagnetism and electromagnetic induction (Ch. 10) are based upon the totally false assumption of the 'conventional' current, which in a mathematical sense is supposed to flow in the opposite direction to that of the electrons.

This and further chapters will therefore discuss both electromagnetism and electromagnetic induction on the basis of _electron flow only,_ in an attempt to eliminate much of the confusion that undoubtedly exists at present in many people's minds. Some caution is therefore required when studying these subjects from other books, as they may invoke the 'conventional' current for their rules. Differences in the two approaches are explained in the Insights where appropriate.

9.4 MAGNETIC FIELD DUE TO A STRAIGHT WIRE

The presence of a magnetic field around a current-carrying conductor was first discovered by Oersted when passing

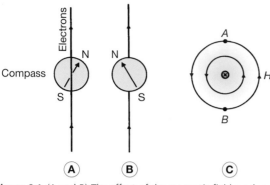

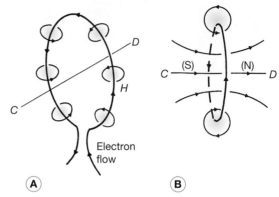

Figure 9.1 (A and B) The effect of the magnetic field produced by the electrons flowing in the wire upon a magnetic compass. (C) If we look along the wire in the direction of electron flow, then the field is an anticlockwise direction (⊗ means that the electrons are flowing away from the eye of the observer).

Figure 9.2 The magnetic field around a coil of wire carrying a current. Note the similarity to the field around a small bar magnet.

a current through a straight wire placed near a magnetic compass, as illustrated in Figure 9.1.

If the wire is aligned in a north–south direction (i.e. along the direction of the compass needle), then an electric current through the wire causes deflections of the compass, as shown in Figure 9.1: *clockwise* when the wire is above the compass (A) and *anticlockwise* when the wire is below the compass (B). This is only possible if the lines of magnetic force are circular and in an anticlockwise direction when viewed along the same direction as the movement of the flowing electrons. We may therefore use the following convention.

Convention

Each moving electron produces an *anticlockwise* magnetic field about itself when viewed along the direction of its motion.

This convention is illustrated in Figure 9.1C, where the symbol ⊗ means that electron flow is away from the eye (and ⊙ is towards the eye). The arrows on the lines of force are in an anticlockwise direction, in accordance with our convention, and give the direction in which a north pole would move if placed in that position. Thus, a weightless north pole would, if released, travel round and round the wire indefinitely in an anticlockwise circle.

9.5 MAGNETIC FIELD DUE TO A CIRCULAR COIL OF WIRE

Figure 9.2A shows a circular coil of wire in which an electric current is made to flow. Now, each individual moving

electron produces anticlockwise magnetic lines of force about itself, as illustrated in Figure 9.2A. The closeness of the lines of force to each other represents the total magnetic effect (i.e. the magnetic flux density, as described in Sect. 8.2). The addition at a point of all the magnetic flux densities represented by the lines of force produces the total magnetic flux density at that point. Note that, within the coil, the lines of force all tend to be in the direction C to D, while outside the coil, they are from D to C. A top view of the coil (Fig. 9.2B) shows the pattern of the overall lines of force so obtained. It is interesting to note the similarity of these lines of force to those of a short bar magnet (see Fig. 8.1), where they emerge from the north pole end and travel around the magnet to the south pole end and back again. Here we have the reason for the 'atomic magnets', where (on a tiny scale) the coil would be equivalent to the net flow of electrons around a particular atomic nucleus, producing lines of force as in Figure 9.2B and hence the magnetized atom.

9.6 MAGNETIC FIELD DUE TO A SOLENOID

A solenoid consists of several coils joined together, and so produces magnetic lines of force, as shown in Figure 9.3A, similar to a bar magnet.

The effect of a piece of soft iron within the solenoid is to increase the magnetic flux density many times because of the induced magnetism within the soft iron. This effect is reflected by an increase in the number of lines of force in Figure 9.3B compared to Figure 9.3A. The combination of solenoid and soft iron in this manner is known as an electromagnet. The coils in an AC transformer act as a solenoid inducing a magmatic flux in the core of the transformer.

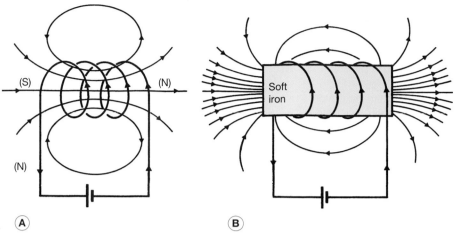

Figure 9.3 (A) The magnetic field produced by a current-carrying solenoid. (B) The large increase in the magnetic field produced when using a soft iron bore in the solenoid.

Insight

A general method of calculating the magnetic flux from any general shape of current-carrying conductor is due to Biot and Savart. The formula shown in Figure 9.4 can be used to calculate the magnetic flux density for any general shape of conductor. (Table 9.1 shows some of these examples.)

The effect of aligning atoms is to produce a total flux density, B, within the sample which is greater than that in the air alone, such that:

$$B = \mu H$$

where μ is the permeability of the medium. Here, the magnetizing force, H, is regarded as the *cause* of the magnetic flux density, B, in a medium of permeability, μ.

Rearranging the equation in Figure 9.4:

$$H = \frac{B}{\mu} = \text{constant} \times \frac{IL}{r^2}$$

so that the units of the magnetic field strength (or magnetizing force) H are in amperes per metre.

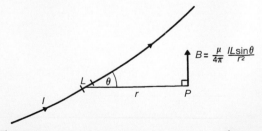

Figure 9.4 Biot and Savart's law for determining the magnetic flux density due to any shape of current-carrying conductor.
(Table 9.1 shows some of these examples)

Table 9.1 Magnetic flux density from different shapes of current-carrying conductors

CONDUCTOR	MAGNETIC FLUX DENSITY, B (TESLA)
Infinite straight wire	$B = \dfrac{\mu_0 I}{2\pi r}$
Circular coil	$B = \dfrac{\mu_0 I}{2r}$
Infinite solenoid	$B = \mu_0 I$ (air only) $B = \mu n I$ (where n = number of turns/metre)

Summary

In this chapter you should have learnt the following:

- Atomic magnetism is caused by electrons orbiting atomic nuclei. Electromagnetism is caused by isolated moving particles (e.g. free electrons) (see Sect. 9.3).

- Negative and positive charges may flow in a vacuum, gas or liquid, but only negative charges (electrons) may flow in a solid. This is because the atomic nuclei (which contain the positively charged protons) are not free to move in a solid (see Sect. 9.4).

- Circular magnetic fields exist around moving charges: anticlockwise around negative charges and clockwise around positive charges when viewed along the direction of motion (see Sect. 9.5).

- The magnetic flux density due to a current-carrying solenoid may be increased many times by inserting within it a material of high permeability, e.g. soft iron, since $B = \mu$. The magnetic domains become aligned with the direction of H, so adding to the overall magnetic flux density (see Sect. 9.6).

FURTHER READING

Ball, J.L., Moore, A.D., Turner, S., 2008. Ball and Moore's Essential Physics for Radiographers, fourth ed. Blackwell Scientific, London (Chapter 8).

Bushong, S.C., 2004. Radiologic Science for Technologists: Physics, Biology and Protection. Mosby, New York (Chapter 8).

Dowsett, D.J., Kenny, P.A., Johnston, R.E., 1998. The Physics of Diagnostic Imaging. Chapman & Hall Medical, London (Chapter 2).

Chapter | **10** |

Electromagnetic induction

10.1 AIM

This chapter considers the laws of electromagnetic induction. The direction of the induced current will be identified. The concepts of mutual induction and self-induction will be discussed in preparation for Chapter 14, where the application of these will be considered in transformer design.

10.2 INTRODUCTION

In Chapter 9, we covered the topic of electromagnetism and this chapter deals with the topic of *electromagnetic induction*. As can be seen from the definitions below, one is just the reverse of the other. They may each be defined as follows:

Definitions

Electromagnetism is the production of a magnetic field by the passage of an electrical current (see Ch. 9).

Electromagnetic induction is the production of electricity by the interlinking of a conductor with a changing magnetic field, or moving a conductor relative to a stationary magnetic field (also known as the generator effect).

10.3 CONDITIONS NECESSARY FOR ELECTROMAGNETIC INDUCTION

Consider the simple experiment depicted in Figure 10.1. A solenoid L is joined to a meter that can measure both the magnitude and the direction of the current flowing through the solenoid. The following effects are observed:

- No current flow is observed on the meter if the magnet is *stationary* with respect to the solenoid (Figure 10.1A and C).
- A current flows through the meter whenever the magnet is *moved* towards or away from the solenoid (Figure 10.1B and D).
- The *magnitude* of the induced current is *greater* if the magnet is moved faster.
- Reversing the direction of the movement of the magnet reverses the direction of the induced current (Figure 10.1B and D).
- Reversing the pole of the magnet, which is closer to the solenoid, reverses the direction of the induced current for a given movement.

From this simple experiment, we can conclude that *only a changing magnetic field relative to the conductor* is able to induce electricity in the conductor. We can also see that

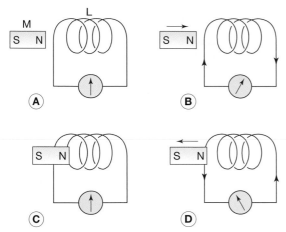

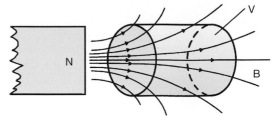

Figure 10.2 The magnetic flux linkage associated with a volume *V*.

Figure 10.1 An example of electromagnetic induction. A current flows only when there is relative movement between the bar magnet (*M*) and the solenoid (*L*).

the amount of electricity produced is in some way related to the *rate of change of the magnetic field* relative to the conductor. Finally, we can conclude that the *direction of movement of the magnetic field* influences the direction of the induced current. These concepts will be discussed in more detail in the following sections of this chapter.

10.4 FARADAY'S LAWS OF ELECTROMAGNETIC INDUCTION

Faraday produced two laws of electromagnetic induction that cover some of the observations we made in the previous section. These may be defined as follows:

1. A change in the magnetic flux linked with a conductor induces an electromotive force (EMF) in the conductor.
2. The magnitude of the induced EMF is proportional to the rate of change of the magnetic flux linkage.

In order to understand Faraday's laws, we need to have a clear understanding of *EMF* and *magnetic flux linkage*.

EMF was considered in Section 7.6 and can be considered as the force which is capable of causing electrons to flow (i.e. EMF will cause a current to flow in a complete circuit). It is important to note that Faraday's laws do not specify whether or not the conductor is connected to an external circuit but, in either case, an EMF will be induced in it.

Magnetic flux and *magnetic flux density* are discussed in Chapters 8 and 39. The magnetic flux through a volume *V* can be visualized as being proportional to the number of lines of flux passing through that volume (Fig. 10.2). Thus, if a magnetic flux of 10 weber passes through *V*, then the magnetic flux linkage with *V* is also said to be 10 weber. If the magnet in Figure 10.2 is moved to the left

of the page, then the number of lines of *flux* (or the flux linkage) in the volume *V* will be reduced.

We now see that moving the magnet relative to the solenoid will alter the flux linkage between the magnet and the solenoid and so an EMF will be induced – Faraday's first law. Also, a rapid movement of the magnet increases the rate of change of flux linkage and so increases the size of the induced EMF – Faraday's second law.

Changing the magnetic flux linkage associated with a particular conductor may be achieved in two ways:

1. By moving the conductor relative to a stationary magnet – this principle is used in the alternating current (AC) generator or dynamo (Sect. 10.9).
2. By varying the magnitude of the magnetic *flux* while the conductor is stationary – this principle is used in the AC transformer (see Ch. 14).

10.5 LENZ'S LAW

In our initial observations regarding the induced current (Sect. 10.3) we noted the direction as well as the size of the current. Faraday's laws apply to open or closed circuits but, as Lenz's law concerns the direction of the induced current, it can only be applied to *closed* circuits. The law can be stated as follows:

> **The** direction of *the induced* current *in a conductor caused by a changing magnetic* **flux is such that its own magnetic field opposes** *the changing magnetic* **flux.**

Insight

Lenz's law is an example of the application of the law of conservation of energy (Sect. 3.3). If the direction of the induced current was such that its magnetic field helped the changing magnetic field, then we would be getting something for nothing so we could establish perpetual motion of the conductor and the magnetic field. This would be in defiance of the law of conversation of energy.

When the north pole of a bar magnet is moved towards a solenoid (Figure 10.1B), the current will *flow* in the solenoid in such a direction that it produces a north pole at the end closest to the magnet. This has the effect of producing a force of repulsion between the bar magnet and the solenoid and so *work* must be done against this force in order to keep the magnet moving towards the solenoid. Thus, *mechanical energy* is transformed to *electrical energy* and the law of conservation of energy is maintained. The reverse occurs when the magnet is withdrawn.

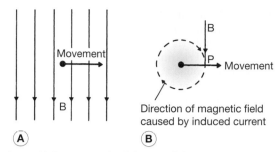

Figure 10.3 An example of the use of the convention described in the text for establishing the direction of the induced current.

10.6 SIGN CONVENTION FOR THE INDUCED CURRENT

When current *flow* was considered as the flow of positive charge, this was determined using Fleming's right-hand rule. As we now know that current flow *is* a flow of electrons, Fleming's hand rules are liable to cause confusion and so the direction of current flow will be determined using the convention shown in Figure 10.3.

Convention

Consider a situation similar to that shown in Figure 10.3A. Here a conductor is moved at right angles to a magnetic field (Fig. 10.3B) – the direction of the movement and the direction of the magnetic field are as shown in the diagram. We wish to determine whether the induced electron flow along the conductor will be either into the page or out of the page. This can be determined as follows:

1. Mark the position of the conductor and draw a line to indicate the direction of movement.
2. Draw a second line (B) to represent the permanent magnetic field direction to intersect the first line at the point P (Fig. 10.3B).
3. Now, draw a circle with the conductor at its centre such that its circumference passes through the point P.
4. This circle represents the magnetic field that will be caused by the current induced in the conductor. The direction of this magnetic field is the same as the direction of the permanent magnetic field at the point P – the field is in a clockwise direction.
5. As we learnt in Section 9.4, *the magnetic field around a current-carrying conductor is anticlockwise when the electrons are travelling away from us*. Thus, because of the clockwise magnetic field, we can conclude that the electrons (of the induced current) are travelling towards us.

10.7 MUTUAL INDUCTION

If a changing current is passed through one conductor, then this will produce a changing magnetic field around this conductor (see Ch. 9). If a second conductor is placed within this changing magnetic field, then (by Faraday's laws) an EMF will be generated in the conductor and a current will flow in it if the conducting loop is complete (Fig. 10.4).

By Lenz's law, this current will be in the opposite direction to the original current. The size of this secondary current will vary with the magnetic field – it will be a current of changing magnitude, as there is a changing magnetic field. This changing secondary current will produce its own changing magnetic field, which will induce an EMF and current in the first conductor. Thus, *each conductor induces electricity in the other* and the effect is known as *mutual induction*.

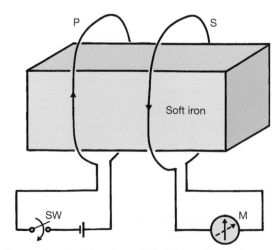

Figure 10.4 Principles of mutual induction. A changing current in coil *P* (the primary coil) induces a current in coil *S* (the secondary coil) and vice versa. The soft iron core magnifies the effect by improving the magnetic flux linkage between the coils. M, ammeter; SW, switch.

Consider Figure 10.4. When the switch, SW, is closed, electrons will flow from the negative pole of the battery to its positive pole via the coil P. During the time while the rate of flow of electrons builds up, there is a changing magnetic field around P. This is linked to S via the iron core (the iron core greatly enhances the flux linkage) and so an EMF and current flow will occur in S. The direction of the pointer on the ammeter, M, indicates that this flow of electrons in S is in the opposite direction to that in P, verifying Lenz's law. After a short time, the current in P is constant and so S is no longer influenced by a *changing* magnetic field. As a result, no EMF is generated in S (Faraday's first law). If the switch, SW, is now opened, the magnetic field around P collapses and so an EMF is again generated in P, but this time it is in the opposite direction. If a more powerful battery is now used, this produces a greater current in P, thus a greater magnetic field and consequently a greater EMF in S (the magnitude of the induced EMF is proportional to the rate of change of the magnetic flux). Finally, if we undertake the experiment with the iron bar present, and then with the iron bar removed, we find that the EMF produced in the coil S is greatest when the iron bar is present. This is because of improved magnetic flux linkage (Faraday's second law).

From this experiment, we can show that the EMF induced in the secondary winding E_S is:

- proportional to the rate of change of the current in P (the primary)
- dependent on the detailed design of the two conductors and the flux linkage between them. This is called the *mutual inductance* (M).

Thus:

Equation 10.1

$$E_s = M \times \text{rate of change of primary current}$$

The greater the mutual inductance, M, the greater the mutual effect between the two conductors. M is measured in henrys, and may be defined as:

Definition
A mutual inductance of 1 *henry* exists between two conductors if 1 volt is induced in one conductor where there is a current change of 1 ampere per second in the other.

10.8 SELF-INDUCTION

Consider the solenoid in Figure 10.5A. If the switch, SW, is closed, current flow starts to build up in the solenoid. As this current increases, each turn of the solenoid produces a changing magnetic flux, which is linked to

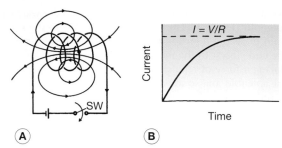

Figure 10.5 Principles of self-induction. The changing magnetic flux produced by the current flow through the solenoid when the switch, SW, is closed links with all the turns of the coil. This produces a back-electromotive force, which slows down the rate of growth of current in the coil.

the other turns of the solenoid (the flux from one turn is shown in Fig. 10.5A). Thus, from Faraday's and Lenz's laws, an EMF in the opposite direction to the EMF from the battery will be induced in the solenoid. This is known as a back-EMF. This effect is known as *self-induction* and, if the self-induction is large, the current in the coil will take an appreciable time to build up to its maximum value. The self-induction in an electrical system is defined in a very similar manner to the mutual induction and is given by the equation:

Equation 10.2

$$E_B = L \times \text{rate of change of current}$$

Here E_B is the back-EMF and L is the self-inductance, measured in henrys. Thus, we can say that:

Definition
A conductor has *a self-inductance* of 1 *henry* if a back-EMF of 1 volt is induced when the current flowing through it changes at 1 ampere per second.

A graph of the current flowing through the solenoid is shown in Figure 10.5B. As can be seen, the induced back-EMF slows down the rate of growth of the current and so it takes an appreciable time to reach its maximum value, determined by Ohm's law. If the wire of the solenoid were unwound to become a straight conductor, then there would be no magnetic flux linkage and consequently no back-EMF. Thus, the current would rise to its maximum value very quickly.

As in the case of mutual induction, a soft iron bar placed in the solenoid will enhance the self-induction as the magnetic flux linkage between the coils is improved.

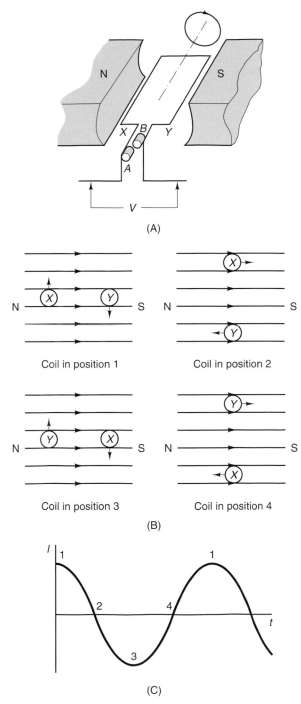

Figure 10.6 (A) Simplified diagram of an alternating current generator; (B) four positions of the coil relative to the magnetic field; (C) the current waveform produced when the coil moves through positions 1, 2, 3, 4 and returns to 1. A complete turn of the coil will produce one cycle of current. See text for further details.

10.9 THE AC GENERATOR

Electric power is produced from an AC generator. This is an example of a situation where mechanical energy is converted to electrical energy. The basic components of such a generator are shown in Figure 10.6A. A permanent magnetic field exists between the poles of the magnet, and coils of copper wire rotate through this field. For simplicity, only one coil is shown in the diagram. The EMF generated in the device is collected at brushes positioned at A and B.

Now consider the situation where the coil shown is rotated in a clockwise direction. Thus, from the initial position, side X of the coil will move upwards through the magnetic field and side Y will move downwards (Fig. 10.6B). At this point in its movement, the coil is cutting the maximum number of lines of flux as it is moving at right angles to the flux lines, and so the maximum EMF will be generated. If we use the convention discussed earlier (see Sect. 10.6) to establish the direction of electron flow, we can see that electrons will travel towards us on side X and away from us on side Y. Thus, an excess of electrons will exist at brush A and a shortage of electrons will exist at brush B: brush A is negative and brush B is positive. This situation is shown as position 1 on the graph in Figure 10.6C. Now consider the situation when the coil has turned in a clockwise direction from its initial position through 90°: this is the second position of the coil shown in Figure 10.6B. In this position, both side X and side Y of the coil are moving parallel with the lines of magnetic flux and so no current is generated – this is again shown as position 2 in Figure 10.6C. In position 3, the coil has rotated through 180° from its original position. Side X of the coil is now moving downwards through the magnetic field and side Y is moving upwards. As in position 1, a maximum number of lines of flux are being cut as the conductor is moving at right angles to the flux, and so, again, the maximum EMF will be generated. The polarity of A and B is now the reverse of position 1. In position 4, the conductor is again moving parallel to the lines of flux so no EMF is generated. The conductor then returns to position 1 and so one cycle is complete. The process is then repeated. The type of current shown in Figure 10.6C is known as AC and will be the subject of Chapter 11.

In cases where there is no external circuit connected, then no current is able to flow and only sufficient work to overcome the frictional resistance is necessary to keep the rotational movement at the same speed. As soon as an external circuit is connected, then a current is able to flow in the circuit and in the winding.

It should come as no surprise to discover that this current will flow in such a direction as to oppose the motion of the coil (remember Lenz's law). This means that mechanical work must be performed to overcome this resisting force, i.e. mechanical energy is converted into electrical energy.

The effect of suddenly increasing the electrical load demanded from the generator (e.g. when making an X-ray exposure) is suddenly to increase the opposition to its rotation. Hence, the generator slows down momentarily, the induced EMF (which depends on the speed of rotation) is reduced. We find that, in times of increased demand on the generators, there is a drop in the voltage they supply. In X-ray units, this is taken into account by the inclusion of a *mains voltage compensator* on the unit.

Summary

In this chapter you should have learnt the following:

- That an EMF is induced in a conductor if it is linked with a changing magnetic field (see Sect. 10.3).
- Faraday's first and second law of electromagnetic induction (see Sect. 10.4).
- Lenz's law, which determines the direction of the current flowing as the result of the induced EMF (see Sect. 10.5).
- The sign convention for the direction of the induced current (see Sect. 10.6).
- The meaning and a simple application of mutual induction (see Sect. 10.7).
- The meaning and a simple application of self-induction (see Sect. 10.8).
- The mode of operation of an AC generator (see Sect. 10.9).

FURTHER READING

Ball, J.L., Moore, A.D., Turner, S., 2008. Ball and Moore's Essential Physics for Radiographers, fourth ed. Blackwell Scientific, London (Chapter 9).

Dowsett, D.J., Kenny, P.A., Johnston, R.E., 1998. The Physics of Diagnostic Imaging. Chapman & Hall Medical, London (Chapter 1).

Ohanian, H.C., 1994. Principles of Physics. W W Norton, London (Chapter 22).

Thompson, M.A., Hattaway, R.T., Hall, J.D., Dowd, S.B., 1994. Principles of Imaging Science and Protection. W B Saunders, London (Chapter 5).

Chapter | **11** |

Alternating current (AC) flow

11.1 AIM

This chapter introduces the reader to alternating current (AC) flow. The various parameters used to measure such a current will be discussed. Simple AC circuits and three-phase power supplies will be considered.

11.2 INTRODUCTION

Direct current (DC) electricity (Ch. 7) is representative of a flow of electrons in one direction only. This chapter deals with the situation where electrons flow through a circuit first in one direction and then in the other (due to the changing polarity of the ends of the circuit) – this is known as an AC flow.

11.3 TYPES OF DC AND AC

Figure 11.1 shows different types of DC and AC in graphical form – the magnitude of the current (the dependent variable) is plotted on the vertical axis against time on the horizontal axis.

Figure 11.1A is a case where the number of electrons passing a point per second in the circuit is constant producing a horizontal straight line. This is an example of the type of DC described in Chapter 7. Figure 11.1B is a case where the electrons always move in the same direction but the number of electrons passing a point varies with time – the electrons move as a series of pulses and this is known as pulsatable or pulsating DC. In Figure 11.1C there is no discernable pattern in the flow of electrons, except to say that they flow in both directions at different times. This is an example of an irregular AC waveform. Figure 11.1D shows a situation where the number of electrons travelling in one direction is constant for a short period of time and then the same number of electrons travel in the opposite direction for the same period of time. This is an example of a square waveform. Figure 11.1E shows an example of a sinusoidal AC wave form. This is the most common AC waveform and will be discussed in detail in the remainder of the chapter.

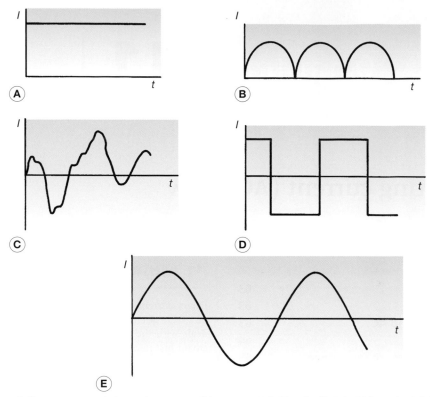

Figure 11.1 Types of direct current and alternating current: (A) constant DC; (B) pulsatile DC; (C) irregular AC; (D) square waveform AC; (E) sinusoidal AC.

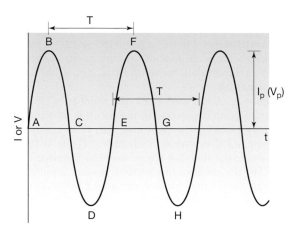

Figure 11.2 A sinusoidal current or voltage waveform.

11.4 SINUSOIDAL AC

The sinusoidal AC waveform is shown in more detail in Figure 11.2, together with some of the quantities used to measure it.

Definitions

One cycle: One complete waveform starting at a point and continuing until the same point on the pattern is reached. This is usually measured from zero to zero (ABCDE) or from peak to peak (BCDEF).

Period (T): The time taken to complete one cycle, measured in seconds.

Frequency (f): The number of cycles which occur in 1 second, measured in cycles per second or hertz (Hz).

Amplitude: The maximum value of positive or negative current (or voltage) on the waveform. This may be referred to as the peak value.

There is a simple relationship between the period (*T*) and the frequency (*f*) which can be seen if we consider the following situation. Suppose we have a frequency of 10 Hz (10 cycles per second). Since the waveform is regular, each cycle must last for 0.1 second. Thus, we can say:

Equation 11.1

$$f = \frac{1}{T}$$

For a sinusoidal current, this equation may be rewritten as:

Equation 11.2

$$I_t = I_p \sin 2\pi f t$$

where I_t is the current at a time t and I_p is the amplitude or the peak value of the current. A similar equation can be produced for the voltage.

11.4.1 Peak current (or voltage)

The peak current is the same as the amplitude, i.e. it is the *maximum positive or negative value of the current*. Similarly, the peak voltage is the maximum value of the voltage. In radiography, the peak voltage across the tube, when the anode is positive and the cathode is negative, is usually quoted. If an X-ray tube is operating at 75 kVp then the peak potential difference between the anode and the cathode is 75 kV. The reasons for quoting the tube voltage as kVp will be considered later in this chapter.

11.4.2 Average current (or voltage)

As we can see from Figure 11.2, the average current flowing in one cycle of a sinusoidal waveform is zero, as the current flowing in one direction during the positive half-cycle has the same overall value (but of the opposite sign) during the negative half-cycle. The same conclusion applies to any number of complete cycles. A similar argument suggests that the average voltage for a sinusoidal waveform is also zero. Thus, for a sinusoidal waveform:

Equation 11.2

$$I_{AV} = 0$$
$$V_{AV} = 0$$

However, if the waveform is *rectified* (or made unidirectional; Ch. 28) then a value of the average current (or voltage) is obtained. The voltage waveform produced for *half-wave rectification* is shown in Figure 11.3A. This results in a pulsating voltage which (assuming a complete external circuit) results in a net electron flow in one direction –

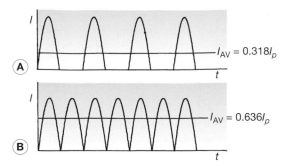

Figure 11.3 Forms of rectified sinusoidal alternating current: (A) half-wave rectification; (B) full-wave rectification.

this allows us to consider average values of voltage and current which are not zero.

The voltage waveform for a *full-wave rectified* circuit is shown on the same scale in Figure 11.3B. Again, a pulsating voltage is produced where the average value is twice that for the half-wave rectified circuit as there are twice as many peaks in unit time.

Thus, we can say for half-wave rectification:

Equation 11.3

$$I_{AV} = 0.318 I_p$$
$$V_{AV} = 0.318 V_p$$

and for full-wave rectification:

Equation 11.4

$$I_{AV} = 0.636 I_p$$
$$V_{AV} = 0.636 V_p$$

11.4.3 Effective (or RMS) current or voltage

If an AC supply is connected across a resistor, then electrons will flow in one direction during the first half-cycle and in the opposite direction during the second half-cycle. As there is no net movement of electrons for any given number of complete cycles, the average current is zero.

This does not mean that the net heating effect is zero. Electrons will produce heat within a resistor irrespective of their direction of travel. The average current is therefore a quantity, which is not suitable for determining the energy or power expended in a circuit which is connected to an AC supply. The quantity of importance is the effective or root mean square (RMS) value of the current and may be defined as:

Definition
The *effective current* is that value of constant current which, flowing for the same time, would produce the same expenditure of electrical energy in a circuit as the alternating current.

The effective value of the current is also known as the RMS value, for reasons which we will consider below. The effective or RMS voltage is defined in a very similar manner:

Definition
The *effective voltage* is that voltage which, being present for the same time, would produce the same expenditure of energy in a circuit as the alternating voltage.

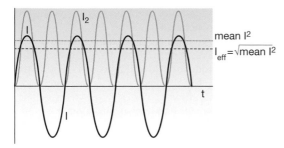

Figure 11.4 Graphic representation of an effective (root mean square or RMS) value of current.

Insight

Consider the graphs shown in Figure 11.4. The AC *I* has an average value of zero because each positive value is matched by an equal and opposite negative value. Thus the peak positive value is matched with a peak negative value. If we take these peak values and square them, we can get rid of the negative sign and so it is possible to get an average value of the peak current (or voltage) squared. If we take the square root of this value, we now have the root of the mean of the square of the peak value. This is the effective value of the current (or voltage):

$$I_{RMS} = \frac{I_p}{\sqrt{2}}$$

In Section 7.9.3 it was shown that the general equation for electrical power was $W = V \times I$, where W is expressed in watts, V in volts and I in amperes. In an AC circuit, both V and I are constantly changing and so it is the effective or RMS value of each that must be taken into account when using the above equation:

Equation 11.5

$$W = V_{RMS} \times I_{RMS}$$

Here, W is the *average* power generated in the circuit, taking into account at least one half-cycle of AC. We can manipulate Equation 11.5 in a similar way to Equation 7.16 to get:

Equation 11.6

$$W = I_{RMS}^2 \times R$$
$$W = \frac{V_{RMS}^2}{R}$$

Note: we can apply Ohm's law (Ch. 7) to AC circuits provided the same types of units for voltage or current (e.g. RMS) are used throughout the equation.

The RMS values of current or voltage can be related to the peak relationships by the following equations:

Equation 11.7

$$I_{RMS} = 0.707I_p$$
$$V_{RMS} = 0.707V_p$$

and:

Equation 11.8

$$I_p = 1.414I_{RMS}$$
$$V_p = 1.414V_{RMS}$$

Thus, for an AC, the effective value is just over 70% of the peak value.

11.5 AC AND THE X-RAY TUBE

In order to produce X-rays, the X-ray tube requires a high potential difference (voltage) across it and a current flowing through it. The voltage available from the mains supply is far too low for use directly across the X-ray tube so a means of increasing it to the high values of thousands of volts is required. This is relatively easy to accomplish using an AC transformer (Ch. 14). Since this transformer increases the voltage, it is known as a step-up transformer. The filament of the X-ray tube requires a low voltage supply so that it can produce the electrons that form the mA through the tube, and so the mains voltage passes through a step-down transformer before being applied to the filament. Thus, an alternating voltage may either be increased using a step-up transformer or decreased using a step-down transformer.

In AC circuits, the voltages or currents are usually expressed in terms of their effective values unless otherwise stated. When considering the X-ray circuit, the following conventions apply:

- The voltage across the tube (kV) is expressed in terms of the peak voltage, i.e. kVp.
- The current flowing through the tube (mA) is expressed in terms of the average current.
- The mains voltage and current to the X-ray generator are expressed as effective or RMS values.

11.5.1 Voltage across the X-ray tube (kVp)

The potential difference across the X-ray tube is expressed in terms of the peak value for the following reasons:

- The maximum energy of X-ray photons emitted by the anode is the same value in keV, i.e. an X-ray tube operated at 100 kVp will emit X-ray photons with a maximum energy of 100 keV. (This will be explained in more detail in Ch. 21.)

- The voltage rating of the high-tension cables must be able to withstand the maximum voltage applied to them. This occurs during the peak value of the voltage.

If the voltage applied to the X-ray tube is a constant potential (Ch. 28), then this is effectively a DC supply so the peak and the effective values are the same.

11.5.2 Current through the X-ray tube (mA)

The mA display is designed to measure the *average* current flowing through the X-ray tube during an exposure. The intensity of the radiation beam is proportional to the average current. If we take the average current (mA) and multiply this by the exposure time in seconds, we get the mAs for that exposure. This represents the total charge that has passed through the X-ray tube during the exposure. The quantity of X-rays produced during the exposure is proportional to the mAs.

11.5.3 The mains voltage and current

The electrical mains is the source of power and so it makes sense to quote the mains supply in terms which make the calculations of power most convenient – the effective or RMS values. The mains voltage in the UK has a nominal value of 230 volts$_{RMS}$ and so this gives us a peak value for this voltage of approximately 325 volts (Equation 11.8).

11.6 BASICS OF AC CIRCUITS

Having considered the different measures that can be made of an alternating current or voltage, we are now ready to look at the consequences of passing this current through some basic circuits.

11.6.1 Phase difference

So far in this chapter we have only considered the case where the peak voltage occurs at the same time as the peak current. The current and voltage are then said to be in phase. This is not necessarily true for all types of AC circuits and we can get situations where a phase difference exists between the current and the voltage. Examples of phase differences are shown in graphical form in Figure 11.5. In Figure 11.5A, the current (I) lags behind the voltage (V) – a waveform displaced to the right occurs later than, and therefore lags behind, the waveform with which

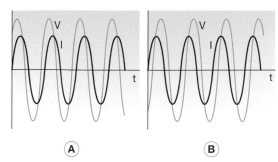

Figure 11.5 Phase differences between current and voltage waveforms: (A) I lags behind V; (B) I leads V.

it is being compared. Also, in Figure 11.5B, we have a situation where I leads V.

The angle between the two waveforms is expressed as the *phase angle* where 360° is equivalent to one cycle.

11.6.2 Reactance and impedance

When we considered the opposition to the flow of direct current in a circuit, we found that this opposition consisted of resistance and was measured in ohms (see Ch. 7). There are two additional measures of AC resistance in a circuit: *reactance* and *impedance*. Both are measured in ohms as in DC resistance but measure different quantities.

To summarize, resistance, reactance and impedance all represent opposition to the flow of current and are all measured in ohms. They are expressed by the ratio of volts to amperes but the voltage vector is different in each case – it is *in phase* with the current for *resistance*, at *right angles* to the current for *reactance* and at the *phase angle* to the current for *impedance*. Impedance is thus the general term for opposition to current flow, and reactance and resistance form separate components of this.

11.7 SIMPLE AC CIRCUITS

In a simple AC circuit containing only resistance, the opposition to current flow rises through Ohm's law which can be applied to calculate power consumption in the same way as in DC circuits. When capacitors and inductors are introduced in an AC circuit we need to consider the opposition to current flow caused by capacitors and inductors. This opposition, reactance, is in addition to the opposition to current flow rising from resistance.

The combination of resistance and reactance of an AC circuit, the impedance, can be calculated. However, these calculations can be quite complex and fall into the realm of electronic engineering, not radiography, and so will not be covered in any detail in this chapter.

11.8 THREE-PHASE AC

The basis of the generation of electricity was explained in Section 10.9. However, the requirements for electrical power vary widely depending on the machinery used. Any national electrical supply must be able to cope with a wide variation in the demand for electrical power. This is made possible by the winding geometry of three-phase AC generators. These have three symmetrical windings, making three *phases* of AC available as shown diagrammatically in Figure 11.6. The windings, W_1, W_2 and W_3 in Figure 11.6A, are on single a rotor, but are separated by an angle of 120° and, as the rotor is rotated, each winding moves through a magnetic field in turn.

Each set of windings has a sinusoidal alternating voltage induced in it (see Sect 10.9) but these voltages are out of phase with each other because of the different times they encounter the strongest regions of the magnetic field within the generator. These voltages (V_1, V_2 and V_3 from the windings W_1, W_2 and W_3) are known as *phase voltages* and are separated by 120° from each other, as shown in 11.6B. Thus a phase difference of 120° exists between each phase voltage. These voltages are now increased by the use of a step-up transformer for transmission over long distances and are then stepped down for use in industry, hospitals, homes, etc., using suitable star and delta connections of the phase voltages, as outlined below.

11.8.1 Star and delta connections

Star and delta connections of the phase voltages are shown in Figure 11.7. If we assume that an RMS voltage of 230 volts is induced in each winding of the generator, then three sets of 230-volts supply are available from the delta connection. The centre of the star connection is

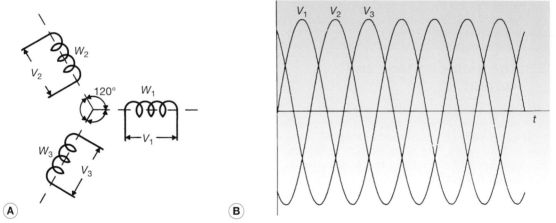

Figure 11.6 Three-phase electrical generation. (A) Diagrammatic representation of three sets of windings in the alternating current generator; (B) graphical representation of the three voltage phases against time showing the 120° separation between each phase.

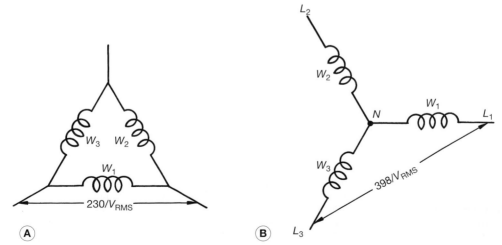

Figure 11.7 Three-phase electrical generation: (A) delta connection; (B) star connection.

called the neutral and is kept as near earth potential as possible by equalizing the power outputs from the three phases. This allows the possibility of six voltages from the star connection:

- Three phase voltages of 230 volts are possible if a connection is made to the neutral and to one end of a winding.
- Three line voltages of 398 volts are possible by making connections to the ends of two of the windings – one such connection is shown between W_1 and W_3.

Note that the line voltage is 398 volts and not 460 volts as would be expected, as each phase voltage is 230 volts. This is because of the phase difference between the phase voltages. It may be shown (see Insight below) that the line voltage is also sinusoidal and has a magnitude which is a factor of $\sqrt{3}$ greater than the phase voltage.

The transfer of power from the generating station to a city, which makes use of delta and delta transformers, is shown diagrammatically in Figure 11.9. The four wires L1, L2, L3 and N are distributed to domestic, hospital and industrial users and the appropriate voltages (phase or line) are available; phase voltages for domestic use and both phase and line voltages for hospital and industrial use. The star connection is often referred to as a *three-phase four-wire supply*, for obvious reasons.

11.8.2 Three-phase circuits in radiography

There are two main uses for three-phase supplies used in radiography:

1. The line voltage from a three-phase supply is used to ensure that a 398-volt supply is available for most static X-ray sets. This means that the turns ratio

---

Insight

The difference between the voltages across L_1 and L_3 in Figure 11.7 is the difference between the voltages across L_1–N and L_2–N. If we consider a situation where the potential of N is zero, L_1–N is 10 volts and L_3–N is 4 volts, then the potential difference between L_1 and L_3 is $10 - 4 = 6$ volts. Thus, we may use the vector diagram shown in the Figure 11.8.
Now $\sin 60° = \sqrt{(3)}/2$

$$= \frac{(L/2)}{V_1} \text{ (from Figure 11.8)}$$
$$\therefore L = \sqrt{(3)}V_1$$

Thus the *line voltage* is $\sqrt{3}$ times the phase voltage. In the UK, the phase voltage is 230 volts (RMS) and so the line voltage is 398 volts (RMS).

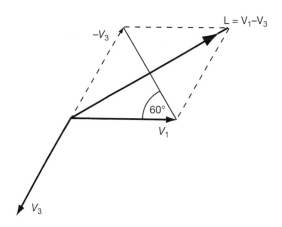

Figure 11.8 Vector diagram used to calculate the line voltage (L) across V_1–V_3.

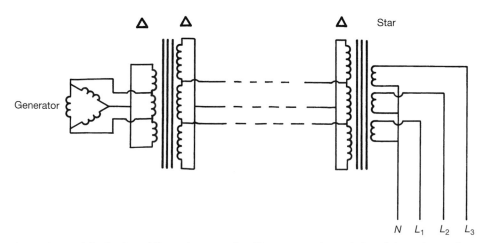

Figure 11.9 Generation and distribution of three-phase supplies. The consumer has a choice of three phase voltages (e.g. L_1–N) or three line voltages (e.g. L_1–L_2).

(see Ch. 14) required in step-up transformers is less than that required for a 230-volt supply.

2. The induction motor used to rotate the anode of the X-ray tube uses three phases. This is further discussed in Chapter 30.

Summary

In this chapter, you should have learnt the following:

- Sinusoidal AC is described mathematically by the formula $I = I_p \sin 2\pi ft$ and $V = V_p \sin 2\pi ft$ where I_p and V_p are the peak current and voltage and f is the frequency of the AC supply in hertz (see Sect. 11.4).

- One cycle is one complete waveform; the period is the time for one cycle; the frequency is the number of cycles per second; and the *amplitude* is the maximum value of voltage or current (see Sect. 11.4).

- The frequency (f) and the period (T) are related by the equation $f = 1/T$ (see Sect. 11.4).

- For a sinusoidal waveform, the average current (or voltage) is = 0. For half-wave rectified AC, the average current (or voltage) is = 0.318 × peak current (voltage). For full-wave rectified AC, the average current (or voltage) is = 0.636 × peak current (voltage) (see Sect. 11.4.2).

- The definition of the RMS current as that value of constant current which, acting over the same time, would produce the same expenditure of electrical energy in a circuit as the AC. All AC voltages and currents are quoted in RMS values unless otherwise stated. $I_{RMS} = 0.707 \times I_p$; $V_{RMS} = 0.707 \times V_p$ (see Sect. 11.4.3).

- Voltages across the X-ray tube are expressed in peak voltages (kVp); current through the tube is expressed in average value (mA), and mains supply is expressed in RMS values (see Sect. 11.5).

- Three-phase circuits consist of three sinusoidal waveforms 120° apart. These may be connected by *star* or *delta* configurations (see Sect. 11.8).

- The *phase voltage* is that across individual windings; the *line voltage* is that obtained across each of the three connections of the star and delta connections. For a delta connection, the line and phase voltages are equal; for a star connection, the line voltage is $\sqrt{3}\times$ the phase voltage (see Sect. 11.8.1).

FURTHER READING

Ball, J.L., Moore, A.D., Turner, S., 2008. Ball and Moore's Essential Physics for Radiographers, fourth ed. Blackwell Scientific, London (Chapter 10).

Chapter | 12 |

The motor principle

12.1 AIM

The aim of this chapter is to consider the motor principle. The application of this principle to the direct current (DC) motor and the alternating current (AC) induction motor will be considered, as will the magnetic deflection of electrons. Finally, the relevance of these to radiography will be discussed.

12.2 INTRODUCTION AND DEFINITION OF THE MOTOR PRINCIPLE

In Chapter 9, we considered the topic of electromagnetism where a magnetic field was produced by an electric current. This chapter considers what happens when an electromagnetic field is created in the presence of another magnetic field. If we consider two bar magnets lying in close proximity to one another, then (depending on their orientation) a force of repulsion or attraction will exist between them (see Ch. 8). If one of the bar magnets is now replaced by a solenoid (see Sect. 9.6), we would expect a force between the solenoid and the bar magnet when an electric current is passed through the solenoid, since it behaves like a bar magnet under these circumstances. This force will cause the solenoid to move if it is free to do so. When the current is switched off, the magnetic field due to the solenoid disappears and so does the force between it and the magnet. This interaction between electromagnetism and another magnetic field is known as the *motor principle* (or motor effect) and may be formally defined:

Definition
A current-carrying conductor will experience a force when placed within a magnetic field.

The principle of the electric motor is that it converts electrical energy into kinetic energy (mechanical energy) through the interaction of the two magnetic fields.

12.3 DIRECTION AND MAGNITUDE OF THE FORCE ON THE CONDUCTOR

Consider a length L of straight wire which is carrying an electric current I, the whole wire being placed in a uniform magnetic flux density B, as shown in Figure 12.1. In this diagram, it is assumed that the direction of B and of the wire are both in the plane of the paper. Experimentally, the following results are observed:

- The *direction* of the force on the wire is always into or out of the paper, i.e. at *right angles* to the direction of B and I.
- The *direction* of the force on the wire is *reversed if the current is reversed*.
- The *magnitude* of the force is proportional to:
  - the magnetic flux density, B
  - the magnitude of the electric current, I
  - the length of the wire, L
  - the sine of the angle between the direction of B and I, i.e. $\sin \theta$ in Figure 12.1. Thus, the force on the wire is at its maximum when the wire is at right angles to the field ($\sin 90° = 1$) and zero when the wire is parallel to the field ($\sin 0° = 0$).

Combining the factors in the last bullet point above, we have:

Equation 12.1

$$F = BIL \sin \theta$$

where the force, F, is in newtons, B in tesla, I in amperes and L in metres.

The findings discussed above may be used to define the *tesla* as follows:

Definition
A magnetic flux density of 1 *tesla* (T) exists if the force on a straight wire of length 1 *metre* is 1 *newton* when the wire carries a current of 1 *ampere* and is placed at *right angles* to the direction of magnetic flux.

The direction of the force on the current-carrying conductor may be obtained using the appropriate rule or convention. As we saw before, in Chapter 10, Fleming's right- and left-hand rules were produced to deal with 'conventional current' and not electron flow. To avoid confusion, a different convention will be presented to calculate the direction of the force on the current-carrying conductor.

12.4 CONVENTION FOR THE DIRECTION OF THE FORCE

Consider the situation shown in Figure 12.2A. Here a wire is carrying an electric current such that the electrons are flowing away from the eye of the observer into the paper. The magnetic field, H, produced by this current is in an anticlockwise direction, as shown. If an external magnetic field, B, is applied to the wire as shown, it is found that the wire experiences a force, F, which pushes it to the right. Figure 12.2B shows the convention which will be used to determine the direction of the force – this is similar in many ways to the convention used in Section 10.6 to determine the direction of the induced current. The direction of the force can be determined as follows:

1. Mark the position of the wire, and draw the direction of electron flow and the magnetic field around it. In Figure 12.2B, this is an anticlockwise magnetic field as the electrons are flowing away from us.
2. Align one of the lines of force from the external magnetic field (B) so that it touches the field around the wire at the point where both fields are in the same direction. This occurs at point A in Figure 12.2B
3. Now draw a line from this point through the wire (AF). The direction in which you draw this line indicates the direction of the force acting on the wire. This line is drawn from left to right in this case, agreeing with the previous findings.

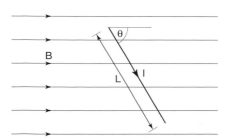

Figure 12.1 The interaction of the permanent magnetic field, B, with the magnetic field caused by the current, I, flowing through the wire causes a force to act on the wire – the motor principle.

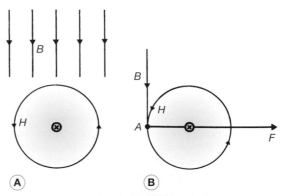

Figure 12.2 Convention for establishing the force acting on a current-carrying conductor placed in a magnetic field. For an explanation of how to use the convention, see the text.

This procedure can be applied to any direction of current and any orientation of the wire and the magnetic field. In some cases, however, the applied magnetic field is not exactly perpendicular to the wire and so cannot be made to line up to the field produced by it, as described so far. In this situation, the applied magnetic field may be split into two components: one parallel to the wire (which produces no force on the wire) and one perpendicular to the wire (which will produce a force on the wire according to the above convention). The following examples should help to clarify the above points.

Examples

a. The situation of the wire and the external magnetic field is shown in the left-hand diagram below. In the right-hand diagram, the observer is looking along the wire (as if looking from the bottom of the page). The convention described previously can now be applied, giving an upward direction of force.

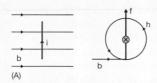
(A)

b. In this case, when we draw the right-hand diagram, the electrons will be flowing towards the observer and so the magnetic field around the wire will be in a clockwise direction. By applying the convention, it can be found that the force is downwards into the paper (the opposite of the previous situation).

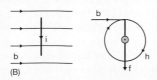
(B)

c. In diagram C, the wire and the lines of flux are parallel and so no force will be experienced by the wire when current flows through it.

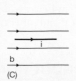
(C)

d. In the situation shown in diagram D, the wire is not at 90° to the lines of flux and so these must be split into two components, B_0, which is parallel to the wire and B_{90}, which is at right angles to it. This is

shown in the right-hand diagram. As described in the previous example, the field, which is parallel to the wire (B_0), will have no effect on it and so can be ignored. Application of the convention now shows that the force acting on the wire will be in an upwards direction, as in the first example.

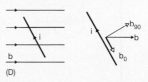
(D)

12.5 INTERACTION OF TWO ELECTROMAGNETIC FIELDS

So far in this chapter we have seen that a force exists on a current-carrying conductor when it is in the presence of a magnetic field and that this is known as the motor principle. It is immaterial whether the magnetic field interacting with the conductor is from a permanent magnet or whether it is produced electromagnetically. In this way, if two current-carrying solenoids are held close together, they behave in the same way as two bar magnets with a north pole at one end of the solenoid and a south pole at the other. Thus, the solenoids will attract or repel each other depending on the orientation in which they are placed: like poles repel and unlike poles attract.

12.5.1 Two parallel wires of infinite length

This rather improbable situation is used in the International System of Units (SI) system to define the ampere and so will be considered here.

Figure 12.3 (see page 74) shows two parallel wires C and D carrying currents I_C and I_D respectively. Figure 12.3A shows the plan view of the wires while Figure 12.3B is the view obtained by looking along the wires towards C and D where the electron flow is into the paper for both wires. The magnetic field around each wire will consist of a series of concentric circles with the field being in an anticlockwise direction. We will now consider how the magnetic field of one wire will interact with the magnetic field of the other. The magnetic field from wire C (B_C) is 'upwards' at wire D while the field from wire D (B_D) is 'downwards' at wire C. If we now apply our convention to this situation, we can see that we get forces F_C and F_D, as shown in Figure 12.3B. Thus, there is a mutual force of attraction between the wires. This situation is used as the basis of the definition of the ampere in the SI system:

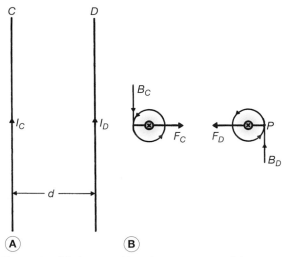

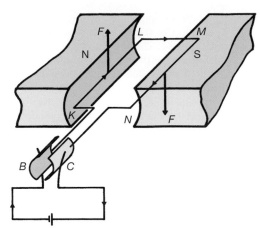

Figure 12.4 The direct current electric motor. See text for details.

Figure 12.3 (A) The mutual force between two parallel current-carrying wires of infinite length. (B) The same wires rotated through 90° so that the flow of electrons is into the paper. This arrangement is used for the definition of the ampere.

Definition

A current of 1 *ampere* flows in one infinite straight wire if an equal current in a similar wire placed 1 meter away in a vacuum produces a mutual force of 2×10^{-7} newton per meter.

12.6 THE DC ELECTRIC MOTOR

The electric motor is, of course, the prime example of the motor principle in that it converts electrical energy into mechanical energy. To understand the workings of the electric motor we need to understand the motor principle and also electromagnetic induction (see Ch. 10). A simplified DC electric motor is shown in Figure 12.4, where a battery is connected to a coil of wire *KLMN* via brushes *B* at a commutator *C*. The coil of wire is in the magnetic field of a permanent magnet, the direction of whose field is from left to right in the figure.

When the current is switched on, the electron flow is in the direction indicated in the diagram, and the coil is affected by a clockwise force due to the motor principle (i.e. an *upward* force on *KL* and *a downward* force on *MN*, as may be verified using the convention in Sect. 12.4). The commutator *C* turns with the coil *KLMN* so that the current always flows in the same direction relative to the permanent magnet. Hence, the coil always experiences a clockwise force and keeps turning. Without the commutator,

KLMN would eventually stop at right angles to the permanent magnetic field.

Since a clockwise force is being continuously applied to the coil, it would seem logical to assume that the speed of rotation would continuously increase. This does not, in fact, happen. The speed of rotation increases up to a certain rate and then remains constant. To understand why this happens, we need to look at electromagnetic induction. We have a conductor *KLMN* which is moving relative to a magnetic field, i.e. undergoing a change of magnetic flux, so an electromotive force (EMF) and current must be induced according to Faraday's and Lenz's laws (see Sects 10.4 and 10.5). The faster the coil rotates, the greater is the induced EMF and current because the rate of change of flux linkage increases (Faraday's second law). The direction of the induced EMF is in the opposite direction to the applied EMF so this opposes the motion of electrons along *KLMN*. Thus, the faster the coil rotates, the smaller is the net current that flows. Thus, for a free-moving, frictionless motor the rotational speed becomes such that no current at all flows because the forward- and back-EMFs cancel each other out. It is for this reason that an electric motor does not rotate more and more quickly; it achieves a steady speed of rotation due to the back-EMF induced in the windings.

When the motor is under load – performing mechanical work – then the rotational speed reduces so that a net current may flow and electrical energy may be transformed into mechanical and other types of energy.

12.7 THE AC INDUCTION MOTOR

The type of motor commonly used in an AC circuit is an AC induction motor, so called because it works on the principle of electromagnetic induction (particularly Lenz's law). The principle of such a motor may be understood by considering

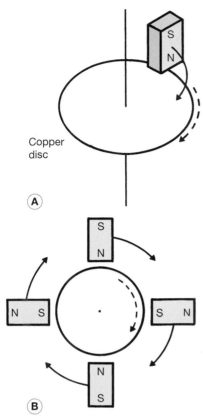

Figure 12.5 An elementary explanation of the induction motor. Rotating the magnets in (A) and (B) will cause the disc to rotate in the same direction because of eddy current formation in the copper.

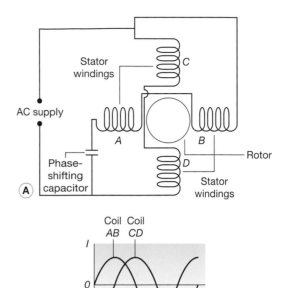

Figure 12.6 (A) Cross-section showing the typical arrangement of stator coils and rotor in an induction motor; (B) current waveform produced by the two pairs of coils because of the influence of the phase-shifting capacitor. Note that the current from one pair of coils is at its maximum when the current from the other pair is at zero.

the simple experiment depicted in Figure 12.5A where a bar magnet is moved around the rim of a supported copper disc. It is found that the disc follows the movement of the magnet. The sequence of events is as follows:

- A moving magnetic flux from the magnet is linked with the conductor – the copper disc.
- From Faraday's laws we know that an EMF will be induced in the disc. From Lenz's law we can deduce that a current will be induced in the disc in such a way as to oppose the change producing it.

The disc thus moves in the same direction as the magnet in order to reduce the relative motion between them, so opposing the change producing the current, as required by Lenz's law. In a frictionless system, the disc would eventually move at the same speed as the magnet so that there would be no relative motion and no induced currents.

A more efficient system is shown in Figure 12.5B where more magnets are used and so a higher magnetic flux linkage is obtained. The copper disc follows the direction of rotation of the magnets for the reasons outlined above. It is not necessary to use permanent magnets since current-carrying solenoids will act as magnets.

The arrangement of the coils for such a motor is shown in Figure 12.6. The current through *AB* will be 90° out of phase with the current through *CD*. This produces a magnetic field which appears to rotate at the same frequency as the AC mains supply (50 Hz) and so the disc will also rotate at the same speed (50 revs per second (r.p.s.) = 3000 revs per minute (r.p.m.).

Insight

An AC induction motor is used to cause the rotation of the anode in the rotating anode X-ray tube. The anode assembly is attached to a rotor and these devices are contained within the glass envelope. The stator coils (which produce the rotating magnetic field) are fixed around the outside of this envelope, but the magnetic fields can penetrate the glass and cause the anode to rotate. This will be discussed further in Chapter 30.

12.8 MAGNETIC DEFLECTION OF AN ELECTRON BEAM

There are a number of situations in radiography where we wish to deflect a beam of electrons, e.g. a beam of electrons

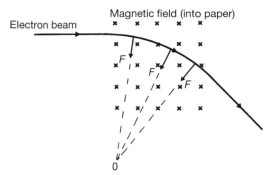

Figure 12.7 The deflection of an electron beam due to a magnetic field. The electrons enter the magnetic field from the left and are deflected on a circular path with 0 as the centre of the circle. The electrons continue on a straight path when they leave the influence of the magnetic field.

12.9 THE MOTOR PRINCIPLE IN RADIOGRAPHY

The motor principle is relevant to radiography whenever electrical energy is transformed into mechanical energy via magnetic energy. Obvious examples of this include the use of electric motors to drive mobile X-ray machines and the use of motors to tilt or elevate X-ray tables. The motor principle is also utilized in rotating the anode of the rotating anode X-ray tube. Finally, the motor principle is applied to allow scanning of the electron beam in television cameras and monitors.

is made to scan the face of a television monitor to produce an image or in the bending magnet of a linear accelerator.

Figure 12.7 shows an electron beam travelling in a vacuum and passing through such a magnetic field. It can be seen that the path taken by the electron beam when it passes through the magnetic field is circular since the direction of the deflecting force is always at right angles to the direction of travel. Thus, the electrons are deflected when they pass through the magnetic field. After leaving the magnetic field, the beam again travels in a straight line.

The angle of deflection increases as the magnetic flux density increases, so that the direction of the beam can be controlled by varying the magnetic flux density. Thus, by placing magnetic deflection coils on either side of a television monitor we can scan the electron beam in a pattern (known as a *raster*) across the face of the monitor.

Summary

In this chapter, you should have learnt the following:
- The definition of the motor principle (see Sect. 12.2).
- The factors affecting the direction and magnitude of the force acting on a current-carrying conductor in a magnetic field (see Sect. 12.3).
- A convention to establish the direction of the force on a current-carrying conductor in a magnetic field (see Sect. 12.4).
- The interaction between two electromagnetic fields and how this is applied to two parallel wires (see Sect. 12.5).
- The operation of the DC motor (see Sect. 12.6).
- The operation of the AC induction motor (see Sect. 12.7).
- The factors influencing the magnetic deflection of an electron beam (see Sect. 12.8).
- The applications of the motor principle in radiography (see Sect. 12.9).

FURTHER READING

Ball, J.L., Moore, A.D., Turner, S., 2008. Ball and Moore's Essential Physics for Radiographers, fourth ed. Blackwell Scientific, London (Chapter 8).

Ohanian, H.C., 1994. Principles of Physics. W W Norton, London (Chapter 21).

Thompson, M.A., Hattaway, R.T., Hall, J.D., Dowd, S.B., 1994.

Principles of Imaging Science and Protection. W B Saunders, London (Chapter 5).

Chapter | **13** |

Capacitors

13.1 AIM

The aim of this chapter is to introduce the subject of capacitors and capacitance. It then considers the factors that influence the performance of a capacitor, how capacitors can be linked to other components and how capacitors are used in radiography.

13.2 INTRODUCTION

In Chapter 11, we considered the influence of a capacitor on the current and voltage in an alternating current (AC) circuit. We were able to do this without an understanding of the construction or the operation of a capacitor. There are circumstances where capacitors are used and where we need to understand either the construction and/or the operation of the capacitor to understand its function within the piece of equipment. This chapter deals with the physics of the capacitor, which is a device for storing electrical charge. It has many applications in radiography as it can be charged and discharged quickly unlike a battery.

13.3 ELECTRICAL CAPACITY (CAPACITANCE)

We have previously shown in Chapter 6 that when a body has a net positive or negative charge it also possesses an electrical potential, because work must be done in moving a unit positive charge from infinity to the body. This potential is positive if the charge on the body is positive and negative if the charge on the body is negative.

The *electrical capacity* or *capacitance* of the body is the relationship between the charge put on the body and its potential:

Equation 13.1

$$\text{capacitance} = \frac{\text{charge}}{\text{potential}}$$

$$\text{or} \quad C = \frac{Q}{V}$$

13.3.1 Definitions and unit of capacitance (farad)

The definition of capacitance varies slightly depending on the type of body holding the charge. When a body consists of *one surface* only (e.g. a sphere) the following definition applies:

Definition
The capacitance of a body is the ratio of the total charge on the body to its potential.

If the body consists of *two surfaces* close together, we must consider the *potential differences* between the surfaces rather than the potential on each. This leads to the following alternative definition of capacitance:

Definition
The capacitance of a body is the ratio of the total charge of one sign on the body to the potential difference between its surfaces.

It is important to remember that capacitance involves both charge and potential and so it is not correct to think of capacitance as the 'amount of charge a body can hold' unless we add the phrase 'per unit potential difference'. The International System of Units (SI) unit of capacitance is the *farad* and may be defined as:

Definition
An electrical system has a capacitance of 1 *farad* if a charge of 1 coulomb held by the body results in a potential (or potential difference) of 1 volt.

Thus, Equation 13.1 may be expressed as:

Equation 13.2

$$\text{farads} = \frac{\text{coulombs}}{\text{volts}}$$

Definition
An alternative definition of capacitance, and one that is often more useful in radiography, is to consider capacitance in terms of the *change* of charge divided by the corresponding *change* in potential.

If a capacitor starts with a charge Q and a potential difference, then by definition:

Equation 13.2A

$$C = \frac{Q}{V}$$

If an extra charge, ΔQ is added to the plates and an extra potential difference ΔV, results, then:

$$C = \frac{(Q + \Delta Q)}{(V + \Delta V)}$$

i.e. *capacitance is the total charge divided by the total potential difference*.

By cross-multiplying the above equation, we get:

Equation 13.2B

$$CV + C\Delta V = Q + \Delta Q$$

However, we can say from Equation A that:

$$CV = Q$$

Thus, Equation B can be rewritten:

$$C\Delta V = \Delta Q$$
$$\therefore C = \frac{\Delta Q}{\Delta V}$$

This gives the alternative definition of capacitance, which can be used in radiography for calculations involving capacitor discharge circuits, etc.

For practical purposes, the farad (F) is rather a large unit in which to measure capacitance and so it is more commonly expressed in units of *microfarads* (μF) or *picofarads* (pF), where:

$$1\mu F = 10^{-6} F$$

and

$$1 pF = 10^{-12} F$$

13.4 CAPACITANCE OF A PARALLEL-PLATE CAPACITOR

Figure 13.1 (see page 79) shows a parallel-plate capacitor with two plates of equal area, separated by a distance, d. The plates are made of electrical conductors so that charge may flow in and out of each plate. If the capacitor is *charged* – e.g. by connecting it across a battery as shown – then a charge of $+Q$ will exist on one plate and a charge of $-Q$ on the other. If the battery is disconnected, the charge will continue to be stored on the plates of the capacitor as the positive charge on one plate attracts the negative charge on the other. This is why a capacitor is often described as a device for storing charge. (A large capacitor will retain this

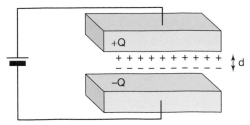

Figure 13.1 A parallel-plate capacitor charged by a battery.

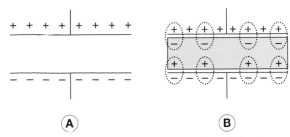

Ⓐ　　　　　Ⓑ

Figure 13.2 (A) Parallel-plate capacitor with no dielectric between the plates. (B) Capacitor after a dielectric has been introduced between the plates. The induction of charge in the dielectric 'cancels' some of the charges stored on the plates (shown as ringed charges). This means that the battery can now place more charge on the plates of the capacitor.

charge for a long period of time after it has been disconnected from the source of electromotive force (EMF). For this reason, it should be treated *with extreme care* as *severe electric shock* may result from touching the plates or the electrical connections to the capacitor.)

When the capacitor is fully charged, a potential difference equal to that of the battery exists across the plates. Thus, the capacitance of the parallel-plate capacitor is given by the equation $C = Q/V$ where Q is the charge of one sign on one of the plates and V is the potential difference between the plates.

Certain characteristics of the capacitor will affect its capacitance and these will now be considered.

13.4.1 Area of the plates

If the area of the plates (A) is increased, then more charge will be able to flow onto the plates from the battery until the charge per unit area is the same as before. It can be seen that if the area of the plates is doubled then the amount of charge which they will hold, to give the same charge per unit area, will also be doubled. In this situation, V remains unaltered, as it is the same as the potential difference from the battery and $Q \propto A$. Since $C = Q/V$, we can say that:

$$C \propto A$$

Note: If the plates are not directly opposite each other, then the area taken for this calculation of capacitance is the effective area, i.e. the area of the plates which are in direct opposition to each other.

13.4.2 Separation of the plates

If the rest of the capacitor remains unaltered but the plates are brought closer together, then the charges on opposite plates will experience a greater force of attraction so that the battery will be able to 'push' more charge onto the plates. Once again, V is constant, but $Q \propto 1/d$. Since $C = Q/V$ we can then say that:

$$C = \frac{1}{d}$$

13.4.3 Dielectric constant of material between the plates

A material with a high dielectric constant is an insulator where it is relatively easy to induce a charge on its surface (see Sect. 6.7.2). The effect of placing such a material between the plates of a charged capacitor is shown in Figure 13.2. The close proximity of the charges on the plates and on the dielectric results in some 'cancellation' of charges (as shown ringed in Figure 13.2B). If this capacitor is now reconnected to the battery, it will be seen that more charge will flow onto the capacitor. Thus, once again, V is the same value but Q has increased and so the capacitance of the capacitor increases with the dielectric constant (K), so we can say:

$$C \propto K$$

This leads to the definition of the *dielectric constant.*

Definition
The *dielectric constant* of a material is the ratio of the capacitance of the capacitor with the dielectric to the capacitance without the dielectric (i.e. with a vacuum between the plates of the capacitor).

From this, it can be seen that the dielectric constant of a vacuum is unity (1). If we take the above three components together we get:

$$C \propto \frac{KA}{d}$$

By the addition of a constant of proportionality (ε_0), this now becomes:

Equation 13.3

$$C = \frac{\varepsilon_0 KA}{d}$$

13.5 CHARGING A CAPACITOR THROUGH A RESISTOR FROM A DC SUPPLY

Consider the situation illustrated in Figure 13.3A. Here a battery is connected across a resistor R and a capacitor C in series. When the switch S_1 is closed, electrons will flow onto one of the plates of the capacitor and away from the other plate, as shown in the illustration. The potential difference across the capacitor, V_C, therefore increases due to the charge on the plates. However, it does not increase indefinitely, but settles to a value that is the same as (but of opposite polarity) to that of the battery. To understand why this is the case, consider the forces acting on an electron at the point P. When the switch S_1 is initially closed, a complete circuit is made and, due to the EMF from the battery, a force is exerted on the electron, pushing it towards the capacitor. However, as soon as the plate starts to build up electric charge, it in turn exerts a force on the electron at P in the opposite direction, which slows down the rate of flow of charge onto the plate. Eventually the two opposing forces on the electron will become equal and there is no further flow of electrons through the circuit. At this stage, the potential across the capacitor is equal and opposite to the potential across the battery. This situation is shown in Figure 13.3B where there is an initial rapid rise in potential (V_C) when S_1 is closed, but this slows down and approaches V_B relatively slowly.

The effect of the resistance R is to limit the electron flow rate so that V_B is approached more slowly for large values of R than for small values of R, as shown in Figure 13.3B.

From this, it can be seen that *a capacitor does not pass direct current* (DC), for, after the short time required to charge the capacitor, all further electron movement (flow of current) ceases.

13.6 DISCHARGING A CAPACITOR THROUGH A RESISTOR

In Figure 13.4A, a charged capacitor with a potential V_C across its plates is allowed to discharge through the resistor R when the switch S_2 is closed. When this happens, electrons travel from the negative plate of the capacitor, through resistor R and onto the positive plate and the charge on the plates and the potential between them (V_C) is reduced. The reduction in V_C means that there will be less 'push' on the electrons in the next time interval (see Sect. 13.7) resulting in a smaller drop in V_C. This situation continues, as shown in Figure 13.4B, until the capacitor is discharged and the potential difference is zero. Again, the effect of R is to slow down the current and so the rate of fall of V_C.

13.7 THE TIME-CONSTANT FOR A CAPACITOR RESISTOR CIRCUIT

This is an example of the exponential law (see Ch. 20) and this can be seen by comparing the graphs in Figures 13.3 and 13.4 with those in Chapter 20. The potential difference between the plates of a discharging capacitor can be calculated from the equation:

Equation 13.4

$$V_C = V_0 e^{-t/RC}$$

where V_0 is the potential difference between the plates before discharging the capacitor, t is the time of the discharge (in seconds), R is the resistance in ohms and C is the capacitance in farads. The quantity RC is called the *time-constant*. After a discharge time of 1 time-constant, the potential difference across a discharging capacitor has dropped to $1/e$ of its initial value, i.e. 0.37 of its initial value. If the original potential difference is 6V, the value after 1 time-constant is $0.37 \times 6 = 2.2$V. After 2 time-constants, the value will be reduced to a further 0.37, i.e. $0.37 \times 2.2 = 0.8$V. Note that this is very similar to the

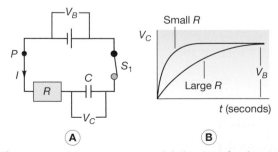

Figure 13.3 Charging a capacitor. (A) The circuit for charging a capacitor (C) though a resistor (R). (B) Graph showing the effect of using different resistors on the rate of charge.

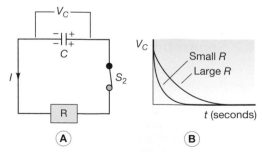

Figure 13.4 Discharging a capacitor. (A) Circuit for discharging capacitor (C) through resistor (R). (B) Graph showing the effect of different resistors on the rate of discharge.

concept of half-life discussed in Chapter 20 since both are examples of exponential decay.

If we consider a capacitor being charged, then the equation for the potential across it is:

Equation 13.5

$$V_C = V_0(1 - e^{-t/RC})$$

V_0 is the charging source EMF. Again, RC is the time-constant. After 1 time-constant the potential across the capacitor will be $1 - 1/e$, which is 0.63. Thus, for a charging capacitor, after 1 time-constant the potential across its plates will be 0.63 of its final value (the final value will be the same as the charging source EMF).

13.8 CAPACITORS AND ALTERNATING CURRENT

We have already shown in this chapter that a capacitor will eventually possess the same potential difference as the electrical supply connected across it. If the potential difference of supply is changed, a new equilibrium will become established where, once again, the two values of potential difference are equal. Thus, if an alternating supply is connected across the capacitor, the potential of the capacitor 'follows' the potential of the supply. Thus, it can be said that a *capacitor passes AC* since the potential difference (PD) on the capacitor changes continually, in sympathy with the PD of the supply.

As we have already seen in Chapter 11, when a capacitor is introduced to an AC circuit, the PD across the plates lags 90° behind the current. The effect of this phase difference must be taken into account for many of the uses of capacitors in AC circuits.

13.9 CAPACITORS IN RADIOGRAPHY

The ability to store electrical charge on the plates of a capacitor has important practical consequences in radiography. Some of the practical uses of capacitors in radiography are the following:

- Capacitor discharge mobile units.
- Voltage smoothing.
- Phase splitting for AC induction motors.
- Electronic timers.

There is insufficient space in this text to describe all these uses in detail and so only a brief overview of each will be given. The applications of capacitors in electronic timers will be studied in more detail in Chapter 29.

13.9.1 Capacitor discharge mobile units

Figure 13.5 shows the basic principles of such a circuit. When an exposure is made on a mains-dependent

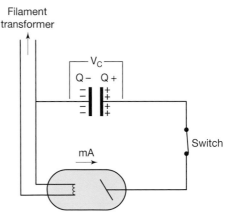

Figure 13.5 Simplified diagram of the principles of a capacitor discharge X-ray circuit.

mobile unit, a large current (around 30 A) is drawn from the mains during the exposure. This large current can cause large power losses in the mains cables (remember, $P = I^2R$). The capacitor discharge mobile works on the principle that a small current is drawn from the mains to charge a capacitor before the X-ray exposure, and this capacitor is allowed to discharge through the X-ray tube during the exposure. Since the electrical energy to the tube comes from the capacitor, no significant stress is applied to the mains supply during the exposure.

Figure 13.5 shows the basic principles of such a circuit. With the switch open, the capacitor is initially charged until the required potential (V_C is the same value as the kV which will be applied to the tube) is established across its plates. On closing the switch, electrons flow from the negative plate of the capacitor to the positive plate via the X-ray tube. This means that a potential difference (kV) is applied across the tube and charge (mAs) flows through it, comprising a radiographic exposure. At the end of the exposure, the switch is opened.

As a result of the exposure, the capacitor loses some of the charge on its plates and so the potential difference at the end of the exposure is less than the initial potential difference. However, when long exposures are made, there is a significant drop in the energy of the X-ray beam during the exposure as the energy stored in the capacitor falls. This must be taken into account when selecting exposure factors on such a unit.

13.9.2 Voltage smoothing

When an alternating voltage is full-wave rectified (see Ch. 28) and applied to a component, the voltage waveform will be as shown in Figure 13.6A. Thus, during each half-cycle a potential difference ranging from the peak voltage to 0 V is applied across the component. This difference between the peak and the trough in the voltage is known as the *voltage ripple*. In this case, the ripple is

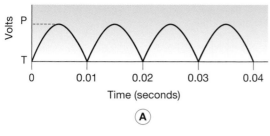

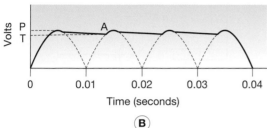

Figure 13.6 (A) Voltage waveform from a single-phase transformer after it has been rectified. (B) The same waveform after capacitor smoothing, where *P* represents the peak and *T* the trough. The difference between the peak and the trough is known as the ripple. Note how capacitor smoothing reduces the voltage ripple.

100%. There are some situations where it is beneficial to reduce this ripple. This is done by connecting a capacitor (or sometimes two capacitors) in parallel with the component so that the voltage supply is smoothed by the capacitor before it is applied to the component. The result of capacitor smoothing of the voltage is shown in Figure 13.6B. The broken line shows the voltage waveform from the rectification circuit. Initially the capacitor charges so that the potential between its plates is the same as the peak potential from the rectification circuit. As this supply voltage drops, the capacitor discharges through the component so that the potential difference between its plates slowly drops. When this potential has dropped by a small amount, the potential from the supply 'catches up' with it (point A on the graph) and charge will once again flow on to the capacitor so that it reaches its peak potential difference at the same time as the supply voltage.

This application is important in medium-frequency rectification systems as, by using capacitors that are suitably matched to the components being supplied with electrical energy, the voltage ripple can be reduced to less than 1%.

13.9.3 Phase splitting for AC induction motors

When a capacitor is introduced into an AC supply, it causes a phase shift between the current and voltage. This is utilized in the AC induction motor. The detail of the operation of this motor is given in Section 12.7. The role of the capacitor is to produce a current in one pair of coils that is 90° out of phase with the current in the other pair. This produces a magnetic field, which *appears* to rotate at the same speed as the mains frequency and so produces rotation of the motor rotor.

13.9.4 Electronic timers

The ability to store electrical charge on the plates of a capacitor has important practical consequences in radiography. These will be discussed in Chapter 29.

Summary

In this chapter, you should have learnt the following:
- The meaning of the term *electrical capacitance* (see Sect. 13.3).
- The definition of the farad – the unit of capacitance (see Sect. 13.3).
- The factors affecting the capacitance of a parallel-plate capacitor (see Sect. 13.4).
- The definition of the term *dielectric constant* (see Sect. 13.4).
- The consequences of charging a capacitor from a DC source through a resistor (see Sect. 13.5).
- The definition and the uses of the *time-constant* for a capacitor/resistor circuit (see Sect. 13.7).
- The effect on the voltage and the current in an AC circuit when a capacitor is introduced to the circuit (see Sect. 13.8).
- Some of the applications of capacitors in radiography (see Sect. 13.9).

FURTHER READING

Ball, J.L., Moore, A.D., Turner, S., 2008. Ball and Moore's Essential Physics for Radiographers, fourth ed. Blackwell Scientific, London (Chapter 7).

Chapter | **14** |

The AC transformer

14.1 AIM

The aim of this chapter is to discuss the main concepts that govern the operation of the step-up or the step-down alternating current (AC) transformer. In addition to this, two forms of specialist transformers are discussed, namely the autotransformer and the constant-voltage transformer. Finally, there is an overview of the factors that affect transformer rating and how these factors relate to radiographic exposures.

14.2 INTRODUCTION

An AC transformer has an electrical input and an electrical output. For the transformer to function, the input is an AC supply. The electrical output potential difference may be either greater or smaller than the electrical input voltage. If the output voltage is greater than the input voltage, then the transformer is a *step-up* transformer; if it is less, then the transformer is a *step-down* transformer. A transformer is thus a device that changes ACs or voltages from one level to another.

The transformer has a wide range of applications in radiography. The mains voltage is too low to be applied directly across the X-ray tube and so it is increased using a step-up transformer (the high-tension transformer). On the other hand, the mains voltage is too high to be connected directly across the filament and so it is reduced in the filament transformer – an example of a step-down transformer. Two other types of transformer are encountered in radiography and so will be discussed in this chapter. These are the *autotransformer* and the *saturated core* or *constant-voltage* transformer.

14.3 THE IDEAL TRANSFORMER

Let us start by defining this device:

Definition
An *ideal transformer* is one whose output electrical power is equal to its input electrical power – there is no power 'lost' in the transformer itself.

There is, of course, no such thing as the ideal (or perfect) transformer, although real transformers with efficiencies of 98% or more are not uncommon. Although not a practical reality, the concept of the ideal transformer is a useful one in that it simplifies the mathematics which can be used to describe the behaviour of transformers.

Consider such an ideal transformer, shown in Figure 14.1, where two isolated sets of windings share a common core – there are a number of other configurations of core and windings but the one shown in Figure 14.1 is the simplest. The input or *primary* side of the transformer consists of n_p turns around the core and has an alternating voltage V_P across it. The output or *secondary* side of the transformer consists of n_s turns and has a voltage V_s induced in it. This is a case of mutual induction, as discussed in Section 10.7. The sequence of events is as follows:

- The alternating voltage in the primary winding V_P causes an AC to flow through the winding.
- This AC, I_p, produces *a changing magnetic flux density (B)* in the soft iron *core*.
- The *changing magnetic flux density* is linked to the secondary winding so that an electromotive force (EMF), V_s, is induced in it according to Faraday's and Lenz's laws of electromagnetic induction (see Sects 10.4 and 10.5).

As already mentioned in the introduction to this chapter, an AC supply is essential for the operation of the transformer since no EMF will be generated in the secondary if the magnetic flux is constant (Faraday's first law).

The purpose of the soft iron core is to contain all the magnetic flux within it so that the magnetic flux linkage between the primary and the secondary is as near perfect as possible. The core is able to do this because of its strong induced magnetism, resulting from its high magnetic permeability (see Table 14.1).

The mathematics of the ideal transformer are relatively simple if we first consider the effect of the magnetic flux on a single turn of wire around the core. Since we are assuming that the transformer is ideal, there is no magnetic

Table 14.1 A summary of the losses associated with a particular transformer

TRANSFORMER LOSS	COMMENTS
Copper losses	Caused by the resistance of the copper windings. Also known as I^2R losses
Iron losses	Losses produced in the transformer core
Imperfect magnetic flux linkage	Very small loss flux
Eddy currents	Caused by electromagnetic induction within the core of the transformer – reduced by core lamination
Hysteresis	Caused by the work required to move the magnetic domains – reduced by the appropriate choice of core material (e.g. stalloy)
Regulation (a consequence of all the above losses)	Output voltage decreases with increased current load because of the increased losses due to the resistance of the windings

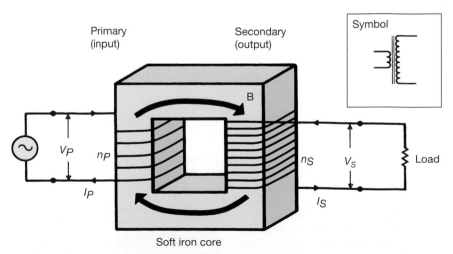

Figure 14.1 An 'ideal' transformer showing the core and the primary and secondary windings. In practice, the core is laminated, as shown in Figure 14.2. As there are more turns on the secondary winding than on the primary winding, this is a step-up transformer. The symbol for a step-up transformer is also shown. See text for details.

flux loss and the EMF induced is independent of the position of the wire. Thus, the same voltage will be induced in each turn of the primary and in each turn of the secondary. If we call this voltage v, then we can say that the total primary voltage is the voltage in each turn multiplied by the number of turns. Thus:

$$V_p = v \times n_p$$
$$\text{or} \quad \frac{V_p}{n_p} = v$$

Similarly, for the secondary:

$$V_s = v \times n_s$$
$$\text{or} \quad \frac{V_s}{n_s} = v$$

Thus, we can combine the two equations above to get:

$$\frac{V_p}{n_p} = \frac{V_s}{n_s}$$

By cross-multiplying this equation, we get the formula:

Equation 14.1

$$\frac{V_s}{V_p} = \frac{n_s}{n_p}$$

Note: This equation is true for either peak or root mean square (RMS) values of the voltage, provided V_s and V_p are both expressed in the same units.

The ratio V_s/V_p is known as the *voltage gain* of the transformer. This is greater than unity for a step-up transformer and less than unity for a step-down transformer.

The ratio n_s/n_p is known as the *turns ratio* of the transformer. Again, if this is greater than unity, we have a step-up transformer and if it is less than unity, we have a step-down transformer.

If we have a transformer with a turns ratio of 200:1, we know that there are 200 times as many turns on the secondary as on the primary and that the voltage across the secondary is 200 times that of the primary.

The *current* flowing in the secondary of the transformer may be calculated from the power in the primary winding and secondary winding (for simplicity, in the following discussion, RMS values are assumed). In the ideal transformer, the power in the primary and the power in the secondary are equal. Thus:

$$V_p \times I_p = V_s \times I_s$$
$$\therefore \frac{I_p}{I_s} = \frac{V_s}{V_p}$$

From Equation 14.1 we know:

$$\frac{V_s}{V_p} = \frac{n_s}{n_p}$$

Thus, for an ideal transformer, we can say:

Equation 14.2

$$\frac{I_p}{I_s} = \frac{n_s}{n_p}$$

14.4 FARADAY'S LAWS AND LENZ'S LAW APPLIED TO TRANSFORMERS

We have already considered Faraday's laws of electromagnetic induction (Sect. 10.4) and Lenz's law (Sect. 10.5) and we can now look at how these are applied to transformers.

As discussed in the previous section, there is a changing magnetic flux produced by the alternating supply connected to the primary and, since this is linked to both the primary and secondary windings, by Faraday's laws, an EMF is produced in each of the windings. Assuming we have an ideal transformer, the magnitude of the EMF in each turn of the primary winding is equal to the magnitude of the EMF in each turn of the secondary.

Lenz's law may be used to determine the direction of the induced current in the secondary. As it acts to oppose the changing magnetic flux, it will be in the opposite direction to (180° out of phase with) the current in the primary. The eddy currents induced in the core (these will be discussed later in this chapter, as they are part of the transformer 'losses') will also be in the opposite direction to the primary current.

Insight

Some find it surprising that it is the current drawn from the secondary of a transformer that determines the primary current, especially as the secondary voltage for a given transformer is determined by the primary voltage. The explanation of this fact is as follows.

Consider a situation when the secondary winding is open circuit (it is not connected to anything), so no current can flow through it, although an EMF is induced across it. If we assume that we have an ideal transformer, then the same EMF will be induced by this magnetic flux in the primary winding and, by Lenz's Law, this will be in the opposite direction to the forward-EMF. Thus, no current flows in the primary winding when the secondary current is zero.

If the secondary is now connected across an external circuit so that some current flows through it, this current, by Lenz's law, will oppose the magnetic flux in the core. The core flux is reduced and so the back-EMF in the primary is reduced. The forward-EMF in the primary is now greater than the back-EMF and so a current flows. Thus, a current in the secondary has caused a current to flow in the primary, the relative magnitudes of each being given by Equation 14.2.

14.5 TRANSFORMERS IN PRACTICE

It is not possible to construct an ideal transformer, as there are always power 'losses' within the transformer itself. This means that the power in the secondary is always less than the power in the primary by an amount equal to the transformer losses. The efficiency of a transformer may be defined as follows:

Definition
The *efficiency* of a transformer is the ratio of the output power to the input power.

Note: It is often convenient to express the transformer efficiency as a percentage. For example, if a transformer is 95% efficient and 100 watts of power is supplied to the primary of that transformer, then 95 watts is produced in the secondary. In this case, 5% of the power is 'lost' because of power loss in the windings and core, i.e. this 5% is not available as useful electrical power.

Equation 14.1 gives a reasonable estimate of the voltage change in practical transformers but Equation 14.2 no longer applies because of the power losses in practical transformers. This may be illustrated by the following example.

Example

A transformer has a turns ratio of 100:1 and an efficiency of 95%. If a current of $5\,A_{RMS}$ flows in the primary when a voltage of $10\,V_{RMS}$ is applied across it, what is the output RMS voltage and output RMS current?
From Equation 14.1 we get:

$$\frac{V_s}{V_p} = \frac{n_s}{n_p}$$

$$\therefore \frac{V_s}{10} = \frac{100}{1}$$

$$V_s = 1000\,V_{RMS}$$

We also know that efficiency is the ratio of the output power to the input power. Thus:

$$\text{efficiency} = \frac{(V_s \times I_s)}{(V_p \times I_p)}$$

$$\therefore \frac{95}{100} = \frac{(1000 \times I_s)}{(10 \times 5)}$$

$$\therefore I_s = \frac{(50 \times 95)}{(100 \times 1000)} \quad \text{(by cross-multiplication)}$$

$$= 47.5\,mA_{RMS}$$

Note that an ideal transformer would have produced the same secondary voltage but the secondary current would be $50\,mA_{RMS}$.

14.6 TRANSFORMER LOSSES

A detailed analysis of the sources of transformer losses is considered in this section. These are summarized in Table 14.1 (See page. 84) and discussed below.

14.6.1 Copper losses

The term *copper* refers to the copper wire of the windings of the transformer, which has a small but finite resistance. If we consider a current I_{RMS} flowing through a resistance R, then there is a power of $(I_{RMS})^2 R$ watts produced within the resistor. (The copper loss is often referred to as the $I^2 R$ loss of the transformer.) The copper loss produces a small heating effect within the coils of the transformer.

We wish to keep the copper loss as low as possible and, as it is related to $I^2 R$, it makes sense to keep R low when I is large. As we saw in Chapter 7, the resistance of a conductor is inversely proportional to its cross-sectional area. For this reason, the winding of the transformer, which carries the larger current, is made of thicker wire. In the step-up transformer, this is the primary winding while in the step-down transformer it is the secondary winding.

14.6.2 Iron losses

The term *iron losses* refer to the losses that occur in the soft iron core of the transformer. These take three forms, as outlined below.

14.6.2.1 Magnetic flux losses

If the iron core is magnetically saturated, then all of the magnetic flux will not be contained within the core. This means that magnetic flux will be produced by the primary, which is not linked with the secondary. The EMF induced in the secondary and the output electrical power will be lower than if the flux linkage were perfect. By the appropriate design of the transformer core, in practice this loss is made very small indeed and so can be neglected for most practical purposes.

14.6.2.2 Eddy currents

From Faraday's and Lenz's laws, we know that when a changing magnetic flux is linked with a continuous conductor, an EMF and current are induced in the conductor. Also, the direction of the induced current opposes the effect of the changing magnetic flux linkage. The iron core of the transformer is a continuous electrical conductor and so the varying flux passing through the core will induce electric currents within the core itself in such a direction as to oppose the changing magnetic flux within the core. This principle is shown in Figure 14.2A (see page 86) where the direction of the eddy currents in the core is

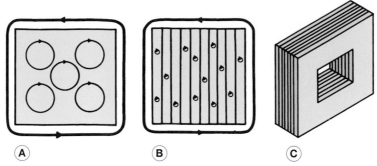

Figure 14.2 (A) Flow of eddy currents in an unlaminated transformer core. If the core is laminated, as shown in (B) and (C), then the eddy current flow is restricted and so the eddy current losses are limited.

in the opposite direction to the current in the winding. The effect of these currents is two-fold:

1. The flow of electrical current through the core causes heating of the core due to the electrical resistance of the core.
2. The magnetic flux associated with the eddy currents is in the opposite direction to the flux from the winding and so there is a reduction in the flux interlinking with the secondary – flux which interlinks with the secondary is the flux produced at the primary minus the eddy current flux. This constitutes a power loss within the transformer core.

Eddy currents may be reduced but not entirely eliminated by *lamination* of the core, as shown in Figure 14.2B and C. The laminated sheets of soft iron are bolted together to produce the required cross-sectional area. Each lamination is insulated from its neighbours by the application of a thin layer of insulation (e.g. polyester varnish) to its surface. This means that the eddy currents produced in the core are now confined to the small cross-sectional area of each lamination. As resistance is inversely proportional to cross-sectional area, lamination produces an increase in resistance and a consequent reduction in the size of the eddy current. There is, however, some eddy current present and this causes heating of the transformer core. Because of this, the transformer core requires to be cooled either by air or by immersing the transformer in oil, the latter acting as both a coolant and an insulator.

14.6.2.3 Hysteresis losses

Hysteresis is the lagging-behind of the induced magnetism in a ferromagnetic material when the applied magnetic field changes. Consider the changes which will occur in a transformer core during 1½ cycles of AC. The magnetizing force H changes with the current (see Fig. 14.3A, page 88). This produces changes in the magnetic intensity I as shown in Figure 14.3B. This graph is referred to as *a hysteresis loop* and the shape and size of this loop are important in the function of the transformer. The shape of this loop is explained as follows.

Consider a situation where the core is initially unmagnetized. As the magnetic domains are in randomized directions, there is no magnetic intensity within the core. This represents the origin O on both of the graphs. The current increases until it reaches its peak value at point A. The magnetizing force increases with the current and so initially does the magnetic intensity. This, however, flattens as magnetic saturation of the sample occurs so that the line is horizontal at point A on the hysteresis graph. The current now follows the curve AB and, as the magnetizing force decreases, so the magnetic intensity reduces along the curve AB on the hysteresis graph. Note that at point B, the magnetizing force is zero but there is still some magnetic intensity left in the ferromagnetic core sample. This magnetic intensity is known as the *remanence* in the core. To get rid of this remanence – so completely demagnetizing the core – a *coercive force*, represented by OC, must be used. Because the current has been reversed, the magnetizing force is also reversed and this continues until magnetic saturation is again produced at D. This occurs at the negative peak value of the current. As the current is reduced, the magnetizing force is again reduced and it is zero when the current is at point E on the graph of current. At this point on the hysteresis graph, there is again a remanence represented by OE (equal and opposite to OB) and this must be destroyed by the coercive force OF. The magnetizing force now continues to its positive peak, A, and the magnetic intensity follows the curve FA. The hysteresis loop is now complete.

The *area of the hysteresis loop* is important as it represents the work done in taking the sample through a complete hysteresis cycle. In considering the transformer core, the smaller the amount of work done, the smaller the iron loss from hysteresis. This should become clearer if we consider the hysteresis loops for soft iron and for steel.

Figure 14.4 (see page 89) shows the differences in the hysteresis loops for soft iron and steel. These differences may be summarized as follows:

- The saturation of soft iron occurs at much lower values of magnetizing force than the saturation of steel.

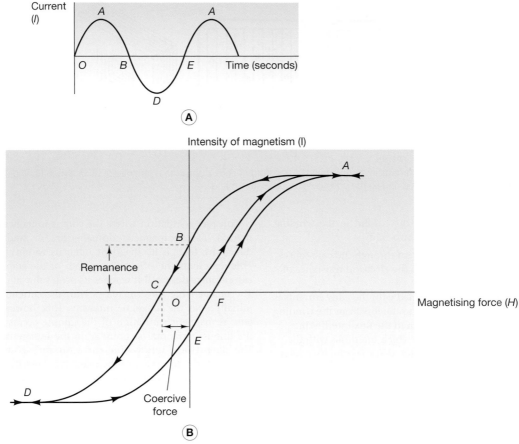

Figure 14.3 (A) Typical alternating current supply for a transformer winding; (B) hysteresis loop for a ferromagnetic sample. For an explanation of the connection between the two, see the text.

- The value of the coercive force is much greater for steel than for soft iron.
- The area of the hysteresis loop is much greater for steel than for soft iron.

Soft iron is therefore suitable for situations where a strong induced magnetism is required with the minimum expenditure of energy, and where the induced magnetism may be switched off at will. Note that, although the remanence is greater for soft iron than for steel, the coercive force is so small that a slight agitation of the sample will cause it to demagnetize. Suitable applications for soft iron are transformer cores (used as an alloy – stalloy).

Steel is a more suitable material for permanent magnets since it has a higher coercive force than soft iron and is thus more difficult to demagnetize. The high coercive force and the large area of the hysteresis loop make it unsuitable for use in the transformer core.

Subsidiary **hysteresis loops**. It is not necessary to take a ferromagnetic sample around a complete hysteresis loop, i.e. from magnetic saturation one way to magnetic saturation the other. In such cases, *subsidiary hysteresis loops* result, as shown in Figure 14.5 (see page 89). This is the type of hysteresis loop produced in most transformers – the exception being the saturated core transformer, which produces a complete hysteresis loop. The material with the hysteresis loop with the smallest area is still the most appropriate core material for a transformer.

The material usually selected for transformer cores is *stalloy* or *permalloy* as their small hysteresis loops limit the hysteresis 'loss'. The power loss due to hysteresis in the core increases the kinetic energy of the atoms of the core and so manifests itself in the form of heat.

14.6.3 Regulation

Regulation in a transformer is a consequence of the resistance of the windings. If the electrical load drawn from the secondary is *increased* – a higher current is made to flow in the secondary – it is found that the potential difference across the secondary is *decreased*. This effect is termed transformer regulation.

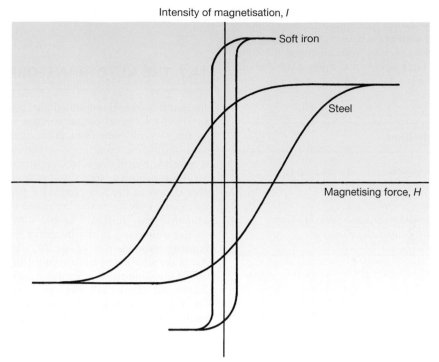

Figure 14.4 A comparison of the hysteresis loops for soft iron and steel.

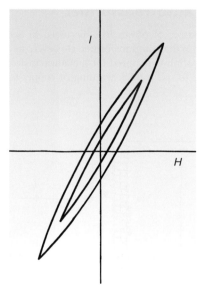

Figure 14.5 Subsidiary hysteresis loops where the ferromagnetic sample is not taken to full magnetic saturation.

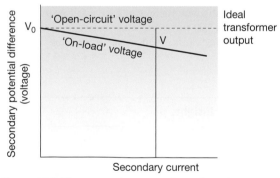

Figure 14.6 The greater the current drawn from the secondary winding of the transformer, the smaller becomes the potential difference across it. This effect is caused by the resistance of the transformer windings and is known as transformer regulation.

Regulation occurs in any source of electricity which contains an internal resistance. In the case of the transformer, the internal resistance is the resistance of the secondary winding. Figure 14.6 shows a graph of the voltage output from a given transformer for differing secondary currents. The output current is zero when the secondary is open circuit. This corresponds to the open-circuit voltage (V_0 in Fig. 14.6). In this condition, the transformer has zero regulation, it behaves as an ideal transformer and so Equation 14.1 may be used to calculate the secondary voltage. When the secondary of the transformer is connected to a load, current will flow in the secondary winding and the output voltage falls linearly with the secondary current. The transformer regulation therefore varies with the transformer load and so the output current is usually quoted with the regulation, e.g. 'a transformer has a regulation of 2% when the secondary current is 400 mA'. The regulation is often expressed as a percentage and may be defined as follows:

Definition

The *percentage regulation* at a given load can be calculated by:

$$100 \times \frac{\text{(open-circuit voltage} - \text{on-load voltage)}}{\text{open-circuit voltage}}$$

In Figure 14.6:

$$\text{percentage regulation} = 100 \times \frac{V}{V_0}$$

Most transformers used in radiography have a low percentage regulation and so the on-load voltage is close to the open-circuit voltage. In the case of the high-tension transformer, however, there must be a correction for this regulation, otherwise there would be a fall in the kVp if the tube mA was increased. Such corrections are made by *compensating circuits*, which are beyond the scope of this text.

Insight

The primary winding of a step-up transformer has such a low resistance that its effect on regulation may be ignored. If an EMF of V_0 is induced in the secondary and the secondary resistance is r, then a current I will produce a voltage drop of Ir (Ohm's law: $V = IR$) across the internal resistance r. This means that the potential difference which is available to the external circuit has been reduced by an amount Ir. Thus:

$$V = V_0 - Ir$$

This formula should explain why the regulation is linear with the current, as shown in Figure 14.6. It should also be noted that when the secondary is 'open-circuit' then the secondary current is zero and so the voltage drop

because of the internal resistance is zero. In such a situation, $V = V_0$.

14.7 THE AUTOTRANSFORMER

The autotransformer permitted the operator to manually select a range of output voltages values whose values not very different from those of the input voltage (usually differing by a factor of between 0.5 and 2.0). Its principle function was to compensate for these slight variations, providing stable operating conditions for the other circuits of the X-ray generator. For this reason it is more commonly known as 'the mains compensator'. The autotransformer consisted several turns forming single winding connected to the incoming mains supply. The changing magnetic flux of the AC supply produces an EMF in the winding which is evenly distributed over every turn of the winding. In accordance with Lenz's Law (see Chapter 10) a back EMF is also produced the position of S_2 in Figure 14.7 permits the operator to select a limited number of turns on the winding tapping the back EMF which has been produced in accordance with Lenz's Law, thus producing a secondary voltage Vs and secondary current I_s.

14.7.1 Losses and regulation in the autotransformer

All the sources of power loss discussed in Section 14.6 also apply to the autotransformer. However, the less severe design constraints required for the autotransformer make it possible to use a thick winding of copper wire with a

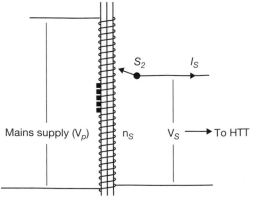

Figure 14.7 A circuit diagram for an autotransformer. It operates on the principle of self-induction. The number of secondary turn of the transformer can be varied at S_2. Thus the output from transformer to the X-ray generator and high-tension transformer can be varied.

consequent reduction in winding resistance. Therefore, the copper losses and the regulation are lower for the autotransformer than for the conventional transformer as both these losses are dependent on the resistance of the windings. One practical consequence of this is that there is not a great deal of heat generated in the autotransformer and so it is air-cooled.

14.8 THE CONSTANT VOLTAGE TRANSFORMER

Because it was manually operated the autotransformer has been replaced by the constant-voltage transformer. This will now be discussed in more detail.

The constant-voltage transformer is designed in such a way that there can be considerable variation in the input voltage to the transformer but the output voltage remains relatively constant. For reasons which will be discussed in Chapter 30, the output from the X-ray tube is sensitive to the temperature of the tube filament and so some units use a constant voltage transformer to ensure a well-stabilized voltage supply to the filament. Figure 14.8A gives a diagrammatic representation of the construction of such a transformer. Figure 14.8B shows a graph of the input and output voltages.

This transformer operates on the principle that the secondary limb of the core, B, is magnetically saturated during normal operation. The magnetic flux produced at the primary core, A, passes through two other magnetic circuits, the much thinner secondary core, B, and a central path of high magnetic resistance in core C – this high magnetic resistance is caused by the fact that there is an air gap between one end of C and the rest of the core (remember, air is less permeable than iron). The thinner core, B, is rapidly brought to magnetic saturation and the excess magnetic flux then passes through C. As can be seen from the graph, once B is saturated then an increase in input voltage does not produce any more magnetic flux in B and so the output voltage from the transformer remains fairly constant. Magnetic saturation occurs at an input voltage of X, and Y on the graph represents the normal operating input voltage of the transformer. Note that a large fall in the input voltage (say to Z on the graph) can result in the limb B becoming unsaturated with a resultant fall in the output voltage.

14.9 TRANSFORMER RATING

For transformer rating, the term *rating* means the maximum combination of factors that a system can withstand

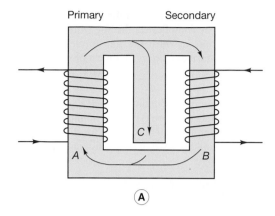

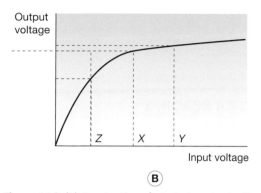

Figure 14.8 (A) Construction of a typical constant voltage transformer; (B) graph of the input and the output voltage for such a transformer.

without damage. If the rating is exceeded for a transformer, this may cause damage to the electrical insulation of the windings because of overheating or it may cause electrical breakdown.

The transformers in an X-ray unit are energized when the X-ray exposure is made. There are basically two types of exposure in radiography:

1. Fluoroscopy – this uses a low amount of power for a relatively long time.
2. Radiographic exposures – these use a relatively large amount of power for a short time.

Each of the above produces heat in the high-tension transformer and this transformer thus requires oil cooling. In particular, a long exposure must be made at a relatively low current (and therefore low power), otherwise the heat generated in the transformer will not be convected away sufficiently quickly by the oil and the transformer will overheat. Short exposures may use higher current values since the total energy deposited in the windings will still be low enough to cause no damage.

The detailed specification of the rating of any one transformer may be complicated, dealing with all the conceivable situations in which the transformer may be used. There are three main factors that must be considered:

1. The maximum kVp that the secondary winding may produce.
2. The maximum continuous current the transformer may supply that would be used in fluoroscopy.
3. The maximum current supplied for short exposures – (that) would be used during radiographic exposures.

Summary

In this chapter, you should have learnt the following:
- The concept of an ideal transformer and the equations for voltage and current produced from such a transformer (see Sect. 14.3).
- How Faraday's laws and Lenz's law apply to transformers (see Sect. 14.4).
- The types of losses that occur in a practical transformer and how these are minimized (see Sect. 14.6).
- Transformer regulation and its effect on the output voltage from a transformer (see Sect. 14.6.3).
- The operating principles and main functions of an autotransformer in an X-ray set (see Sect. 14.7).
- The operating principles of a constant voltage transformer (see Sect. 14.8).
- The factors to be considered for transformer rating in radiography (see Sect. 14.9).

FURTHER READING

Ball, J.L., Moore, A.D., Turner, S., 2008. Ball and Moore's Essential Physics for Radiographers, fourth ed. Blackwell Scientific, London (Chapter 10).

Chapter | 15 |

Semiconductor materials

15.1 AIM

This chapter introduces the reader to semiconductors and semiconducting devices that are important to radiography. This is a very large field, and the chapter concentrates on the barrier layer rectifier, which has made a major impact on radiographic science. After an overview of the development and manufacture of integrated circuits. the chapter concludes with an overview of the used of semiconductor devices in radiography.

15.2 INTRODUCTION

The use of semiconductor materials and the associated technology play an increasingly important part in our everyday lives as well as in radiographic science. Today it is possible to produce millions of electronic circuits on a small silicon chip using ultra-large-scale integration (ULSI) techniques. This has enabled the production of microprocessors that are capable of being programmed to perform specific tasks. Such devices are cheap and easy to program. They can perform a wide range of functions and are very reliable. Because of this, microprocessors are found in devices from wristwatches to aircraft flight systems and it is not surprising to learn that they are used in many devices in diagnostic imaging and radiotherapy departments.

However, the microprocessor is a complicated solid-state device and a detailed description of its operation is beyond the scope of this text.

Other, simpler, solid-state devices are widely used in X-ray circuitry and are suitable for inclusion in this chapter after a general description of the properties of semiconductor materials.

93

15.3 INTRINSIC SEMICONDUCTORS

An intrinsic semiconductor is a chemically pure semiconductor, which is also assumed to have perfect regularity of atoms within its crystalline structure or lattice. The concept of semiconducting materials was briefly introduced in Section 7.3.2 where the properties of conductors, insulators and semiconductors were compared in terms of the energy band model for the orbiting electrons. This was illustrated in Figure 7.2 and this diagram is reproduced here as Figure 15.1 (below). As shown in Figure 15.1B, one of the characteristics of semiconductors is that there is a small energy gap (up to a few eV) between the top of the valence band and the bottom of the conduction band. At very low temperatures, all the outer electrons have energies near the bottom of the valence band, and no electrons are able to take part in electrical conduction, as there are no free electrons in the conduction band. As mentioned in Chapter 7, increasing the temperature of a semiconductor increases its conductivity. At normal room temperatures, many electrons are able to gain sufficient energy (because of the increased kinetic energy of the atoms) to jump up to the conduction band and so take part in electrical conduction.

15.3.1 Positive holes

Associated with each electron which is able to jump up to the conduction band is a 'vacancy' in the valence band, referred to as a positive hole or just hole. This hole may be filled by an electron from the valence band of a neighbouring atom, but in doing so the electron leaves a hole in the valence band of that atom. In this way, a hole may appear to move around the crystal lattice of a semiconductor (behaving like a positive charge) until eventually an electron drops down from the conduction band to fill the hole and remove it from the valence band. This process is referred to as recombination. At any one moment in time, all three of the above processes are occurring:

1. Electrons are being excited into the conduction band creating holes in the valence band.
2. There is movement of electrons in the conduction band and holes in the valence band.
3. There is a recombination of electrons in the conduction band with holes in the valence band.

The overall conductivity of such an intrinsic semiconductor is the sum of the effects of the movements of the electrons in the conduction band and the holes in the valence band.

Insight

Consider the situation depicted in part A of the diagram below, where there is a row of ball bearings at the base of a box, with no available space between them for sideways movement to take place. If we now lift ball bearing C onto the lid of the box, it is possible for ball bearing D to move to the left to fill the space once occupied by C. In doing so, D has now created a space to its right, i.e. the hole may be considered as moving in the opposite direction to the ball.

Now consider the above situation as it refers to the valence and conduction bands of a semiconductor. No net movement is initially possible in the valence band because it is full of electrons. When an electron is raised to the conduction band, movement within the valence band is possible. Thus, if an electron moves from right to left within the band, it leaves a hole in its starting position, i.e. the hole appears to move from left to right. If an electron is removed from the valence band of an atom, then the atom is positively charged since the protons in the nucleus now outnumber the orbiting electrons; the hole is referred to as a positive hole. If a semiconductor is passing a current such that the electron flow in the conduction band is from left to right, there will also be an effective flow of positive charge associated with the movement of positive holes in the valence band in the opposite direction.

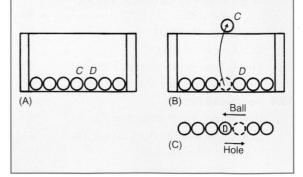

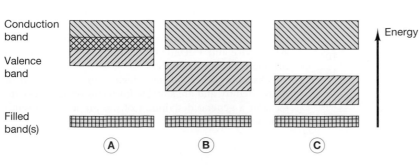

Figure 15.1 Energy level bands for (A) a conductor, (B) a semiconductor and (C) an insulator.

15.3.2 Silicon

Silicon is currently the most widely used general semiconductor material. It has an atomic number of 14 and has 14 protons in its nucleus and 14 electrons orbiting that nucleus (see Ch. 18). This means that the two inner shells (*K*- and *L*-shells) are completely full and contain two and eight electrons respectively. The next shell out from the nucleus is the *M*-shell and this exhibits a stable configuration when it contains either eight or 18 electrons (see Ch. 18). In this case, it contains four electrons and so may be regarded as an incomplete shell in the solitary silicon atom. However, in the silicon crystal there is a regular arrangement of atoms in which each silicon atom shares its outer electrons with four neighboring atoms so that each atom appears to have eight electrons in its *M*-shell and thus stability (see Fig. 15.2). Such electron bonds are known as *covalent bonds* and the electrons are termed *valence electrons* and inhabit the valence energy band of the atom. The covalent bonds give the crystal its regularity by inhibiting the movement of any particular atom. At room temperature, these bonds are being continuously broken and reformed as some of the valence electrons are gaining sufficient energy to reach the conduction band (bond broken) and electrons from the conduction band fall back into the valence band (bond reformed). The eight-electron configuration of the *M*-shell behaves like a full shell and so the valence band is effectively full until an electron moves up to the conduction band. As previously explained, when this happens, electron flow in the conduction band and positive-hole flow in the valence band are both possible.

Intrinsic semiconductors, which we just considered, have very limited practical use, due to their low conductivity. If small amounts of specific impurities are added to them (by a process called *doping*), they are then known as *extrinsic semiconductors* and have properties which allow

us to use them as rectifiers and integrated circuits (ICs), all of which are found in most X-ray generators. Extrinsic semiconductors will now be discussed.

15.4 EXTRINSIC SEMICONDUCTORS

The addition of small amounts of specific impurities to silicon or germanium is the basis on which most extrinsic semiconductors are produced. The doping may be heavy or light, depending on the component being produced. A typical concentration is one part of impurity to 10 million parts of pure silicon. The electrical conductivity of the extrinsic semiconductor is much greater than that of an intrinsic semiconductor and the level of conductivity can be controlled by altering the ratio of doping material to pure material. The impurity atoms within the silicon crystal lattice are the source of this greatly increased electrical conductivity. This is because the type of impurity is chosen either to enhance electron flow in the conduction band (this gives an *N*-type semiconductor) or to enhance the flow of positive holes in the valence band (a *P*-type semiconductor). These two types of extrinsic semiconductor will now be considered.

15.4.1 *N*-type semiconductors

As we have seen, single atoms of intrinsic semiconductors have four valence electrons. To produce an *N*-type extrinsic semiconductor, a *pentavalent impurity* (one with five valence electrons) is used as the doping material. Arsenic, antimony and phosphorus are examples of pentavalent elements that are suitable. Figure 15.3 (See page 96) illustrates the effect of introducing an atom of phosphorus into the crystalline structure of silicon. Four of the valence electrons in the phosphorus form covalent bonds and the fifth electron is unbonded. This electron has an energy level which is just below the bottom of the conduction band (see Fig. 15.3B). At normal room temperatures, it is therefore virtually a free electron since it is easily lifted into the conduction band and can take part in electrical conduction if a potential difference is applied across the crystal.

Since such pentavalent atoms provide a 'spare' electron, they are known as *donor impurities*. It must be remembered that some electrons from the valence band will also be able to jump into the conduction band due to the normal vibrational energy within the atom at room temperature (this is similar to the intrinsic semiconductor; see Sect. 15.3). Positive holes will also be produced in the valence band and add to the conductivity. At normal room temperatures, this effect is much less than the effect produced by the donor atoms. In the case of an *N*-type semiconductor, the *majority carriers* are the electrons in the conduction band and the *minority carriers* are the holes in the valence band.

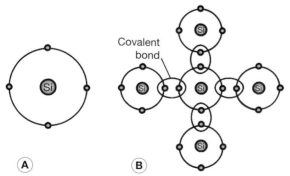

Figure 15.2 Pure silicon as an example of an intrinsic semiconductor. (A) A silicon atom showing the four electrons in its valence shell; (B) the covalent bonds formed in a pure silicon crystal by each silicon atom sharing electrons with four neighbouring silicon atoms.

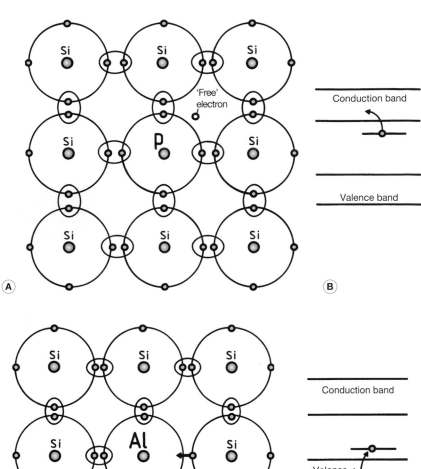

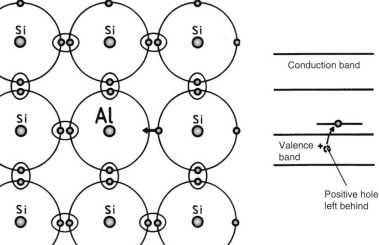

Figure 15.3 An example of an N-type extrinsic semiconductor. (A) The introduction of a pentavalent impurity produces a 'free' electron which does not take part in the covalent bond formation; (B) the energy of such free electrons is close to the conduction band so that they can readily be enabled to take part in electrical conduction.

Figure 15.4 An example of a P-type extrinsic semiconductor. (A) The addition of a trivalent impurity produces a 'hole' in the outside electron shell; (B) such acceptor atoms take an electron from the valence band, leaving a positive hole capable of flowing through this band.

15.4.2 P-type semiconductors

As discussed in the previous section, the N-type semiconductor has enhanced conductivity because of the movement of electrons (negative, hence the N) so it is logical to assume that the P-type semiconductor functions because of the movement of positive holes. In the case of intrinsic semiconductors, we saw that holes were in the valence band, and that this allowed the movement of electrons within this band, giving the appearance of positive-hole movement (see previous Insight). In the P-type semiconductor, the movement of electrons within the valence band is encouraged by the creation of more positive holes within this band.

Figure 15.4 illustrates the result of introducing a trivalent material (one with three valence electrons) into a silicon crystal lattice. The material used in this case is aluminium, and it results in a broken covalent bond between it and the silicon atoms as there are not sufficient electrons in its outer shell to form the four covalent bonds. The energy level of this broken bond is only just above the valence band (Fig. 15.4B) and so, at normal room temperatures, electrons have sufficient energy to leap this small gap. Thus, the electrons, which have left the valence band of the silicon, leave positive holes behind them and so there is an increase in the number of positive holes in the valence band because of the trivalent impurity. This type of impurity

Table 15.1 Summary of the properties of semiconductors

	INTRINSIC SEMICONDUCTOR	EXTRINSIC SEMICONDUCTOR	
Typical material	Pure silicon or germanium	Silicon or germanium with added impurities	
Type of impurity	None	Pentavalent	Trivalent
Term for impurity	–	Donor	Acceptor
Conductivity	Low	High	High
Majority carrier	Electrons and positive holes in equal numbers	Electrons in conduction band	Positive holes in valence band
Minority carrier	–	Positive holes in valence band	Electrons in conduction band
Effect of temperature	Increases both the number of electrons and the number of positive holes	Increases number of minority carriers (positive holes) only	Increases number of minority carriers (electrons) only

is known as an *acceptor impurity* since it accepts electrons from the silicon atoms, creating holes in the valence band.

The *majority carriers* in the P-type material are positive holes in the valence band and the *minority carriers* are electrons that have sufficient energy to rise to the conduction band at room temperature, as in pure silicon (see Sect. 15.3.2).

Table 15.1 summarizes the main points we have considered so far regarding intrinsic semiconductors and the N-type and P-type of extrinsic semiconductor. Note that an increase in temperature does not affect the conductivity due to the majority carriers, but only that due to minority carriers. This is due to the increased numbers of electrons able to reach the conduction band from the valence band as the temperature increases.

15.4.3 Diagrammatic representation of *N*- and *P*-types

When we discuss the *PN* junction in the next section, we need to form a mental picture of what occurs when an N-type and a P-type semiconductor are fused together. This is made easier if we have a simple symbolic representation of each, as shown in Figure 15.5. In the N-type, the majority carriers are the free donor electrons, represented by the minus (−) sign. Each nucleus of the donor impurity has an excess positive charge because of the loss of its outer electron. These fixed positive charges are represented by the circles enclosing the + sign. In the P-type, the positive holes are free and so are shown as a plus (+) sign while the electrons captured by acceptor atoms give these an overall negative charge. Since these atoms form part of the crystal lattice, they are not free to move so the minus sign is shown enclosed in the circles. Thus,

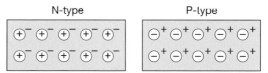

Figure 15.5 A diagrammatic representation of *N*- and *P*-type semiconductors. In both illustrations the ringed charges represent the fixed charges while the unringed charges represent the free charges which form the majority carriers (electrons for the N-type and positive holes for the P-type).

in both the diagrams the ringed charges are fixed and the unringed charges are free or mobile.

Note that in both the diagrams there are minority carriers caused by the elevation of electrons from the valence band to the conduction band. Since these play little part in the electrical properties of the material, they have been omitted from the diagrams for simplicity.

Before considering the *PN* junction in the following section in which the *PN* junction is discussed as a rectifier, let us first remember that the term *diode* applies to any two-electrode electrical device. The X-ray tube is an example of a thermionic diode as it has two electrodes – an anode and a cathode. Other examples of solid-state diodes used in radiography are light-emitting diodes (LEDs), which have replaced bulbs as indicators. LEDs operate in a forward-bias mode (see Sect. 15.5.2), while the photodiode is a semiconductor diode which converts light into electrical current in a reverse-bias mode (see Sect. 15.5.3), and has replaced the photo-multiplier valve in many applications where its smaller size, low power consumption and high current output are important, e.g. computed tomography (CT) scanners.

15.5 THE *PN* JUNCTION

When *P*- and *N*-types are heat-fused together to form *PN* junctions, interesting effects appear. Examples of the *PN* junction include the junction diode, the transistor and the thyristor, which have one, two and three *PN* junctions respectively.

If we use the diagrammatic representation that we have just discussed, then the *PN* junction may be shown as in Figure 15.6. When *P*- and *N*-types are brought together and heat-fused in intimate contact, free electrons from the *N*-type and free positive holes from the *P*-type are able to penetrate across the boundary between them. This diffusion of charge across the barrier results in recombination of the positive holes and the free electrons (the free electrons drop into the positive holes so that their charges are cancelled; see Sect. 15.3.1). Thus, for a short distance on either side of the *PN* junction (about 0.5×10^{-6} m), no free carriers exist – this is known as *a depletion layer*. However, a net charge exists on either side of the junction because the *N*-type has lost electrons and the *P*-type has lost positive holes (Fig. 15.6B), resulting in a negatively charged area just within the *P*-type region and a positively charged area just within the *N*-type region. The two peaks of charge shown in Figure 15.6 increase in size until no further net flow of majority carriers takes place. For example, a free electron from the *N*-type will only be able to pass over to the *P*-type if it has sufficient energy to overcome the repulsion of the negative peak at the *PN* junction.

The charge distribution produces its own potential difference, as depicted in Figure 15.6C. The height of *CD* is known as the potential barrier since it acts in opposition to the flow of majority carriers from either side of the barrier. For a silicon *PN* junction, this potential barrier is about 0.4 eV, so free carriers of energy lower than 0.4 eV cannot overcome this barrier.

15.5.1 Minority carriers at the *PN* junction

The above discussion concerned only the effect of the *PN* junction on the majority carriers. For majority carriers, a potential barrier is formed which prevents any further flow. However, this barrier actually aids the transport of minority carriers between the materials. Consider the potential gradient between *D* and *C* (Fig. 15.6). If a free electron (the minority carrier in a *P*-type material) is in position *D*, it is strongly attracted by the positive potential of the *N*-type material and rapidly moves to *C*. At equilibrium, of course, there are equal numbers of minority carriers moving in both directions.

Minority carriers are dependent on temperature, since an increase in temperature increases the number of electrons which can jump from the valence to the conduction band. Thus, *the flow of minority carriers across a PN junction increases with temperature*. This affects the behaviour of the *PN* junction under conditions of reverse bias, as will be explained later in this chapter.

15.5.2 Forward bias

If a source of potential difference (e.g. a battery) is connected across a *PN* junction, as shown in Figure 15.7A,

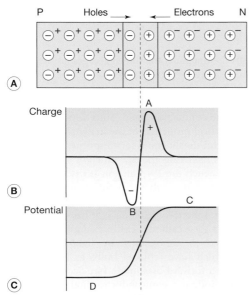

Figure 15.6 The *PN* junction. (A) The diffusion of electrons across the *PN* junction in one direction and positive holes in the other forms a charge barrier, which prevents further flow. (B) Gain in charge across the junction and (C) potential difference established across the barrier.

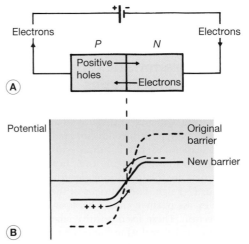

Figure 15.7 (A) The *PN* junction connected in forward bias. The potential from the battery lowers the potential barrier and allows current to flow across the junction. (B) The position of the barrier before connection into the circuit and after the device is connected, as shown in (A).

then a current will flow across the junction because the potential barrier is lowered. This is shown graphically in Figure 15.7B (See page 98). The negative side of the battery reduces the positive potential of the N-type and the positive side of the battery reduces the negative potential of the P-type. The original height of the barrier is lowered and energetic free carriers from either side are able to surmount the barrier. A steady electrical current is set up as long as the battery is connected. This type of connection, which produces current flow across the PN junction, is called forward bias. The removal of the battery results in the full height of the barrier being re-established and so no further current can flow.

15.5.3 Reverse bias

If the source of potential difference is now connected in the opposite orientation, as shown in Figure 15.8A, then this is known as *reverse bias*. No current flows through this circuit due to the increase in the potential barrier at the PN junction. The graph in Figure 15.8B shows that the negative side of the battery increases the negative potential of the P-type and the positive side of the battery increases the positive potential of the N-type. Thus, no current flows, as none of the majority carriers has sufficient energy to surmount this higher barrier. In fact, when a PN junction is connected in reverse bias, the depletion layer extends further into each semiconductor on either side of the PN junction.

The discussion so far has been regarding majority carriers. However, as discussed earlier, a small electrical current due to the thermally generated minority carriers is able to flow.

The PN junction can act as a one-way valve (a diode) which allows current only to *flow* in one direction. For this reason, PN junctions are used to create *solid-state rectifiers* or PN *junction diodes*. The symbol for such a device is shown below.

15.5.4 The *PN* junction as a diode

In our discussion in the last two sections we have shown that current will readily flow through a PN junction when it is forward biased, but very little current will flow through the junction when it is reverse biased. Thus, the PN junction can act as a one-way valve (a diode) allowing current to flow in only one direction. For this reason, PN junctions are used to create *solid-state rectifiers* or PN junction diodes. The symbol for such a device is:

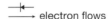 electron flows

Note that electrons may only flow through the diode against the direction of the arrow or bar of the symbol. Such devices have replaced thermionic diodes for the following reasons:

- They contain no filament and thus have a longer life, consume less power and produce less heat.
- They are smaller in size than thermionic diodes, thus enabling the production of a more compact X-ray unit.
- They have a smaller forward voltage drop than thermionic rectifiers and are more efficient rectifiers enabling a higher kVp to be applied to the X-ray tube (see Ch. 30).

15.5.5 PN Junction characteristics

If the current flowing through a PN junction is plotted against the potential difference across it, then the graph produced is referred to as the characteristic curve for the device. Such a graph is shown in Figure 15.9. As the potential difference across the diode is increased in a forward direction, so the current through it increases, as shown by OA on the figure. If we compare this with the forward-bias characteristic for the vacuum diode, we can note that, in this case, there is no saturation current. However, passing too high a current through a PN junction diode can cause irreparable damage.

A normal reverse bias produces only a very low reverse current due to the flow of minority carriers that happen to move into the vicinity of the PN junction and so get swept across it. As already discussed, this reverse current is very sensitive to temperature as this alters the production of minority carriers due to thermal excitation. If the reverse bias is further increased, then the reverse current increases dramatically (see BC in Figure 15.9 (See page 100)). This is called the *zener voltage* or *breakdown voltage* and at this

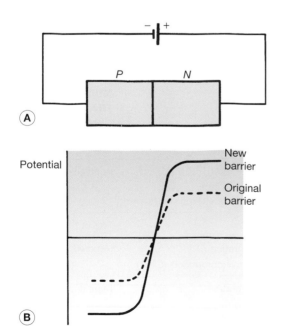

Figure 15.8 (A) The *PN* junction connected in reverse bias. The potential from the battery raises the potential barrier, as shown in (B), and further prevents electrical conduction.

value of reverse bias the diode ceases to act effectively as a rectifier. At this negative bias, the minority carriers that cross the potential barrier gain enough energy to ionize atoms with which they collide. This results in the liberation of additional electrons and hence the large current. This phenomenon is also referred to as *solid-state multiplication* or *electron avalanching*.

A *zener diode* is a type of diode that permits current not only in the forward direction like a normal diode, but also in the reverse direction if the voltage across it is larger than the breakdown voltage. This is known as *zener knee voltage* or *zener voltage*. The zenner diode acts as a protective device by limiting the output voltage to components on its output side while the zenner voltage is passed to earth.

15.6 INTEGRATED CIRCUITS

This section gives an overview of the history and production of a 'typical' integrated circuit (IC). The concept of the IC was proposed by Godffrey Dummer of the Royal Radar Establishment of the British Ministry of Defenses in 1952, although the first working ICs were not produced until 1959 by two Americans. By current standards these circuits were very crude as they contained many discrete components such as miniaturized transistors, resistors and capacitors. By the early 1960s, extensive use of semiconductors had replaced many circuits which had previously used thermionic valves.

As technology improved, the number of components on ICs or 'chips' increased leading to dedicated chips such as counters, adders and amplifier chips. ICs of this type are still available and used in some applications today.

15.6.1 The development of ICs

Table 15.2 gives a brief outline of the development of the integrated circuit. For more details, the reader is advised to consult specialized texts on integrated circuits.

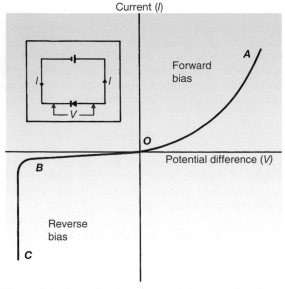

Figure 15.9 The *PN* junction characteristic. For explanation, see text.

Table 15.2 The development of the integrated circuit

YEAR PRODUCED	ABBREVIATION	NAME/FEATURES	NUMBER OF TRANSISTORS IN CIRCUIT
Early 1960s	SSI	Small scale integration	Tens
Late 1960s	MSI	Medium scale integration Resistors, capacitors and inductances added to wafer as part of etching stages	Hundreds
1970s	LSI	large scale integration	Tens of thousands
1980s	VLSI	Very large scale integration Possible to produce microprocessors (CPUs)	Hundreds of thousands
Early 1990s	ULSI	Ultra large scale integration Increased CPU speeds	More than a million
Late 1990s	ULSI	Ultra large scale integration dual core processors Increased CPU speeds	Hundreds of millions

15.6.2 The manufacturing process

Hundreds of ICs are made at the same time on a single, thin slice of silicon and are then cut apart into individual IC chips. The manufacturing process takes place in a tightly controlled environment known as a clean room. Since some IC components are sensitive to certain frequencies of light, even the light sources are filtered.

Manufacturing processes vary depending on the integrated circuit being made. The following process is typical. The process commences with a chemically pure cylindrical ingot of silicon about 100 mm in diameter, and then thin, round wafers of silicon are cut off the ingot by a wafer slicer. Each wafer is about 0.1 mm thick. The surface on which the integrated circuits are to be formed is polished. The surfaces of the wafer are then coated with a layer of silicon dioxide to form an insulating base and to prevent any oxidation of the silicon which would cause impurities.

15.6.2.1 Masking

The complex and interconnected design of the circuit components is prepared in a process similar to that used to make printed circuit boards. For ICs, however, the dimensions are much smaller and there are many layers superimposed on top of each other. These layers can contain components such as resistors, capacitors and inductances. The design of each layer is prepared on a computer-aided drafting machine, and the image is made into a mask which will be optically reduced and transferred to the surface of the wafer. Each layer has its own mask which is opaque in certain areas and clear in others. It has the images for all of the several hundred integrated circuits to be formed on the wafer.

The wafer is first coated with a layer of photo-resist and is then baked to remove the solvent. It is then irradiated with light. Because the spaces between circuits and components are so small, ultraviolet light, which has a very short wavelength, is used as it can pass through the tiny clear areas on the mask. Beams of electrons or X-rays are also sometimes used to irradiate the photo-resist. The layer is the subjected to chemical etching which 'opens' the clear areas of the mask and the first doping process is carried out to create a layer of P- or N-regions.

15.6.2.2 Doping

Two methods of doping may be used:

1. Atomic diffusion is a method of adding dopants to create a layer of P- or N-regions. In this method, a batch of wafers is placed in a quartz tube oven surrounded by a heating element. Here the wafer is exposed to a temperature between 1816 and 1205 °C; the dopant chemical is then carried in on an inert gas. As the gas passes over the wafers, the dopant is deposited on the hot surfaces left exposed by the masking process. This method is suited to doping relatively large areas, but is not accurate for smaller areas. There are also some problems with the repeated use of high temperatures as successive layers are added.

2. The second method to add dopants is ion implantation. In this method, a dopant gas, such as phosphune or boron trichloride, is ionized to provide a beam of high-energy dopant ions which are fired at specific regions of the wafer. These ions penetrate the wafer and remain implanted. The depth of penetration can be controlled by altering the beam energy, and the amount of dopant can be controlled by altering the beam current and time of exposure. Schematically, the whole process resembles firing a beam in a bent cathode ray tube. This method is so precise that it does not require masking – just point and shoot the dopant where it is needed. However, it is much slower than the atomic diffusion process.

15.6.3 Making successive layers

The existing layer of photo-resist is removed, and another layer of photo-resist is added for the next layer. The process of etching or doping is repeated. Sometimes a layer of silicon dioxide is laid down to provide an insulator between layers or components. The etching and doping process continues for each successive layer until all of the layers are completed. A final silicon dioxide layer seals the surface, and final etching opens up contact points, when a layer of aluminum is deposited to make the contact pads. At this point, the individual ICs are tested for electrical function and any chips failing the test are identified.

15.6.4 Making individual ICs

The thin wafer is like a piece of glass. The hundreds of individual chips are separated by scoring a cross-hatch of lines with a fine diamond cutter on the wafer and then putting it under stress to cause each chip to separate. Those ICs that fail the electrical test are discarded. Further inspection under a microscope reveals chips damaged by the separation process; all faulty chips are then discarded.

The good ICs are individually bonded into their mounting package and the thin wire leads are connected by either ultrasonic bonding or thermocompression. The mounting package is marked with identifying part numbers and other information.

Finally the completed ICs are sealed in antistatic plastic bags to be stored or shipped to the end user.

15.6.5 Hazardous materials and recycling

The dopant substances used – gallium and arsenic among others – are toxic, and their storage, use and disposal must be tightly controlled.

Table 15.3 Applications of semiconductor devices

SEMICONDUCTOR DEVICE	APPLICATIONS
Solid-state diode	Rectification of the high-tension supply to the X-ray tube using multiple *PN* junctions connected in series to form stick rectifiers Rectification of the supply to devices that require a unidirectional supply, e.g. solid-state 'chips'
Transistors	Electronic timing circuits Safety interlocks that avoid exceeding the rating of the X-ray tube
Triacs	Primary switching of the X-ray exposure, i.e. the triac switches the exposure on and off – following the signal from the timer
Integrated circuits (ICs)	ICs have replaced many semiconductor devices, with the exception of HT diodes These can check that a number of functions have taken place in sequence, e.g. they can check that the anode is rotating at the correct speed before an exposure is made
Microprocessors	These have many applications in more sophisticated measurement and controls, e.g. microprocessors can check a certain set of exposure factors to ensure that they are not outside the rating of the selected tube focus

Because IC chips are so versatile, a significant recycling industry has sprung up. Many ICs and other electronic components are removed from otherwise obsolete equipment, tested and resold for use in other devices.

15.6.6 The future

It is difficult to tell with any certainty what the future of the IC is. Changes in technology since the device's invention have been rapid, but evolutionary. Many changes have been made in the architecture, or circuit layout, on a chip, but the IC still remains a silicon-based design.

The next major leap in the advancement of electronic devices (if such a leap is to come) may involve an entirely new circuit technology. Better devices than the very best microprocessor have always been known to be possible. The human brain, for example, processes information much more efficiently than any computer, and some futurists have speculated that the next generation of processor circuits will be biological rather than mineral. At this point in time, such matters are the stuff of fiction. There are no immediate signs that the IC is in any danger of extinction.

15.7 SEMICONDUCTOR DEVICES IN RADIOGRAPHY

Semiconductor devices are used extensively in radiography. This chapter has given a brief overview of some of the types that are used. The development of ICs in the 1960s resulted in the production of complete miniaturized circuits which now perform many of the functions previously carried out by discrete solid-state or by ICs. ICs are produced on a single chip of silicon about 1 mm square and about 0.1 mm thick. This process, using ULSI, is able to produce circuits containing in excess of over 100 million transistors per chip. This technology offers components of very high reliability at very low production costs. There is also significant space saving over electromechanical devices. Both of the above have resulted in many of the circuits in modern X-ray generators containing significant amounts of 'chip technology'.

The microprocessor is another development based on silicon chip and ULSI technology. Using Boolean logic and inbuilt programs, microprocessors are used to monitor and control many pieces of equipment used in radiography.

The full description of the function of such ICs is the subject of a book in its own right and as such is beyond the short introduction in this text.

Table 15.3 outlines some of the applications of semiconductor technology in radiography

Summary

In this chapter, you should have learnt the following:
- A semiconductor has a conductivity between that of an insulator and a conductor, reflecting the small energy gap between the conduction and the valence bands (see Sect. 15.3).
- An intrinsic semiconductor, such as silicon, is a chemically pure semiconductor with a regular arrangement of atoms within its crystal lattice (see Sects 15.3 and 15.3.2).

- Extrinsic semiconductors have carefully measured quantities of impurity added to the intrinsic semiconductor by a process known as doping (see Sect. 15.4).
- An *N*-type semiconductor is produced when a pentavalent or donor impurity is added to the silicon. This gives a supply of free electrons in the semiconductor (see Sect. 15.4.1).
- A *P*-type semiconductor is produced when a trivalent or acceptor impurity is added to the silicon. This gives a supply of positive holes within the semiconductor (see Sect. 15.4.2).
- The majority carrier in the *N*-type material is the free electron and the majority carrier in the *P*-type is the free positive hole (see Sects 15.4.1 and 15.4.2).
- Minority carriers are thermally produced and are present in all types of semiconductor at room temperature. Minority carriers in the *N*-type are positive holes and in the *P*-type are free electrons (see Sects 15.4.1 and 15.4.2).
- A *PN* junction produces a potential barrier to the flow of electrons and holes. The height of this barrier grows when the junction is reverse biased and diminishes when the junction is forward biased. Thus the *PN* junction will allow current to flow in one direction only – electrons can flow from *N* to *P* (see Sect. 15.5).
- The development and production of integrated circuits (see Sect. 15.6).
- Some of the applications of semiconductor devices in radiography (see Sect. 15.7).

FURTHER READING

Ball, J.L., Moore, A.D., Turner, S., 2008. Ball and Moore's Essential Physics for Radiographers, fourth ed. Blackwell Scientific, London (Chapter 13).

Braithwaite, N., Weaver, G. (Eds.), 1990. Electronic Materials. Butterworth, Boston.

Part $|$ 3 $|$

Atomic physics

Chapter | 16 |

The laws of modern physics

16.1 AIM

The aim of this chapter is to introduce the reader to the laws of modern physics. In many cases these are refinements or extensions to the laws of classical physics which were discussed in Chapter 3, and in this chapter reference will be made to the laws outlined in Chapter 3. In other areas, there is disagreement between the classical and the modern laws and these will be identified and discussed.

16.2 INTRODUCTION

The laws of classical physics were discussed in Chapter 3 and these have been sufficient to explain the phenomena outlined in previous chapters of this text. In the following chapters on atomic and radiation physics, some important aspects of modern physics must be introduced in order to explain many of the phenomena discussed. The purpose of this chapter is to describe the laws of modern physics which are relevant to our need in the rest of the text.

16.3 CLASSICAL VERSUS MODERN LAWS

Modern physics started at the turn of the twentieth century with *Planck's quantum hypothesis* in 1900 in which he conjectured that radiation energy could only be absorbed or emitted by a body at discrete values of energy. Other dates of interest to the rest of this text include the *mass–energy* relationship postulated by Einstein in 1905, the *Bohr model of the atom* which was suggested in 1913 and the *de Broglie wavelength of particles* which was introduced in 1924. Since these dates, there have been major technical and theoretical strides, but these form part of the firm experimental foundation upon which modern physics is built.

One of the essential differences between classical and modern physics is the way in which matter is regarded. In classical physics, matter and energy are completely separate entities and so we have the *law of conservation of matter* (see Sect. 3.2) and the *law of conservation of energy* (see Sect. 3.3) with no interconnection being produced between the two laws. In classical physics, matter is supposed to behave in one way – like matter! – and waves are supposed to behave like waves, and one cannot behave like the other; classical physics does not allow for the existence of a particle with a wavelength. There are no such rigid boundaries in modern physics. In particular, the work of Einstein showed that matter can be thought of as being interchangeable with energy if the conditions are right. This principle is known as *mass–energy equivalence* and will be discussed in more detail later in this chapter (see Sect. 16.4.1). In addition, it is found in modern physics that particles of matter do behave like waves and vice versa and this is known as the *wave–particle duality principle* (see Sect. 16.6). In this way, an X-ray beam may be considered as photons (particles) which have a specific energy and so can liberate electrons from atoms of the materials they pass through.

With these concepts in mind, we will now consider the laws of modern physics in more detail in the remainder of this chapter.

16.4 LAW OF CONSERVATION OF ENERGY

This law now states that the *amount of energy in a system is constant*. In the context of modern physics, this can be thought of as the sum of all the energies (rest energies + kinetic energies + potential energies) being a constant for any given system. The phrase 'a system' can be used to define either a very small or a very large area, provided the influence of other bodies outside the system is negligibly small. In the context of modern physics, the use of the term *energy* in the above law embraces the contribution of matter to the total energy of a system under consideration. This concept of mass–energy equivalence will now be discussed.

16.4.1 Mass–energy equivalence

Einstein showed that the mass of a body, m, and its energy, E (excluding potential energy), are related by the formula:

Equation 16.1

$$E = mc^2$$

where c is the velocity of electromagnetic radiation (often referred to as the velocity of light, as light is probably the best known form of electromagnetic radiation). Since c is a constant, the energy of a body is proportional to its mass (and vice versa). If we consider a stationary body with a rest mass, m_0, then the rest energy of this body is given by $E_0 = m_0c^2$. If we now consider this body travelling with a velocity, V, then its energy is now E_V and Einstein's equation is $E_V = m_Vc^2$. Since the energy of the body when moving, E_V, is greater than the energy of the body when at rest, E_0, and since c is a constant, then m_V must be greater than m_0 – a body increases in mass as its velocity increases. The above statement seems to contradict our common experiences (because of the small values of velocity which we can normally produce) but if we take particles and accelerate them until they travel with a velocity close to the velocity of light (3×10^8 m.s^{-1}) then there is a measurable increase in the mass of the particles. The mass which they then possess is known as the *relativistic mass* of the particles. Thus, if we take a car which is travelling at 40 kilometres per hour, we see no measurable increase in its mass, but if we take electrons travelling at high speeds in a linear accelerator then there is a measurable increase in their mass.

The law of conservation of energy, stated earlier, is sometimes referred to as the law of conservation of *mass–energy* because of the concept of equivalence between mass and energy. It is also not uncommon to quote the *rest mass* of subatomic particles, either in units of mass or in units of energy – the rest mass of the electron can be stated as 9.1×10^{-31} kg (mass) or 0.511 MeV (energy).

As we can see from the above discussion, energy and mass can be considered as two manifestations of the same thing, and may be changed from one form to the other in appropriate circumstances, as the following examples show:

- The forces which hold the atomic nucleus together are obtained because some of the mass of the nuclear particles is converted into energy. Because of this, the mass of the nucleus is less than the sum of the masses of the individual nuclear particles.
- If a gamma-ray has an energy greater than 1.02 MeV and passes close to the nucleus of an atom, the ray may spontaneously disappear and create two particles of matter – an electron and a positron. This process is known as *pair production* and will be described in more detail in Chapter 23. The positron created in this interaction will interact with an electron and their mass will be converted into two photons of radiation, each photon having an energy of 0.51 MeV. The positron and the electron will now cease to exist and the radiation is referred to as *annihilation radiation*. The positron can thus be regarded as the antiparticle of the electron. This interaction shows that energy can be converted into mass and that mass can be converted into energy.

16.5 LAW OF CONSERVATION OF MOMENTUM

This law may be stated as the total linear momentum in a system is constant. The word 'system' is used in the same context as for the law of conservation of energy. As we discussed in the section dealing with the laws of classical physics, the momentum of a body is the product of its mass and its velocity. Thus we can say:

sum of all (mass × velocity) = constant for a system

Here, the mass referred to in the equation is the relativistic mass of the body, i.e. its mass when it is moving with the velocity, V. An example of the law of conservation of momentum being applied to modern physics is in Compton scattering (see Ch. 23) when some of the momentum of the incoming photon is given to an electron – the combined momentum of the scattered photon and the ejected electron is the same as the momentum of the incident photon.

16.6 WAVE–PARTICLE DUALITY

Duality simply means two different features of the same thing. As we have just seen, modern physics regards mass and energy as being two manifestations of the same phenomenon. Similarly, modern physics blurs the distinction which exists in classical physics between a particle and a wave.

16.6.1 Waves as particles

Classical physics was very successful in explaining many of the phenomena associated with electromagnetic radiation (e.g. diffraction and interference) by assuming that such radiation was made up of waves travelling at the velocity of light, c. In this case $c = v\lambda$, where v is the frequency of vibration of the radiation and λ is its wavelength. However, phenomena like the Compton effect and photoelectric absorption (both will be discussed in detail in Ch. 23) are not easy to explain using the wave theory. These effects are explained by considering that sometimes electromagnetic radiation behaves as 'packets' of energy which have an associated momentum. Such a packet of energy is called a photon or a quantum and the quantum theory predicts that:

- the quantum will have an energy, E, given by:

Equation 16.2

$$E = hv$$

where h is a constant known as Planck's constant and v is the frequency of vibration of the associated wave. We will frequently use this formula in the chapters which follow on atomic physics!

- the quantum will have a momentum, p, given by:

Equation 16.3

$$p = \frac{hv}{c}$$

The electromagnetic wave may also behave like a particle, possessing energy and momentum.

16.6.2 Particles as waves

Moving particles of matter, whether these are large or very small, have both kinetic energy and momentum. Are there then occasions when they behave as waves? Perhaps the most dramatic example of particles behaving like waves is in the operation of the electron microscope. Here high-energy electrons are passed through or are scattered by a sample. A very highly magnified image of the sample is obtained so that individual large molecules may be seen in materials. The reason for the high degree of magnification is due to the very small wavelength of the electrons. Whether we consider an optical microscope or an electron microscope, the smaller the wavelength of the radiation used, the finer the detail it is possible to see.

De Broglie proposed that the following relationship exists between the momentum, p, of the particle and its associated wavelength, λ:

Equation 16.4

$$p = \frac{h}{\lambda}$$

In such cases, λ is called the *de Broglie wavelength* and the existence of particles behaving like waves can be verified by a number of experiments.

Note the *inverse* relationship between the momentum of the particle and its associated wavelength. The wavelength decreases as the momentum increases and vice versa. For example, the de Broglie wavelength associated with an electron moving at half the velocity of light is about 4×10^{-12} m which is less than the diameter of the hydrogen atom (100×10^{-12} m). When the velocity of the electron is one-hundredth of that of light then the de Broglie wavelength is at the larger value of 240×10^{-12} m, which is now in the X-ray range of wavelengths (see Ch. 17) and so such electrons can be used for X-ray crystallography.

Within the context of radiographic science, it is more common to consider waves behaving as quanta rather than quanta behaving as waves. This is particularly true when we consider the production of X-rays (see Ch. 21) and the interactions of X-rays with matter (see Ch. 23).

16.7 HEISENBERG'S UNCERTAINTY PRINCIPLE

In classical physics it is *possible in principle* to measure exactly a number of quantities concerning the state of a body, e.g. the body's energy, position, and momentum. Furthermore, if it were possible to build measuring apparatus which was infinitely precise, it would be possible to make *simultaneous exact measurements* of several of these quantities.

According to modern physics, it is not possible to treat quantities like mass and energy or matter and waves as being totally independent of each other. *Heisenberg's uncertainty principle* is an extension of the principle of wave–particle duality and concerns the maximum possible precision which may be obtained in ideal circumstances when measuring two quantities simultaneously. The central point of the principle is that *measuring one quantity affects another quantity* so that it is never possible to measure both quantities simultaneously with complete accuracy – if we try to measure the momentum of a particle, this will automatically affect the position of the particle so that it is never possible to measure momentum and position simultaneously with complete accuracy. Effects due to this principle are too small to be observed in everyday life and concern atomic and nuclear systems. This principle is yet another difference between modern and classical physics – in classical physics, it is assumed that perfect instruments produce perfect results.

If we now apply Heisenberg's uncertainty principle to the duality theory, we can say that, although we can demonstrate that waves can behave like particles and that particles can behave like waves, it is not possible to set up a situation where both properties are demonstrated *simultaneously*.

Summary

In this chapter you should have learnt the following:
- The differences which exist between the laws of classical physics and the laws of modern physics (see Sect. 16.3).
- The law of conservation of energy as applied to modern physics (see Sect. 16.4).
- The concept of mass–energy equivalence (see Sect. 16.4.1).
- The law of conservation of momentum as applied to modern physics (see Sect. 16.5).
- The concept of wave–particle duality (see Sect. 16.6).
- The concept that waves may behave as particles and that particles may behave as waves, with examples of each situation (see Sects 16.6.1 and 16.6.2).
- A brief outline of Heisenberg's uncertainty principle (see Sect. 16.7).

FURTHER READING

You may find Chapter 17 of this text and chapters from the following text provide useful further reading.

Ball, J.L., Moore, A.D., Turner, S., 2008. Ball and Moore's Essential Physics for Radiographers, fourth ed. Blackwell Scientific, London (Chapters 14 and 15).

Chapter | 17 |

Electromagnetic radiation

17.1 AIM

This chapter discusses the properties of electromagnetic radiations. The wave–particle duality of such radiations will be further discussed. Having identified the contents of the electromagnetic spectrum, we will finally consider some parts of this spectrum in more detail as these are of particular relevance to radiography.

17.2 INTRODUCTION

As can be seen from Figure 17.3 (p. 114), the electromagnetic spectrum encompasses a wide range of radiation types and we are only sensitive to a small section of these radiations. We can see the world around us because the retinas of our eyes are sensitive to a section of the electromagnetic spectrum which we know as light. Similarly, we can feel heat from the sun because our skin responds to the infrared part of the electromagnetic spectrum. We can also accidentally walk through a beam of X-rays or handle an isotope which is producing gamma radiation because none of our sense organs are able to detect them. It is important to remember, when we consider radiation protection, that although our sense organs are not able to detect the presence of ionizing radiations (X or gamma), they may still be damaged by them.

17.3 PROPERTIES OF ELECTROMAGNETIC RADIATIONS

All electromagnetic radiations exhibit a set of general properties which are listed below:

- The waves are composed of transverse vibrations of electric and magnetic fields. (Transverse vibrations are ones which are oscillating at right angles to the direction of travel.)
- The vibrations have a wide range of wavelengths and frequencies.
- All electromagnetic radiations travel through a vacuum with the same velocity: $3 \times 10^8 \, \mathrm{m.s^{-1}}$.
- All electromagnetic radiations travel in straight lines.
- The radiations are unaffected by electric or magnetic fields.
- The radiations may be polarized so that they vibrate in one plane only.
- The radiations are able to produce constructive or destructive interference.
- All the radiations obey the duality principle (see Sect. 16.6) and so can either be considered as waves or as quanta with energy and momentum.

Table 17.1 Interactions of different electromagnetic radiations with matter

INTERACTION	NOTES
Emission	All bodies will emit electromagnetic radiation in certain circumstances but the most efficient emission is from a 'black body' (see Sect. 5.4.3.1)
Reflection	Reflection of electromagnetic radiation is not possible for the higher energy radiations (X and gamma radiation)
Refraction	Refraction of electromagnetic radiation is not possible for the higher energy radiations (X and gamma radiation)
Transmission	Different materials are transparent to different wavelengths or photon energies
Attenuation	Different attenuation processes are possible depending on the photon energy of the radiation but, if the photons all have the same energy, the attenuation is always exponential. Photoelectric absorption can occur from ultraviolet to gamma radiations. Compton scattering is produced by X and gamma radiations. Pair production is an attenuation process which is possible if the photon energies are higher than 1.02 MeV
Luminescence – fluorescence and phosphorescence	Electron transitions within the material being irradiated cause the emission of photons that have less energy than the incident radiation. A single photon of incident radiation can produce many fluorescent photons

From the above list it is obvious that all electromagnetic radiations have a lot in common, so how can they be used for such widely differing purposes? The answer to this lies in the differences which they exhibit in their interactions with matter. These are outlined in Table 17.1.

As discussed in Chapter 16, there is a wave–particle duality which exists when electromagnetic radiation interacts with matter. This will be discussed further in the following sections.

17.3.1 Wave-like properties

As the term *electromagnetic* suggests, electromagnetic radiation consists of both electric and magnetic fields. These fields are at right angles to each other and to the direction of propagation and are shown diagrammatically in Figure 17.1. As shown in E and B of the figure, both the electric and the magnetic vectors (see Sect. 4.3) vibrate transversely to the direction of propagation of the wave. In addition, the vectors vary in a sinusoidal manner, as shown in the figure. Thus, if we draw the variations of the electric vector (for example), a sine wave results, as shown in Figure 17.2. These periodic variations of the vectors are the reason why electromagnetic radiations are often referred to as *electromagnetic waves* and this was the sole method of explaining the behaviour of such radiations adopted by classical physics (see Sect. 16.6). The same parameters can be used to describe this type of wave formation as can be used for any sinusoidal waves. These are:

- the *cycle* – one complete waveform (this can start from any point on the wave and end at the corresponding point on another wave)

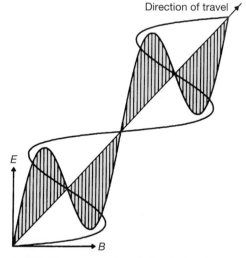

Figure 17.1 Electromagnetic radiation depicted as a wave consisting of alternating electrical and magnetic vectors vibrating at right angles to each other and to the direction of motion of the wave.

- the *wavelength* – the distance travelled in completing one cycle (λ)
- the *frequency* – the number of cycles per second (Hz)
- the *amplitude* – the magnitude of the peak of the wave above the *x*-axis (A).

If we consider Figure 17.2, it should be apparent that we can calculate the distance travelled by the radiation in 1 second by multiplying the wavelength (λ) by the frequency (v).

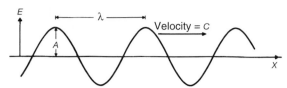

Figure 17.2 An electromagnetic sine wave produced by plotting energy (E) against distance (X). The wave has amplitude of A and a wavelength λ and travels at the velocity of light, c ($3 \times 10^8 \, \mathrm{m.s^{-1}}$).

However, the distance travelled in 1 second is simply the velocity of the radiation (c in a vacuum) and so we have:

Equation 17.1

$$c = v\lambda$$

in a vacuum.

As mentioned earlier, one of the features of electromagnetic radiations is that they all travel with the same velocity ($3 \times 10^8 \, \mathrm{m.s^{-1}}$) in a vacuum. One ray is distinguished from another by the difference in wavelength and frequency – *blue light* has a wavelength of about 400 nm and a frequency of 7.5×10^{14} Hz while *red light* has a wavelength of about 800 nm and a frequency of 3.75×10^{14} Hz. From this, it can be seen that *the greater the frequency, the smaller the wavelength* and vice versa.

In a transparent medium, the waves travel at a velocity V given by the equation $c = nV$, where n is a constant for a given medium and a given incident wavelength and is known as the *refractive index*. The frequency of the radiation is unaltered as it passes through a transparent medium but the wavelength is reduced due to the reduction in the velocity of the wave. If the wavelength in the medium is λ', then Equation 17.1 becomes:

$$V = v\lambda'$$

Substituting the value of V for $c = nV$, we obtain:

Equation 17.2

$$c = nv\lambda'$$

Insight

Chapters 9 and 10 showed that it is possible to produce both a magnetic field from moving electrical charges (electromagnetism) and an electric field from a changing magnetic flux (electromagnetic induction). It can be shown mathematically that a changing electric field can sustain a changing magnetic field, and vice versa, if they both travel at the velocity of light. This is the basis both for the linear propagation of electromagnetic radiations and for the fact that the wave does not gradually diminish in amplitude with time. Electromagnetic radiation can therefore be described as a self-sustaining interaction of electric and magnetic fields travelling with the velocity of light.

---

in a medium of refractive index, n.

Two further properties of electromagnetic radiation which are a consequence of its wave-like nature are polarization and interference.

17.3.1.1 Polarization

A beam of light, from a bulb for instance, consists of many millions of waves whose electric vectors are pointing in random directions with respect to each other. If this light beam is passed through a *polarizing* lens (similar to the one found in polarizing sunglasses), then there is optimum transmission of the waves whose electric vectors are pointing in one direction and complete absorption of those at right angles to this direction (this is the mechanism by which polarizing sunglasses limit the glare due to light reflection from water). The emergent light is said to be plane-polarized – all its vibrations are in the one plane.

17.3.1.2 Interference

Further evidence of the wave-like properties of electromagnetic radiations comes from the phenomenon of interference where the amplitudes of two coherent beams (beams which are in phase with each other) can be added together. If the peaks of the waves coincide, we get constructive interference and this produces bright areas. If the peak of the wave from one source coincides with the trough of the wave from the other source, we get destructive interference and this produces a dark area. Such interference patterns are used in radiographic science to produce holograms, but further discussion on this topic is well outside the scope of this text.

17.3.2 Particle-like properties

In Chapter 16 we discussed how consideration of electromagnetic radiations as quanta or photons having energy and momentum enabled us to explain a number of properties which are not explained by the wave theory. The energy of such a quantum, E, is proportional to the frequency of the associated wave such that:

Equation 17.3

$$E = hv$$

where h is a constant known as Planck's constant and v is the frequency of vibration of the associated wave. Thus, because there is a direct relationship between frequency and the energy of the quantum, as the frequency increases so does the energy. The momentum, p, of the quantum is also proportional to the frequency, and is given by:

Equation 17.4

$$p = \frac{hv}{c}$$

where c is the velocity of electromagnetic radiation in a vacuum.

The photon energy and its wavelength can now be related. If we take Equation 17.3 and substitute $v = c/\lambda$ from Equation 17.1, we get:

Equation 17.5

$$E = \frac{hc}{\lambda}$$

In this equation, h is Planck's constant $(6.62 \times 10^{-34}$ J.s$^{-1})$, c is the velocity of electromagnetic radiation in a vacuum $(3 \times 10^8$ m.s$^{-1})$, λ is the wavelength measured in meters and E is the photon energy measured in joules. For practical purposes, in radiography it is more convenient to measure the photon energy in keV $(1\,keV = 1.16 \times 10^{-16}J)$ and the wavelength in nanometers $(1\,nm = 10^{-9}$m$)$. Because h and c are constants, Equation 17.5 can now be rewritten:

Equation 17.6

$$E = \frac{1.24}{\lambda}$$

This equation gives us an easy link between the energy of the photon in keV and the wavelength of the radiation in nanometres.

Example
If the energy of the X-ray photon is 100 keV, what will be its wavelength in nanometres? Using Equation 17.6: $$E = \frac{1.24}{\lambda}$$ $$\therefore \lambda = \frac{1.24}{E}$$ $$= 1.24/100 \text{ nm}$$ $$= 0.0124 \text{ nm}$$

Lengths as small as 0.0124 nm or 1.24×10^{-11} m are difficult to imagine. This is less than the diameter of an atom

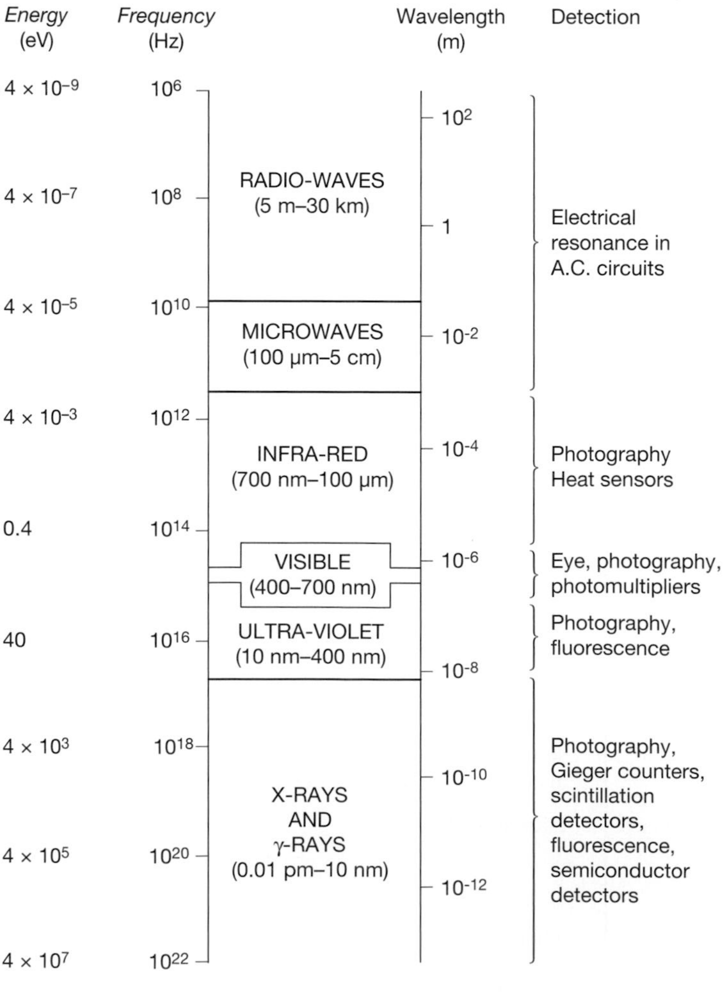

Energy (eV)	Frequency (Hz)		Wavelength (m)	Detection
4×10^{-9}	10^6		10^2	
		RADIO-WAVES (5 m–30 km)		
4×10^{-7}	10^8		1	Electrical resonance in A.C. circuits
4×10^{-5}	10^{10}			
		MICROWAVES (100 μm–5 cm)	10^{-2}	
4×10^{-3}	10^{12}			
		INFRA-RED (700 nm–100 μm)	10^{-4}	Photography Heat sensors
0.4	10^{14}			
		VISIBLE (400–700 nm)	10^{-6}	Eye, photography, photomultipliers
40	10^{16}	ULTRA-VIOLET (10 nm–400 nm)		Photography, fluorescence
			10^{-8}	
4×10^3	10^{18}		10^{-10}	Photography, Gieger counters, scintillation detectors, fluorescence, semiconductor detectors
		X-RAYS AND γ-RAYS (0.01 pm–10 nm)		
4×10^5	10^{20}		10^{-12}	
4×10^7	10^{22}			

Figure 17.3 The electromagnetic spectrum (not drawn to scale). Typical values for wavelengths, frequencies and photon energies for different bands of the spectrum are shown, together with some of the methods used for their detection. (Note: 1 Hz = 1 cycle per second.)

of body tissue (about 10^{-10} m) but is greater than the diameter of the atomic nucleus (about 10^{-14} m).

17.4 THE ELECTROMAGNETIC SPECTRUM

The previous sections of this chapter have shown that electromagnetic radiation may have a very large range of wavelengths, i.e. a *spectrum* of wavelengths (and frequencies). It is convenient to split up such an electromagnetic spectrum into bands which are broadly categorized by their interaction with matter and hence the use to which the bands of radiation may be put. This is illustrated in Figure 17.3, which also shows the wavelengths, frequencies and energies corresponding to the approximate boundaries between the various bands. As we have previously discussed, the table

Insight
At the beginning of this chapter (see Table 17.1) are the types of interactions which are possible between electromagnetic radiations and matter, with brief comments. From this table you will note that refraction is associated with electromagnetic radiations which have wavelengths larger than X-rays. Refraction is a phenomenon associated with an interaction between a photon and the outer electron orbitals of atoms. It is therefore associated with wavelengths which are able to interact with these electrons – ultraviolet and longer wavelengths. Smaller wavelengths become progressively less affected by the outer electron orbitals, and so it is just possible to demonstrate refraction with very large wavelength X-rays but it is not possible to refract X-rays which have shorter wavelengths.

of the electromagnetic spectrum shows that the smaller the wavelength of the radiation, the higher the frequency and the energy.

The common factor which links the interactions between different types of electromagnetic radiations is that *the value of the wavelength determines the size of object with which the radiation will directly interact*. This is illustrated in Table 17.2.

The interactions between X-rays and matter, which are of great relevance to radiographic science, are discussed in detail in Chapter 23 of this book.

17.5 LIGHT AMPLIFICATION BY STIMULATED EMISSION OF RADIATION (LASER)

In the last few years, devices containing a laser source have increasingly become a part of our everyday life and are also increasingly used in radiographic imaging. For this reason, a short section is included here describing the basic physics of laser production and also a section indicating the hazards of lasers if used carelessly.

17.5.1 Basic physics of laser production

Laser is an acronym for light amplification by stimulated emission of radiation. The theory which was first proposed by Albert Einstein in 1917 was further developed in the 1950s and the first laser was produced in 1960. We already know from Section 7.3 that in an atom electrons can exist at various energy levels depending on their position relative to the nucleus. We will also see in Chapters 18 and 24 that electrons can be temporarily raised to a higher energy level by the absorption of photons of

Table 17.2 Common electromagnetic radiations and the type of body with which they will directly interact

TYPE OF RADIATION	BODY WITH WHICH RADIATION DIRECTLY INTERACTS
Radio waves	Transmitted and received by large metallic conductors – aerials
Infrared radiation	Interacts with whole molecules or atoms giving them an increase in their kinetic energy in the form of heat
Visible light and ultraviolet radiation	Interacts with the outer electrons (more loosely bound) of the atom
X-rays and γ-rays	Interact with the inner electron shells or, if they have very high energy, with the nucleus of the atom

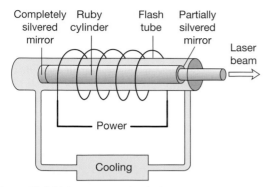

Figure 17.4 Main components of a laser.

energy. In many cases, the electron remains in this excited state for only a few milliseconds and subsequently decays to its lower energy level by the emission of a photon of light (or other energy) – this process is known as fluorescence (see Ch. 24 for a more detailed description). If the light emitted from an atom is incident on another atom which is in an excited state, then the first photon can stimulate the emission of a second photon from this atom. The two photons will be identical in wavelength, phase and direction. This is the basis of laser.

The basic components of a simple laser are shown in Figure 17.4. The excitation of electrons to a higher energy level is achieved by illuminating the material with light of a frequency higher than that which the laser will emit. This light is produced from the flash lamp and is known as optical pumping. The two ends of the laser rod are polished flat and parallel. One end is coated with a completely silvered mirror and the other is coated with a semisilvered mirror. Pulsed light is flashed into the laser at high intensity from the flash lamp and this is reflected within the rods using the two mirrors, thus causing coherent photon emission from the atoms of the rod material. Eventually the high-intensity laser radiation will leave the rod through the semisilvered mirror. The wavelength of the light emitted depends on the design of the laser so the beam may not be visible to the eye.

17.5.2 Potential hazards of lasers

Laser light has several properties which are important when we consider its safe use:

- The light is monochromatic, with its wavelength determined by the design of the laser.
- The light is in the form of a tightly collimated parallel beam, often less than 1 mm in diameter.
- Because the light is in the form of a small, highly collimated area, even lasers of small power can deposit significant amounts of energy on a small area.

Assume that a 10-W laser beam is directed at a material. This does not sound much in terms of power in

that many night lights are rated at 10 W. However, the laser beam is a parallel, very narrow beam. If this beam is 1 mm in diameter then the power deposited on the material is greater than $1000 \, W.cm^{-2}$ – this can ignite paper or cause significant skin burns. If the laser beam enters the eye, the problem is further complicated by the fact that the lens of the eye focuses the beam onto a small area of the retina. Thus, the power deposited on this small area of retina can be increased by a factor of up to 10^5 because of lens focusing. If we consider the original 10-W laser, this will mean a power deposited on a small area of the retina of $10^8 \, W.cm^{-2}$ – compare this to power to the retina of about $10 \, W.cm^{-2}$ if we stare at the midday sun, and it is easy to appreciate how damaging this can be to the eye.

As mentioned earlier, the wavelength of the light from the laser is determined by the laser design. The retina of the eye can detect from about 400 nm to just over 700 nm. Thus, if a laser is operating at, say, 900 nm, we will not be able to see the beam from this laser. However, the beam can still penetrate the lens system of the eye and cause damage to the retina of the eye. For this reason it is important to wear eye protection whenever lasers are in use, e.g. in an operating theatre, even if the laser beam is not visible.

17.6 ELECTROMAGNETIC RADIATIONS AND RADIOGRAPHY

The process of taking a radiograph (using a digital imaging system) results in the emission of radiations whose wavelengths and energies are from different parts of the electromagnetic spectrum, described in the previous section. These are summarized in Figure 17.5. When the anode is bombarded by electrons, it emits both heat and light as well as X-rays. The X-ray spectrum is composed of a continuous or Bremsstrahlung spectrum upon which is superimposed a characteristic or line spectrum from the tungsten target. The absorption processes within the aluminium filter and the lead collimators also produce characteristic radiation from these elements, although these are of fairly low intensity. When the radiation beam passes through the patient, some of the photons are absorbed (A in the diagram) and some are scattered (S in the diagram). The above processes produce a tiny amount of heat and other characteristic radiations from the elements which make up the body tissues. Some of the scattered radiation is absorbed by the grid. When the transmitted X-ray beam (T) strikes the digital imaging system, it produces changes in electron energies which can then be utilized to produce the digital image – this will be discussed in more detail in Chapter 34. Further

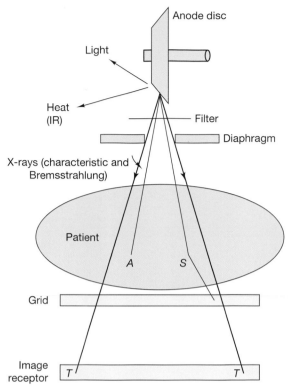

Figure 17.5 The production of radiation from different parts of the electromagnetic spectrum utilized when a digital radiographic image is produced.

examples of electromagnetic radiation relevant to radiography include:

- the emission of light from thin field transistors (TFTs) to produce images on flat-screened imaging devices
- the emission of light from cathode ray tubes and television monitors when the phosphors are bombarded by electrons
- the emission of light from fluorescent tubes to allow us to view hard copies of images
- the emission of gamma-rays from certain radioisotopes which allow imaging or treatment of organs
- the emission of light from sodium iodide crystals (in gamma cameras and computed tomography (CT) scanners) when bombarded with gamma-rays or X-rays
- the emission of light from photostimulable plates when scanned using a laser beam
- the use of a laser beam to 'write' information onto the film in a laser imager
- the use of low-intensity lasers to aid positioning of the radiation beam in radiotherapy.

Summary

In this chapter, you should have learnt the following:
- The properties which are common to all electromagnetic radiations (see Sect. 17.3).
- The different ways in which electromagnetic radiations can react with matter (see Sect. 17.3).
- How electromagnetic radiation can be described as having wave-like properties and how these properties can be used to explain polarization and interference (see Sect. 17.3.1).
- How electromagnetic radiation can be described as having particle-like properties and the equation which links the photon energy and the wavelength of the radiation (see Sect. 17.3.2).
- The various components of the electromagnetic spectrum and the principal interactions of the radiations with matter (see Sect. 17.4).
- A brief description of the physics of laser production and a note of its potential dangers (see Sect. 17.5).
- The electromagnetic radiations which are of importance to radiography (see Sect. 17.6).

FURTHER READING

You will find further information on the methods of X-ray production in Chapter 21 and more information on the mechanisms by which X-rays interact with matter in Chapter 23 of this text. In addition, you may find the chapters of the following text useful:

Ball, J.L., Moore, A.D., Turner, S., 2008. Ball and Moore's Essential Physics for Radiographers, fourth ed. Blackwell Scientific, London (Chapters 14 and 15).

Chapter | **18** |

The elementary structure of the atom

structures are extremely complex and are the subject of a number of textbooks in their own right. Most of the phenomena which we encounter in radiography can be explained using a relatively simple *planetary model* of the atom. In this model, there are solid electrons orbiting a solid nucleus – some phenomena can also be explained using the *quantum physics model* and where this is appropriate this model will be referred to in Insights.

The planetary model of the atom was first described by Rutherford in 1911. It describes an atom consisting of a small, positively charged central nucleus (containing protons and neutrons) around which negatively charged electrons move in defined orbitals. This model can be used to illustrate the carbon atom, as shown in Figure 18.1. As we can see from the diagram, the nucleus

18.1 AIM

The aim of this chapter is to introduce the reader to the key components of an atom. The principal particles which form the nucleus will be identified, as will the factors which determine whether or not the nucleus is stable. The differing electron orbitals and the influence of the electron orbitals on the chemical properties of the material will be discussed. The consequences of transitions of electrons between orbitals will also be identified.

18.2 INTRODUCTION

Any attempt to understand the universe around us must start with the fundamental question: *what is matter made of?* The atom as the fundamental building block of matter has been the subject of a great deal of both theoretical debate and experimental study by physicists. Many of the modern theories concerning atomic and subatomic

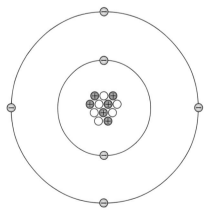

Figure 18.1 The basic structure of a carbon atom. At the centre of the atom is a nucleus which contains six protons (positively charged) and six neutrons (zero charge) – i.e. the nucleus contains 12 nucleons. Six electrons (negatively charged) orbit the nucleus in defined orbitals. As the atom contains equal numbers of positive and negative charges, the whole atom is electrically neutral.

of this atom consists of *12 elementary particles – six protons and six neutrons*. These particles are bound together in a small volume of extremely high density – about three thousand million, million times greater than the density of water. The protons in the nucleus carry a positive charge and the electrons carry an equal negative charge, so this atom is electrically neutral – the neutrons carry no charge. The electrons are arranged in orbitals or shells called *K, L, M* … starting from the orbital closest to the nucleus. The *K*-shell can only contain two electrons and, in the case of the carbon atom, the *L*-shell contains the remaining four. Different atoms contain different numbers of protons and neutrons in the nucleus and different numbers of electron configurations; this will be discussed later in this chapter. The particles which make up the atom are very tiny and the atom consists largely of empty space. For example, if an atom were to be enlarged until it was the size of a house, the size of the nucleus would be about the size of a pinhead, although it contains 99.95% of the total mass of the atom.

The masses and charges of the subatomic particles which will be considered in this and later chapters are summarized in Table 18.1.

Table 18.1 Masses and charges of the main subatomic particles

| PARTICLE | SYMBOL | REST MASS | | REST ENERGY | CHARGE[b] | COMMENTS |
		kg	AMU[a]	MeV		
Proton	p	1.672×10^{-27}	1.007	938	+1	Nucleon, i.e. present in the atomic nucleus
Neutron	n	1.675×10^{-27}	1.009	939	0	Nucleon, i.e. present in the atomic nucleus
Alpha-particle	α	6.645×10^{-27}	4.003	3718	+2	Two protons and two neutrons Ejected in α decay
Electron	e^- or β^-	9.109×10^{-31}	0.00055 or 1/1820	0.511	−1	Form stable discrete orbits around nuclei Ejected from nucleus in β decay
Positron	e^+ or β^+	9.109×10^{-31}	0.00055 or 1/1820	0.511	+1	Antiparticle of the electron – produces annihilation radiation when both meet
Pi meson	π^+	2.480×10^{-28}	0.150	139	+1	Keep the nucleus together (π^0 and π^- also exist)
Neutrino	ν	0	0	0	0	Emitted during β decay and electron capture Very weak attenuation by matter
Photon or quantum	h_v	–	–	–	0	Travels at 3×10^8 m.s^{-1} Forms part of the electromagnetic spectrum

[a]1 amu is 1 atomic mass unit which is one-twelfth of the mass of a neutral $^{12}_{6}$C atom.
[b]A charge of +1 is $+1.602 \times 10^{-19}$ coulomb.

Insight

Rutherford carried out some elegant experimental work connected with the scattering of alpha-particles by atoms. From this, he concluded that the only explanation for the wide scattering angles which he found experimentally was given by assuming that the atom consists of a very heavy positively charged nucleus with orbiting electrons. The alternative model, whereby all the subatomic particles were contained in a very small volume, was unacceptable because it would produce much smaller scattering angles for the alpha-particles.

Similar experiments have recently been carried out by physicists to try to establish whether protons and neutrons can be broken into smaller pieces. Unfortunately, if the energy of the projectile is large enough to break up the proton or neutron, then the energy is great enough to create new particles – remember $E = mc^2$ – and so it is difficult to tell which are fragments of the proton and which have been created as a result of energy being converted into matter. More subtle experiments use high-energy electrons to bombard the protons and neutrons and measure the angle of deflection of these particles. These angles are again over a wide range, suggesting that there are small solid structures within the protons and neutrons. These may be the basic building blocks of the universe; they are known as *quarks* and 18 different types of quark have been identified. Further discussion regarding this search to identify whether there is a smaller structure within the quark is well outside the scope of this text.

18.3 THE ATOMIC NUCLEUS

The number of protons and neutrons in the atomic nucleus determines both the mass and the charge of the nucleus and the configuration of electron orbitals of the atom. There are several important terms, which we will use in this and in following chapters of this text, that require definition at this stage. These terms, which will help us to understand atomic structure, are defined in Table 18.2.

We can now consider the use of some of the terms in the tables. The most common naturally occurring stable isotope of carbon has six protons and six neutrons, as shown previously in Figure 18.1. The *atomic number* (Z) of this isotope is six and the *atomic mass number* is 12. The whole atom can be written as $^{12}_{6}$C. Thus $^{12}_{6}$C is an example of a *nuclide* – one which contains six protons and six neutrons. In general, an element E is written as $^{A}_{Z}$E. An isotope of carbon, which is also naturally occurring but less abundant, has seven neutrons in its nucleus and may be written as $^{13}_{6}$C.

Note that it is not necessarily the case that isotopes of an element are radioactive, as shown by this example; $^{12}_{6}$C and $^{13}_{6}$C are both isotopes of carbon but neither is radioactive.

An isotope of carbon which is radioactive is $^{14}_{6}$C – the well-known *carbon-14*. This again contains the six protons which identify it as a carbon nucleus, but this time it contains eight neutrons. $^{14}_{6}$C is an example of a

Table 18.2 Terms used to describe a nucleus

TERM	SYMBOL	DEFINITION
Nucleon		A proton or neutron within a nucleus
Atomic number	Z	The number of protons in the nucleus
Atomic mass number	A	The total number of nucleons in the nucleus
Neutron number	N	The number of neutrons within the nucleus
Nuclide		A nucleus with a specific value of Z and A
Element	E	A nucleus with a given value of Z
Isotope (of an element)		Any nucleus which contains the same number of protons as the given nucleus but has a different mass number
Isobar		Any nucleus which has the same atomic mass number as another nucleus (i.e. has the same value of A)
Radionuclide or radioisotope		Any nuclide or isotope which is radioactive

radionuclide or a *radioactive isotope*. It decays, as we shall see in Chapter 19, by beta decay to form $^{14}_{7}N$ (nitrogen) as the *daughter product*.

18.3.1 The stability of the nucleus

At first sight the atomic nucleus would appear to be inherently unstable as the neutrons are uncharged and the protons have a positive charge and so would electrostatically repel each other. This would suggest that the nucleus should fly apart because of the electrostatic forces between the protons.

In practice, some nuclei are so stable as to possess no measurable radioactivity ($^{12}_{6}C$ is an example) while others decay with a half-life (see Sect. 20.5) of less than one-millionth of a second. The nucleus must be visualised as a *dynamic* rather than a *static* structure where there are opposing forces acting – forces which tend to hold the nucleus together and forces which tend to disrupt the nucleus. A *stable nucleus* is one where the disruptive forces never win and an *unstable nucleus* is one where they do succeed. This nucleus is said to undergo *radioactive decay*. It is not possible to predict the exact moment when any particular nucleus will decay, as it is a matter of probability rather than certainty. However, if there are a large number of unstable nuclei in a sample, the *law of radioactive decay* (see Sect. 20.3) is obeyed.

The forces which hold the nucleus together are quite unlike the other forces – e.g. gravity – with which we are familiar. They are known as *short-range nuclear forces* and act over distances of about 10^{-15} metres, over which range they are much more powerful than the electrostatic forces between the protons. These forces are shown diagrammatically in Figure 18.2. A strong force of attraction is evident below 10^{-15} m and this changes to a force of repulsion at about 10^{-16} m. The energy expended in keeping the nucleus together is known as the *nuclear binding energy* (NBE). If the NBE is divided by the number of nucleons within the nucleus, then a figure of about 8.4 MeV is obtained for most nuclei. This is known as the *binding energy per nucleon*. The binding energy between the nucleons is provided by the transformation of some of the nuclear mass into energy, as given by Einstein's equation $E = mc^2$. Each nucleon has a mass of approximately 931 MeV per atomic mass unit (amu), of which about 8.4 MeV is used for its NBE to nearby nucleons. Because of this, the mass of the nucleus is always less than the sum of the masses of the nucleons.

Considering the graph in Chapter 19 (Fig. 19.2) it can be seen that, for low atomic numbers, equal numbers of protons and neutrons produce the greatest stability. This leads to the concept of nuclear shells, which suggests that there is a layering within the nucleus, with maximum stability being produced when a shell is complete. Further discussion of this concept is beyond the scope of this text.

Insight

The π-meson is a particle with a mass between that of an electron and a nucleon and is thought to be responsible for the forces holding the nucleus together. The short-range forces are known as exchange forces and result in (for example) an adjacent proton and a neutron changing continually into a neutron and a proton and back again. This interchange may be written as:

$$p_1 + n_1 \rightarrow n_2 + \pi^+ + n_1 \rightarrow n_2 + p_2$$

The π^+-meson has left the original proton p_1, leaving it as a neutron n_2, and then forms a proton p_2 by combining with the original neutron n_1. The proton and the neutron are continuously exchanging their positions. Negative and neutral π-mesons also exist and are exchanged between nucleons.

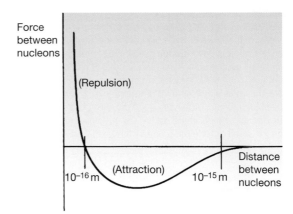

Figure 18.2 If the separation of the nucleons is between 10^{-15} and 10^{-16} metres, then a force of attraction exists between the nucleons which helps to hold the nucleus together. If the separation is greater or less than this distance, then the force is a repulsive force.

18.4 ELECTRON ORBITALS

Consider an atom of hydrogen, as shown in Figure 18.3. It is assumed in the planetary model of the atom that the solitary electron is on a circular path (path 1) around the nucleus. It may be shown that a body moving in a circle of radius r at a velocity V has an acceleration of V^2/r towards the centre of the circle. According to classical physics, such acceleration would result in the emission of electromagnetic radiation from the electron so that the electron is continuously losing energy and would eventually collide with the nucleus (see path 2). Electrons do not behave in this manner, or atoms as we know them would not exist. The electrons orbit in stable paths (path 1) – *discrete electron*

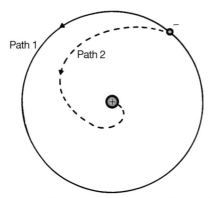

Figure 18.3 A stable, discrete electron orbital (path 1) compared to a 'decaying electron' (path 2), as predicted by the laws of classical physics.

orbitals. Further, these orbitals are grouped in 'shells' where there is a particular number of electrons of approximately the same energy in each orbital. (An explanation of the apparent contradiction of the predictions of classical physics (path 2 and path 1) is given in the 'Insight' below.) The electrons fill up the inner shells first since the energies of the inner shells are less than the outer shells.

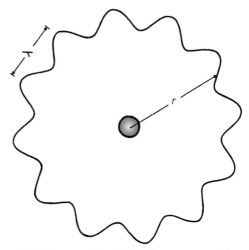

Figure 18.4 The use of the de Broglie wave concept to explain why electrons exist in discrete orbitals.

Insight

The wave–particle duality of matter (see Sect. 16.6) may be used to explain the existence of discrete electron orbitals. Here it is assumed that an orbiting electron has a de Broglie wavelength which is able to fit around the circumference of an orbital an exact number of times (see Fig. 18.4). This fixes the size of each orbital. The condition necessary for this to occur is that $n\lambda = 2\pi r$ where n is a whole number and r is the mean radius of the orbital. Now λ is the de Broglie wavelength of the electron with momentum p and is given by $\lambda = h/p$:

$$\frac{nh}{p} = 2\pi r \text{ or } pr = \frac{nh}{2\pi}$$

But pr is the angular momentum of the electron and this must be a multiple of $h/2\pi$. There is now no question of electromagnetic radiation occurring from an orbital electron. This is an example of a situation where modern physics can be used to describe atomic phenomena which are not explicable by classical physics.

Table 18.3 Numbers of electrons in atomic shells

PRINCIPAL QUANTUM NUMBER OR SHELL NUMBER (n)	SHELL LETTER	MAXIMUM NUMBER OF ELECTRONS	$2n^2$
1	K	2	2
2	L	8	8
3	M	18	18
4	N	32	32

Table 18.3 shows the maximum number of electrons in each shell from the inner K-shell to the N-shell. The shell number, n, starts from $n = 1$ for the K-shell and is known as the *principal quantum number*. The chemical properties of an element are controlled by the electron configuration of its atoms. Atoms with filled outer electron shells are chemically inert – neon ($Z = 10$) has full K- and L-shells, as illustrated in Figure 18.5, and so is a chemically inert gas. Fluorine ($Z = 9$), where the K-shell contains two electrons

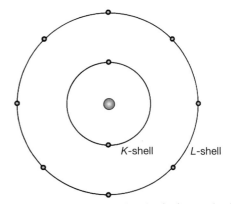

Figure 18.5 An atom of neon, showing both K- and L-shells containing their maximum number of permitted electrons. This means that the neon atom is chemically inert.

and the *L*-shell contains seven, is a chemically active *electron acceptor* (the electron fills the vacancy in the *L*-shell). Sodium ($Z = 11$), where the *K*-shell contains two electrons, the *L*-shell contains eight electrons and the *M*-shell contains one, is a chemically active *electron donor* (the electron in the *M*-shell is donated, resulting in a filled *L*-shell).

The outer electron shells may contain subshells within them. Argon ($Z = 18$) has two electrons in its *K*-shell, eight electrons in its *L*-shell and eight electrons in the *M*-shell. The *M*-shell has a maximum complement of electrons of 18 and yet argon is chemically inert. An outer subshell of eight electrons is particularly chemically stable, a fact which is confirmed by the next inert gas, krypton, which has an electron configuration of 2, 8, 18, 8.

18.5 THE PERIODIC TABLE OF ELEMENTS

If the elements are arranged in order of increasing atomic number, it may be shown that their chemical properties, such as valency, and their physical properties, such as specific heat, tend to occur in a periodic manner. Arranging these elements in these similar groups produces a *periodic table* as shown in Table E (See page 356). Chemical similarities of the elements in each group may be explained by reference to their electron structure as shown in Table F (See page 357), the electron configuration of the elements. It has already been noted that the number of electrons increases with atomic number and that each electron takes an orbital of the lowest possible energy. This means that the inner shells are filled to stable or substable levels before the outer shells accommodate electrons. There are two rules which determine the way in which the electron shells are gradually built up as the atomic number increases:

1. An electron shell, *n*, cannot contain more than $2n^2$ electrons where *n* is the shell number.
2. The outer shell cannot contain more than eight electrons.

These rules are known as the *Bury–Bohr Rules* after their co-discovers and ensure that the orbitals of minimum energy are filled first.

One additional constraint is required in order that electrons may fill orbitals in the correct manner. This is known as the *Pauli exclusion principle* and states that *no two electrons may have precisely the same orbital*. The two *K*-shell electrons of an atom, for example, are not at precisely the same energy level because they orbit the atom in opposing directions and hence have slightly different orbitals. These two electrons complete the *K*-shell so that the electrons must start to fill up the *L*-shell (see lithium in Table F) at a greater distance from the nucleus and so at a higher energy. These *L*-shell electrons all have slightly different energies from each other and the shell is complete when it has eight electrons – neon satisfies these conditions where $n = 2$ and so $2n^2 = 8$.

The *K*- and *L*-shell are thus completed in sequence but the *M*-shell (which from the $2n^2$ formula can contain up to 18 electrons), when it reaches nine electrons (argon), then obeys the rule that the outer shell cannot contain more than eight electrons and the ninth electron is placed in the *N*-shell (see potassium in Table F). This process is repeated each time there are eight electrons in the outer orbital (see rubidium, caesium, fracium, etc.).

As mentioned above, the number of electrons in the outer orbital determines the chemical activity of the element. The ability of one atom to join another is called *valency* and the electron linkage between the atoms is called the valency bond. There are two types valency bond:

1. *Ionic bonds* (see Fig. 18.6A and B): this type of bond is created when one or more electrons are transferred from one atom to another forming charged atoms (or ions) which are attracted towards each other by electrostatic attraction forming the bond. After the electron exchange, the shells of each ion appear to be closed.
2. *Covalent bonds* (see Fig. 18.6C and D): formed by the apparent sharing of electrons such that each atom appears to increase its number of electrons forming an apparently closed shell.

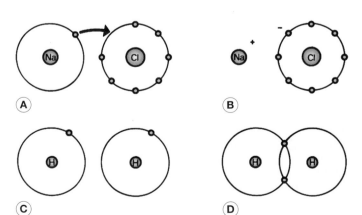

Figure 18.6 An ionic valency bond (or electron valency) is caused by the transfer of an electron from one atom to another – Na to Cl in (A) and (B). A covalent bond (covalency) is formed when two atoms share electrons in the same orbital as shown between two hydrogen atoms in (C) and (D).

18.6 ELECTRON ORBITAL CHANGES

The previous sections of this chapter have shown that electrons may only take up fixed or discrete orbitals around an atomic nucleus. We have also discussed the fact that the inner orbitals are filled before the outer orbitals, since this constitutes the lowest energy state of the whole atom. An atom in this state is said to be in its *ground state*, since it cannot have an electron configuration which will produce a lower energy. However, this is not to say that any particular atom at a given moment of time will be at its ground state, since interatomic collisions or interactions with electromagnetic radiations may have raised the energy of one of its electrons so that it is able to take up an orbital of higher energy – the electron will move further away from the nucleus. This process is called *excitation* of the atom. The excited electron is able to return to its original orbital and releases a quantum of electromagnetic radiation in the process. The energy of this quantum is equal to the energy difference between the excited state and the ground state. Alternatively, an orbiting electron may receive sufficient energy to be able to escape from the atom completely – this might happen as a result of the interaction of a photon with the electron. This process is called *ionization* since the remaining atom will now form a positive ion. Both processes are shown diagrammatically in Figure 18.7.

18.7 BINDING ENERGY OF THE ELECTRON SHELLS

Because the various electron shells are positioned at different distances from the atomic nucleus, they experience different forces of attraction from the nucleus. The *K*-shell is closest to the nucleus and so experiences the greatest force of attraction from the nucleus. It is therefore most difficult to remove an electron from the *K*-shell – the *K*-shell has the highest electron binding energy. The electron binding energy of a shell is the amount of work which must be done to remove an electron from that shell (it is normally stated in KeV or eV). The *L*-shell is further away from the nucleus and so experiences less force of attraction. It also experiences some repulsion from the electrons in the *K*-shell. For this reason, the binding energy of the electrons in the *L*-shell is less than the binding energy of the *K*-shell for a particular atom. Thus we can say that there is a reduction in the binding energy as we move from the *K*-shell to the *L*-shell to the *M*-shell, etc., within a particular atom.

The reason for the existence of the binding energy is the electrostatic attraction between the nucleus and the electrons in the shells. Thus we would expect to find an increase in the *K*-shell binding energy with an increase in the atomic number of the element. This is found to be the case in practice.

A knowledge of the binding energy of the various electron shells in different elements is important in radiation physics for the following reasons:

- A knowledge of the binding energies of the different shells allows us to predict the energies of the characteristic radiations which the atom might produce (see Ch. 21 for further details).
- A knowledge of the binding energies of different electron shells within an atom of an element will allow us to determine the likely position of absorption edges during photoelectric absorption (see Ch. 23 for further details).
- If we know the energy of the characteristic radiation from an element and we know the position of

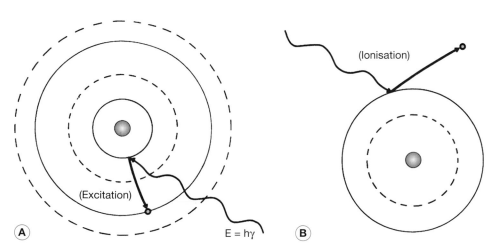

Figure 18.7 An incoming photon interacts with an orbiting electron of an atom. In (A) this photon has sufficient energy to cause excitation and in (B) the photon causes ionization.

absorption edges when radiation is attenuated by this material, then this allows us to explain why elements are relatively transparent to their own characteristic radiation (see Ch. 23 for further details).

Although the binding energy of an electron orbital increases as we move closer to the nucleus, its potential energy reduces. Thus, if an electron moves from the L-shell to the K-shell, it must lose energy (normally in the form of a photon of characteristic radiation). This will be discussed in more detail in Chapter 23.

Summary

In this chapter, you should have learnt the following:
- The main subatomic particle which can be joined together to produce matter (see Sect. 18.2).
- A basic planetary model of the atom which consists of a nucleus containing protons and neutrons and has electrons in specific orbitals around this nucleus (see Sect. 18.2).

- The basic structure of the atomic nucleus and the reasons for its stability or otherwise (see Sects 18.3 and 18.3.1).
- The configuration of electron orbitals for differing atoms and the factors which determine the maximum number of electrons in an orbital (see Sects 18.4 and 18.5).
- The basic structure of the periodic table of elements and the electron configuration of elements (see Sect. 18.5).
- The meaning of the term *ground state* when applied to an atom and the consequences of raising the energy of the electrons above the ground state (see Sect. 18.6).
- An explanation of the term *binding energy* and a brief outline of areas where a knowledge of the binding energy of electron shells is of importance in radiation physics (see Sect. 18.7).

FURTHER READING

Ball, J.L., Moore, A.D., Turner, S., 2008. Ball and Moore's Essential Physics for Radiographers, fourth ed. Blackwell Scientific, London (Chapter 4).

Chapter | 19 |

Radioactivity

19.1 AIM

The aim of this chapter is to discuss the various types of radioactive decay which can occur. Within the chapter the relevance of these processes to nuclear medicine will be considered.

19.2 INTRODUCTION

Chapter 18 referred to various terms which may be used to define nuclear structure. This chapter will examine the changes which may take place in the nucleus during radioactive decay.

The term *radioactive* is applied to nuclei which are unstable. In these nuclei, the forces disrupting the nucleus are stronger than the forces which hold the nucleus together. The instability of the nucleus is demonstrated by the fact that it changes its internal structure to a more stable form, often (but not always) ejecting a charged particle from the nucleus in the process. Each time a nucleus changes its structure it is called a *radioactive disintegration* or a *nuclear transformation* and may result in a change in the atomic number – number of protons in the nucleus – (and therefore element) or a change in the mass number – number of protons and neutrons in the nucleus – or a change of both the atomic number and the mass number.

A pictorial representation of the decay process (see Fig. 19.1) is called a *decay scheme*. In addition to this, it is possible for a nucleus to undergo more than one type of transformation (see Fig. 19.12 later in this chapter) and this type of decay is called a *branching scheme*.

It is impossible to determine the exact time when a particular nucleus will transform, but the laws of probability may be used to determine the behaviour of a large number of nuclei (see Ch. 20 for a discussion of radioactive decay and the exponential law).

The unit of radioactivity is the becquerel (Bq) where 1 becquerel is 1 nuclear disintegration per second.

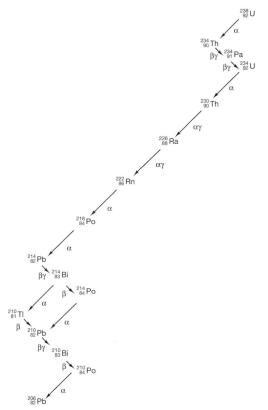

Figure 19.1 The uranium decay series. Note that arrows to the right indicate an increase in the atomic number while arrows to the left indicate a decrease. The downward direction of the arrows indicates that the nucleus loses energy with each transformation (downward direction not drawn to scale).

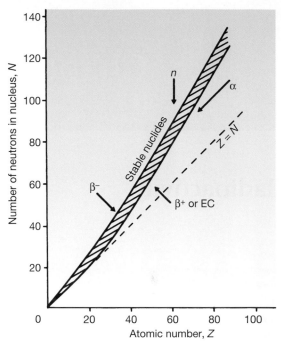

Figure 19.2 A graph of the neutron number (N) plotted against the atomic number (Z) showing the position of the stable nuclides as a shaded band. Note that, as the atomic number increases, a higher proportion of neutrons to protons is required to achieve stability. Also shown are the directions which a nucleus takes for various forms of radioactive decay (these movements are not to scale). EC, electron capture.

Insight

Before the introduction of International System of Units (SI) units, radioactivity was measured in curie (Ci). 1 curie was equal to 3.7×10^{10} nuclear disintegrations per second. Thus, an activity of 1 Ci is the same as an activity of 3.7×10^{10} Bq or 37 GBq. From this it can be seen that the curie was a much larger unit than the becquerel.

It is often useful to know the specific activity of a sample. This is the activity of radionuclide per unit mass of the sample and so is measured in Bq.kg^{-1} or submultiples thereof.

19.3 NUCLIDE CHART

It is often useful to draw a graph, plotting the number of neutrons in a nucleus against the number of protons, as all nuclides may be included in this *nuclide chart*. Such a chart is shown in simplified form in Figure 19.2. Note that isotopes (lines of equal atomic number) are given by any

vertical line on the figure. In such a graph, an angle of 45° to the *x*-axis represents a situation where the nucleus contains equal numbers of protons and neutrons ($Z = N$).

It is found on such a graph that there is a broad band of nuclides with low atomic numbers at about 45° to the *x*-axis and these are all stable or only weakly radioactive. Thus, for the lighter elements, nuclear stability can be produced with equal numbers of protons and neutrons. From the graph it can be seen that, as the atomic number increases, a proportionately larger number of neutrons is necessary to produce nuclear stability. Thus we can say that as the Coulomb repulsion (see Sect. 6.4) between the protons increases, then more neutrons are required to produce the short-range nuclear forces (see Sect. 18.3.1), thus producing the cohesive forces required for a stable nucleus. Nuclei which have atomic numbers greater than 83 (bismuth) are so large that it is impossible to produce a stable nuclear configuration.

Nuclides whose combination of neutrons and protons means that they land outside the band of stability shown in Figure 19.2 have nuclei possessing higher energies than those within the band. As a consequence, such a nucleus is unstable and tends, on decay, to produce a new nucleus of lower energy which is closer to, or within, the stable band. The energy difference between the nucleus before and after decay is emitted either as a charged particle or as a quantum (or quanta) of electromagnetic radiation. The decay scheme towards stability may be in the form of a single step (e.g. $^{14}_{6}$C decays to stable $^{14}_{7}$N[1] by the emission of a beta-particle (see Fig. 19.4) or it may be in the form of a multistage route involving many nuclear transformations (e.g. the decay of $^{238}_{92}$U to $^{206}_{82}$Pb involves at least 14 steps, as shown in Figure 19.1). As a general rule, the greater the mass number of the nuclide, the more complicated the decay path to eventual stability.

The effect of different decay modes is illustrated using arrows on Figure 19.2 The direction of the arrow shows the direction of change of position on the chart before and after the decay process. You may find it helpful to refer back to this chart while studying the decay processes in more detail in the following sections of this chapter.

19.4 ALPHA DECAY OR ALPHA-PARTICLE EMISSION

For the spontaneous emission of an alpha-particle from a nucleus, the nuclide must have an atomic mass number greater than 150. The nucleus must also have *too few neutrons for the number of protons* – a higher neutron-to-proton ratio would be required to produce nuclear stability. The alpha-particle consists of two protons and two neutrons tightly bound together (a helium nucleus). It may be considered as a free particle having high kinetic energy which is trapped in the parent nucleus. Thus the daughter nucleus has two protons and two neutrons fewer than the parent nucleus (see Equation 19.1 below).

The mechanism of production of the alpha-particle is quite complex. As we have already identified (see Sect. 18.3.1), the nucleus depends on a balance of disruptive electrostatic (Coulomb) forces and attractive forces between the nucleons caused by the short-range nuclear forces. In very large nuclei there is a large amount of electrostatic repulsion between the protons which extends across the whole nucleus. This is balanced by the short-range nuclear force which exists between adjacent nucleons. Thus, if the nucleus becomes elongated, the electrostatic forces dominate and the nucleus becomes even more elongated. This process continues until the nucleus divides into two fragments, the daughter nuclide and the alpha-particle.

An example of alpha-decay is the decay of bismuth-212 to thallium-208 with the emission of alpha-particles. This process is shown in the following equation:

Equation 19.1

$$^{212}_{83}\text{Bi} \rightarrow\ ^{208}_{81}\text{Tl} + ^{4}_{2}\alpha$$

Note that there is a reduction of four in the atomic mass number and two in the atomic number between parent and daughter product.

This reaction can also be written as shown in Figure 19.3 (the decay of $^{212}_{83}$Bi also includes the emission of a

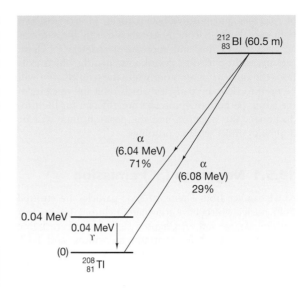

Figure 19.3 An example of alpha-particle emission. The nucleus decreases its atomic number and energy as shown.

beta-particle and is discussed later as an example of a branching programme; for simplicity only the alpha-particle reaction is shown in Fig. 19.3 and the percentages shown refer only to the alpha-particles). Because the daughter product is to the left of the parent nuclide, this shows that there is a reduction in the atomic number. The reaction also shows that the difference in energy between the parent nuclide and the daughter nuclide is 6.08 MeV. If we consider only the alpha-particles emitted, we find that approximately 71% of these have an energy of 6.04 MeV and 29% have an energy of 6.08 MeV. In the case of the first group of alpha-particles, the nucleus is left in an excited state with excess energy of 0.04 MeV which it emits as a gamma-ray.

The ejection of an alpha-particle means that, to preserve momentum, the nucleus must also recoil with an equal and opposite momentum to that of the alpha-particle. The energy of the recoiling nucleus is typically about 2% of that of the emitted alpha-particle. (Recoil also exists for beta-decay but is much smaller due to the tiny mass of the beta-particle.)

Alpha-particles are intensely ionizing but have a very short range in tissue so have little practical application in radiology.

19.5 BETA DECAY OR BETA-PARTICLE EMISSION

In the process of beta decay, a particle, having a mass equal to that of an electron, is ejected from the nucleus. The ejected particles, however, may have either a positive or negative charge and so, although they are known collectively as beta-particles, negative beta-particles (β^{-})

or *negatrons* and positive beta-particles (β^+) or *positrons* both exist. Although the negatron is exactly the same as an electron, in this and subsequent chapters the term *negatron* will be used to describe the particle which exits from the nucleus of an atom while the term *electron* will be used to describe particles which orbit the nucleus of the atom. Because the processes are different for the production of the negatron and the positron, they will be dealt with under separate headings.

19.5.1 Negatron (β^-) emission

As we can see from Figure 19.2, β^--particles are emitted from nuclei which have too many neutrons for nuclear stability. As we saw in Chapter 18, nucleons are being constantly changed from proton to neutron and back within the atomic nucleus. A neutron may be thought of as consisting of a proton and a negatron:

Equation 19.2

$$n \rightarrow p^+ + \beta^-$$

It appears that in nuclei which have too many neutrons, there is a finite possibility that a neutron becomes isolated within the nucleus and then decays to form a proton and a negatron. The proton rejoins the nucleus and the negatron is ejected. This transformation results in the atomic mass number remaining unchanged (the combined number of protons and neutrons is still the same) but the atomic number will increase by one as one extra proton has been added to the nucleus (this results in the formation of a different element with the consequent rearrangement of electron orbitals to suit the new element).

An example of β^--particle decay is shown below, where carbon-14 decays to form nitrogen with the emission of a β^--particle:

Equation 19.3

$$^{14}_{6}\text{C} \rightarrow {}^{14}_{7}\text{N} + \beta^-$$

This can also be illustrated using the methods discussed for alpha-particle emission to show the transformation from parent to daughter product. Such a diagram is shown in Figure 19.4. Note that this time there is an increase in the atomic number so the line is down and to the right. This simple decay process is an example of pure beta emission since no other transformations are involved.

Figure 19.5 shows a more complex emission pattern where the parent and daughter nuclei are separated by an energy difference of 2.81 MeV. The β^--particle has an energy of 0.31 MeV and so the nucleus is left in an excited state – 2.50 MeV above its ground state. The nucleus emits this energy in the form of two gamma-rays, one of energy 1.17 MeV and the other of energy 1.33 MeV. (This will be discussed further when we consider gamma-ray emission in Sect. 19.6.)

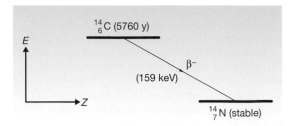

Figure 19.4 An example of pure beta-particle (negatron) emission. The nucleus increases in atomic number and loses energy as shown.

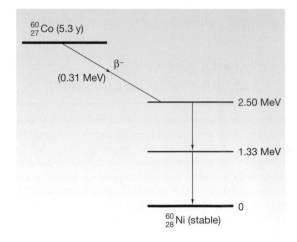

Figure 19.5 The decay of cobalt-60 as an example of beta decay followed by a gamma decay of the daughter nucleus.

19.5.2 Positron (β^-) emission

As mentioned earlier, protons are continuously changing into neutrons and back. In these reactions we can consider a proton as consisting of a neutron and a positron.

Equation 19.4

$$p^+ \rightarrow n + \beta^+$$

If we consider Figure 19.2, we see that positron emission takes place from nuclei which have too many protons to achieve stability. In such cases, protons appear to become isolated within the nucleus and then to decay to form a neutron which rejoins the nucleus and a positron which is ejected from the nucleus. In this reaction, the atomic mass number will remain the same but the atomic number will decrease by one (the total number of protons and neutrons is unchanged but one proton has been converted into a neutron).

An example of such a reaction is the decay of carbon-11 to boron:

Equation 19.5

$$^{11}_{6}\text{C} \rightarrow {}^{11}_{5}\text{B} + \beta^+$$

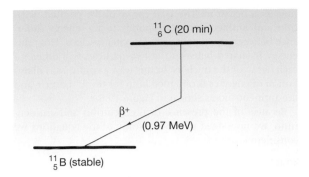

Figure 19.6 An example of positron decay. The nucleus experiences a decrease in the atomic number and loses energy, as shown.

If we consider the energy changes which take place within the nucleus, as shown in Figure 19.6, we see that the situation regarding energy of the β^+-particle is not as simple as it is for the β^--particle. The energy difference between the parent and daughter nucleus in this case is 1.99 MeV. An energy loss of $2mc^2$ is required to create the positron and allow it to escape from the nucleus – where m is the mass of the positron and c is the velocity of electromagnetic radiation. As the mass of the positron is the same as the mass of the electron, then 1.02 MeV is required to create the positron and eject it from the nucleus and any remaining energy (in this case 0.97 MeV) is given to the positron as kinetic energy.

Insight

A negatron or a positron is influenced by the electrostatic forces which exist between it and the nucleus until it is able to escape from the atom. As a result, the kinetic energy of the β^--particle is reduced by the force of attraction which exists between it and the nucleus, while the kinetic energy of the β^+-particle is increased by electrostatic repulsion. Energy and momentum are conserved in this process.

19.5.3 The fate of the positron

An energetic positron emitted by a nucleus will move through the surrounding atoms and will lose kinetic energy because of collisions with them. As its momentum decreases, it is more likely to interact with a free electron in the material. The positron is the *antiparticle* of the electron and when they meet they completely annihilate each other to form two gamma-rays of annihilation radiation. This process is shown diagrammatically in Figure 19.7, where the annihilation radiation consists of two photons, each of energy 0.511 MeV, ejected at 180° to each other. In this way, both energy and momentum are conserved. The mutual annihilation of the electron and the positron is an

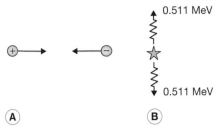

Figure 19.7 (A) A collision between a positron and an electron where both have a minimal kinetic energy. (B) The annihilation radiation where two photons, each of 0.511 MeV, are produced at 180° to each other.

example of the principle of mass–energy equivalence (see Sect. 16.4.1) as given by Einstein's equation $E = mc^2$, and shows that each particle has a mass–energy of 0.511 MeV, in agreement with Table 18.1.

The annihilation radiation produced by the reaction may now interact with neighbouring atoms by the processes of Compton scattering and photoelectric absorption (see Ch. 23) and may produce characteristic radiation and Auger electrons (see Sect. 19.6.3) by processes which will be discussed later in this chapter.

Insight

The positron and the electron may annihilate each other when the positron still has considerable kinetic energy. In this case, the two quanta are not emitted at 180° to each other and each has an energy higher than 0.511 MeV. The excess of energy of the positron is divided equally between each quantum. In each case, energy and momentum are conserved. A diagrammatic representation of the process is shown in the figure.

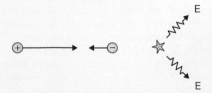

(A) collision between a positron and an electron where the positron has significant kinetic energy; (B) the direction of propagation of the annihilation radiation where the photons have energy in excess of 0.511 MeV each.

19.5.4 The neutrino

Consider the carbon-14 reaction which we discussed earlier. Here the carbon-14 decayed to nitrogen where the difference in energy between the parent and the daughter nucleus was 159 keV. As only beta decay takes place, we could confidently expect that all the β^--particles should have an energy of 159 keV. If we plot a graph of the energy

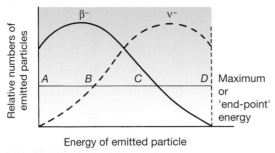

Figure 19.8 The sharing of energy between the beta-particle and the neutrino in beta decay – the case shown is for negatron emission.

of the beta-particles against the numbers emitted, we get a graph similar to the β^- graph shown in Figure 19.8. The maximum or end-point energy of the β^--particles in this case is 159 keV. The graph means that, although only beta decay takes place and although the difference between the parent and the daughter nucleus is 159 keV, some of the β^--particles have energies less than 159 keV. Such a situation would appear to suggest that this does not obey the law of conservation of energy (see Sect. 16.4). This difficulty was overcome by Wolfgang Pauli in 1933 when he postulated that another particle – the *neutrino* – is always ejected with a beta-particle. He suggested that a neutrino (symbol ν) is ejected at the same time as a positron and that an antineutrino (symbol ν^-) at the same time as a negatron. The *total energy* of the emitted negatron and antineutrino corresponds to the energy difference between the parent and daughter nucleus. How this energy is shared between the two particles will differ for each decay of the nucleus. In this way, a continuous distribution of energies is obtained both for the β^--particle and the antineutrino as shown in Figure 19.8.

Because of the presence of the neutrino and antineutrino, we now need to modify some of the equations we considered earlier:

Equation 19.6

$$^{14}_{6}\text{C} \rightarrow {}^{14}_{7}\text{N} + \beta^- + \nu^-$$
$$^{11}_{6}\text{C} \rightarrow {}^{11}_{5}\text{B} + \beta^+ + \nu$$

19.6 GAMMA DECAY OR GAMMA-RAY EMISSION

Gamma-rays are part of the electromagnetic spectrum and are similar in many ways to X-rays. Gamma-rays are emitted from a nucleus which has excess energy whereas X-rays are from electrons as they lose energy (this will be further discussed in Ch. 21). It is possible for gamma-rays to have lower energies than X-rays and vice versa. However, the maximum energy possible from gamma-rays exceeds that of X-rays.

We discussed in this chapter (see Sect 19.5.1) the fact that cobalt-60 decayed with the emission of a β-particle but the daughter nucleus was left in an excited state. The situation for this daughter nucleus is depicted in Figure 19.9A. The figure illustrates the energy states of the daughter nucleus by means of horizontal lines above the thick line representing the ground state of the nucleus. In this case, the $^{60}_{28}\text{Ni}$ nucleus is left at an energy 2.5 MeV above its ground state. It immediately decays to its ground state in two jumps:

1. It decays to 1.33 MeV above its ground state by the emission of a 1.17 MeV gamma-ray.
2. It then drops to its ground state by the emission of a second gamma-ray of energy 1.33 MeV.

Figure 19.9B shows the line spectra of the gamma radiation emitted by the nucleus where each gamma-ray has a precise energy corresponding to the discrete energy transformations within the nucleus.

19.6.1 Metastable states and isomeric transitions

In the case of $^{60}_{27}\text{Co}$ decaying to $^{60}_{28}\text{Ni}$, the nucleus remains in an excited state before the emission of the gamma-rays

---

Insight

Although Pauli postulated the existence of neutrinos and antineutrinos in 1933, the presence of these particles proved difficult to detect until much later. There is now conclusive proof of their existence because of experiments performed using nuclear reactors and particle accelerators. The neutrino and the antineutrino differ in their direction of spin relative to their direction of motion – the neutrino spins anticlockwise and the antineutrino spins clockwise. They are antiparticles and if they are made to collide will produce electromagnetic radiation in the form of annihilation radiation. The reason the particles are so difficult to detect can be seen by considering their three major properties:

1. zero rest mass
2. zero charge
3. extremely small interaction with matter.

Because of these properties, it is extremely difficult to detect the presence of neutrinos (or antineutrinos) – they have a half-value thickness (see Sect. 20.8) of many miles in lead!

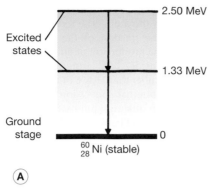

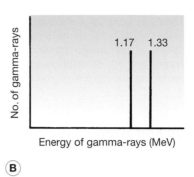

Figure 19.9 (A) The excited states of a nickel-60 nucleus which is left in an excited state as the result of the previous decay of a cobalt-60 nucleus. This decays to its ground state by the emission of two gamma photons, each representing the difference in energy between the excited states. (B) The line spectrum produced by the gamma radiation.

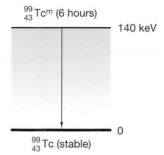

Figure 19.10 An example of the decay of technetium from a metastable to a stable state with the emission of a 140 keV gamma photon.

for a time so short that it is incapable of accurate measurement. However, this is not always the case, and those excited states which last sufficiently long for their durations to be measured are known as *metastable states*. The transition from a metastable state to a more stable state is known as an *isomeric transition*. Such metastable radionuclides prove to be useful in nuclear medicine because of the low dose which they deliver to the patient – the patient gets no dose from β⁻-particles emitted before metastability. Technetium-99m (usually written $^{99}_{43}\text{Tc}^{m}$ or, less commonly, $^{99m}_{43}\text{Tc}$) is a radionuclide which is widely used in nuclear medicine. A simplified decay scheme for it is shown in Figure 19.10 and it will be discussed in more detail Chapter 37 which deals with radionuclide imaging. The half-life of $^{99}_{43}\text{Tc}^{m}$ is 6 hours and it emits a gamma-ray of energy 140 keV when it decays to $^{99}_{43}\text{Tc}$. The half-life of $^{99}_{43}\text{Tc}$ is so long (2.1×10^{5} years) that it can be considered stable for all practical purposes.

The reaction can be written as:

Equation 19.7

$$^{99}_{43}\text{Tc}^{m} \rightarrow {}^{99}_{43}\text{Tc} + \gamma$$

The next section of this chapter considers the possible effects of gamma emission from the nucleus on the whole atom rather than on the nucleus only.

19.6.2 Internal conversion

When a nuclide is decaying by gamma emission, there is a competing process within the atom called *internal conversion*. This process results in electrons with discrete energies (unlike the continuous spectrum of energies of negatrons) being emitted from the atom. The process is a result of a direct interaction between the nucleus and an orbiting electron such that the nucleus is able to drop to its ground state by giving all of its excess energy to the electron.

The innermost electrons of the atom have orbitals which pass close to or even through the nucleus. Thus it is a matter of statistical probability whether the excess energy of the nucleus will result in a gamma-ray emission from the nucleus or electron emission from the inner shells. The *K*-shell is situated closest to the nucleus so is most likely to participate in such a reaction followed by the *L*-, *M*-shells, etc. The *converted electron* escapes from the atom with an energy equal to the energy donated by the nucleus minus the binding energy of that particular electron. This can be stated:

Equation 19.8

$$\text{KE of converted electron} = \\ \text{nuclear energy transition} - \text{BE}$$

where KE is kinetic energy and BE is binding energy of the electron.

The *internal conversion coefficient*, α, is defined as the ratio of the number of nuclear transformations which result in internal conversion to the number which result in gamma-ray emission. Thus, α may take a value between 0, resulting in no internal conversions, and infinity, corresponding to complete internal conversion. This can be illustrated by considering the figures for the decay of

$^{99}_{43}Tc^m$ to $^{99}_{43}Tc$. Approximately 9% of the nuclear transitions result in internal conversions of electrons from the K-shell, 1.1% from the L-shell and 0.3% from the M-shell. This means that 10.4% of the nuclear transitions result in internal conversions and 89.6% result in gamma-ray emission. This gives an internal conversion coefficient (α) for $^{99}_{43}Tc^m$ of 0.116.

19.6.3 X-rays and Auger electrons

If a radioactive decay results in a vacancy occurring within one of the inner electron shells of the atom, then electrons from orbitals further away from the nucleus will perform quantum jumps inwards until there are no inner shell vacancies. Each such quantum jump will result in the emission of electromagnetic radiation from the atom equal to the energy difference between the two shells. For inner-shell transitions, the energy of this electromagnetic radiation may be in the X-ray part of the spectrum. Such radiation is known as *fluorescent radiation* and its energy is characteristic of the atom concerned. If we consider the internal conversion process which we have just described and take a situation where a K-shell electron is removed from the atom, the vacancy thus created in the K-shell may be filled from the L-shell (a K_α transition) or from the M-shell (a K_β transition). Such a quantum jump would be accompanied by the emission of a photon of electromagnetic radiation equivalent to the energy difference between the two shells. If it was a K_α transition, there would now be a vacancy in the L-shell and this might be filled from the M-shell, etc. This would again be accompanied by the emission of a photon of electromagnetic radiation equal to the energy difference between the L- and M-shells. This process continues until the atom is able to capture a free electron to fill the vacancy – usually in one of its outermost shells. Until this occurs the atom contains more protons than electrons and so is regarded as a *positive ion*.

This already rather complex situation is further complicated by the fact that some of the photons emitted by such transitions may have sufficient energy to interact with other electrons in the atom and to remove them from their orbitals and eject them from the atom – this process is called the *photoelectric effect* and may occur if the photon energy is greater than the binding energy of the electron (see Ch. 23 for a more detailed description). The electrons thus ejected are called *Auger electrons* and have discrete energies equal to the photon energy minus the binding energy of the electron. The ejection of an Auger electron from a shell leaves a vacancy in that shell which will be filled by electrons jumping down from orbitals even further away from the nucleus, with the release of more fluorescent radiation and perhaps the release of even more Auger electrons.

From the above we can see that the ejection of an electron from one of the orbitals by internal conversion may result in a complicated sequence of orbital quantum jumps accompanied by the release of photons of electromagnetic radiation and the ejection of Auger electrons from the atom. The term *fluorescent yield* is used to describe the fraction of the electron transitions which result in the production of fluorescent radiation.

If we consider $^{99}_{43}Tc^m$ from the previous discussion, you may remember that 11.6% of the energy from the nucleus results in internal conversion ($\alpha = 0.116$). Of the resulting electron quantum jumps, 80% of the transitions result in fluorescent radiation and 20% result in the production of Auger electrons. Thus the fluorescent yield for technetium is 0.8. Some typical fluorescent radiation energies for $^{99}_{43}Tc^m$ are:

$$K_\alpha = 18.4\,keV, L_\alpha = 2.4\,keV, M_\alpha = 0.2\,keV$$

Note: The fact that the electrons emitted by this process carry discrete amounts of energy makes it easy to distinguish them from negatron emission where there is a continuous spectrum of energies.

Insight

For each decay, the total energies for all the fluorescent radiation and of all the electrons emitted from the shells of the atom equal the energy lost by the nucleus in the nuclear transition. This is because the binding energy of each ejected electron is recovered in the fluorescent radiation emitted in the subsequent cascade of orbital jumps. Thus the whole process obeys the law of conservation of energy (see Sect. 3.3).

19.7 ELECTRON CAPTURE

If a nucleus of low mass number has too few neutrons for stability but has insufficient excess energy ($<1.02\,MeV$) to eject a positron, then an alternative way by which the nucleus may undergo an isobaric transformation and lose energy is *electron capture* (shown in Fig. 19.11). In this process, the nucleus captures one of the orbiting electrons, the most likely being a capture of a K-shell electron. Sometimes the terms 'K capture' and 'L capture' are used to denote the shell from which the electron was captured. A situation where electron capture is the only process involved is shown in Figure 19.11A where $^{131}_{55}Cs$ decays to $^{131}_{54}Xe$.

In the diagram, the atomic number is reduced by one because the capture of an electron by the nucleus results in one of the protons in the nucleus changing into a neutron. Also note that during the process of electron capture, a neutrino is emitted by the nucleus. The processes involved in electron capture may be shown by Equation 19.9:

Equation 19.9

$$p^+ + e^+ \rightarrow n + \nu$$

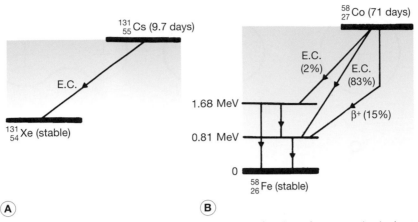

Figure 19.11 (A) Pure electron capture (EC) decay. (B) Electron capture and positron decay occurring in the same nuclide (85% EC and 15% positron decay). Also emitted are the X-rays from the iron-58 atoms and the 0.511 MeV annihilation radiations from the positron–electron annihilations.

In situations where a low-mass nucleus has too few neutrons and an excess energy greater than 1.02 MeV, then the process of electron capture may compete with the process of positron emission. An example of such a competing process is shown in the decay of $^{58}_{27}$Co into stable $^{58}_{26}$Fe in Figure 19.11B.

Note that both the process of electron capture and the process of positron emission involve the conversion of a proton to a neutron. Thus the atomic mass number remains unaltered but the atomic number is reduced by one.

As we mentioned earlier in this chapter (Sect. 19.6.2), creating a vacancy in an inner electron shell will result in the emission of characteristic fluorescent radiation from the atom. It is interesting to note that in the case of electron capture this is characteristic of the *daughter* product. This means that the electron orbitals of the daughter product are established before the consequent electron transitions occur.

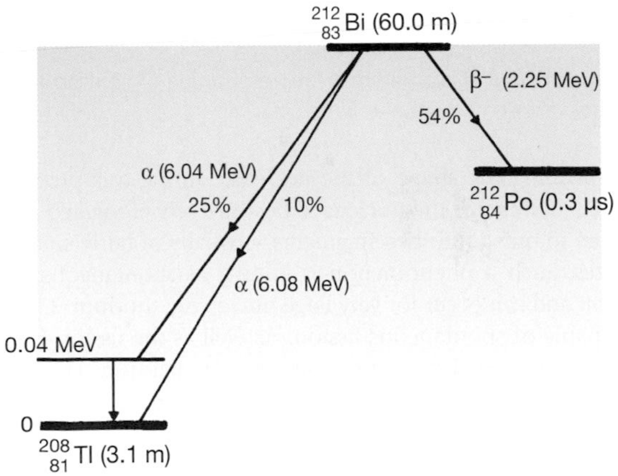

Figure 19.12 A branching decay programme where alpha and beta decay processes compete in the decay of bismuth-212.

19.8 BRANCHING DECAY PROGRAMMES

If the nucleus is very large, it is possible that it may disintegrate in more than one way. We have already encountered this – although it was not described in detail – in the uranium series in Figure 19.2. In this case, $^{214}_{83}$Bi can either decay to $^{214}_{84}$Po by β^--particle emission or it can decay to $^{210}_{81}$Tl by alpha-particle emission.

Another isotope of bismuth, $^{212}_{83}$Bi, decays in a similar branching programme. The decay process for this isotope involves the emission of alpha-particles of energies 6.04 and 6.08 MeV, gamma-rays of energy 0.04 MeV and β^--particles of maximum energy 2.25 MeV. The initial decay scheme for the $^{212}_{83}$Bi nuclide is shown in Figure 19.12. Note that, for

simplicity, only the first disintegrations are shown. As can be seen from the diagram, both $^{208}_{81}$Tl and $^{212}_{84}$Po have short half-lives and so are also radioactive.

19.9 FISSION

As we mentioned in our discussion of alpha decay (see Sect. 19.4), the short-range forces holding the nucleus together exist between adjacent nucleons, whereas the Coulomb forces act across the whole of the nucleus. This fact becomes increasingly important as the size of the nucleus increases. A very large nucleus may be pictured as being rather like a liquid drop in which the nucleons are moving about with very high energy and continuously

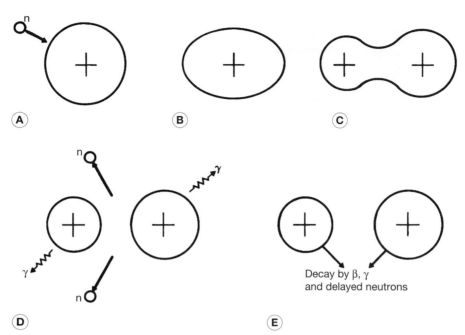

Figure 19.13 A diagrammatic representation of neutron-activated fission. For a fuller explanation of the process, see the text.

deforming the shape of the nucleus. During this process, it is possible for the nucleus to become very elongated and then to break into two fragments – usually of fairly similar sizes. Such a phenomenon is known as spontaneous fission and can occur for very large nuclei, e.g. thorium-232 is capable of spontaneous fission. As well as the fission fragments from such a reaction, one or more neutrons are usually liberated and the whole fission process is accompanied by the release of large amounts of energy.

Neutron-activated fission is a more controllable process than spontaneous fission. This occurs as a result of a heavy nucleus capturing an incoming neutron and then breaking into large fragments in a similar way to spontaneous fission. An example of such a reaction is the disintegration of $^{238}_{92}\text{U}$ into two fission fragments of $^{145}_{56}\text{Ba}$ and $^{94}_{36}\text{Kr}$ if the uranium-238 nucleus is made to absorb a neutron. The fission of the nucleus is normally accompanied by the release of gamma-rays and neutrons. Both of the fissile fragments are extremely rich in neutrons and so each will usually release a neutron. The neutrons from both of the above processes can now react with two $^{238}_{92}\text{U}$ nuclei, resulting in the release of four fissile fragments and four neutrons, and so a chain reaction can be set up. Such a process is accompanied by the release of large amounts of energy (see Insight).

A pictorial representation of the neutron-activated fission process is shown in Figure 19.13. The incoming neutron is captured in Figure 19.13A and delivers sufficient energy to the nucleus (Fig. 19.13B) to elongate its shape into an ellipsoid. As mentioned earlier, the Coulomb forces across the nucleus are now at an advantage over the short-range nuclear forces and the nucleus further

> ### Insight
>
> On average, a uranium-238 nucleus will release an energy of 200 MeV on fission. If we consider the complete fission of a 1-kg mass of uranium (this is about the size of a golf ball), we need to consider the energy released by all the uranium atoms in a 1-kg mass. By applying Avogadro's equation (see Sect. 3.6) to this we can calculate that 1 kg of uranium-238 contains 2.5×10^{24} atoms. If each of these atoms releases 200 MeV of energy, the total energy released will be 5.1×10^{27} MeV. This is the same as 8.1×10^{13} joules of energy.

distorts to form a 'peanut' shape (Fig. 19.13C) and eventually breaks to form two fragments because of the electrostatic repulsion between the two main nuclear masses. The two fragments fly apart (their kinetic energy accounts for about 80% of the total disintegration energy) and several neutrons and gamma-ray photons are usually emitted (Fig. 19.13D). The neutrons emitted by this reaction may now interact with other atoms to cause fission and the release of further neutrons and so a chain reaction is set up, with the consequent liberation of large amounts of energy. The fissile fragments (Fig. 19.13E) are themselves rich in neutrons for their atomic numbers and so will undergo further disintegration to move towards more stable nuclei. This initial process results in the production of β^--particles (with associated gamma-rays) which produces a more stable proton/neutron configuration or, if the nucleus is very excited, the ejection of a neutron from the nucleus. These neutrons are known as *delayed neutrons* to distinguish them from the *prompt neutrons* which are emitted at the moment of fission.

Fission products from any type of nucleus are not always the same and may have different relative sizes on each disintegration. Thus a great range of other decay chains is possible from other fissile fragments.

Insight

It is also possible to initiate fission in the nucleus by bombarding it with protons (or with alpha-particles) or by striking it with high-energy photons. Examples of these are:

- Copper ($^{63}_{29}Cu$), if bombarded with protons, can be made to undergo fission to produce sodium ($^{24}_{11}Na$) and potassium ($^{39}_{19}K$). This process is accompanied by neutron emission.
- Uranium-238 ($^{238}_{32}U$), if it is bombarded by photons of energy equal to or greater than 5.1 MeV, will undergo fission. This latter process is known as *photofission*.

19.10 SUMMARY OF RADIOACTIVE NUCLEAR TRANSFORMATIONS

Table 19.1 is a summary of the types of radioactive decay discussed so far in this chapter. You may find it useful to refer back to this table when considering the production of artificial radionuclides and also in considering the use of radionuclides in medicine in Chapter 37.

Summary

In this chapter you should have learnt:

- The mechanism for alpha decay and alpha-particle emission (see Sect. 19.4)
- Beta decay leading to negatron emission (see Sect. 19.5.1)
- Beta decay leading to positron emission (see Sect. 19.5.2)
- The fate of the positron after emission (see Sect. 19.5.3)
- The fact that a neutrino or an antineutrino forms part of beta emission (see Sect. 19.5.4)
- The mechanism of gamma decay and gamma-ray emission (see Sect. 19.6)
- The meaning of metastable nuclei and isomeric transitions (see Sect. 19.6.1)
- The mechanism of the process of internal conversion (see Sect. 19.6.2)
- The mechanisms involved in the emission of X-rays and Auger electrons from the atoms of radionuclides (see Sect. 19.6.3)
- The mechanism of electron capture and the subsequent changes within the atom (see Sect. 19.7)
- Branching decay programmes (see Sect. 19.8)
- The processes involved in nuclear fission (see Sect. 19.9)
- Summary of radioactive nuclear transformations (See Sect 19.10)

FURTHER READING

Ball, J.L., Moore, A.D., Turner, S., 2008. Ball and Moore's Essential Physics for Radiographers, fourth ed. Blackwell Scientific, London (Chapter 20).

Table 19.1 Summary of the effects of radioactive decay

TYPE OF DECAY	SYMBOL	EFFECT ON NUCLEUS			EFFECT ON ATOM	COMMENTS
		Z	N	A		
Alpha	α	$Z-2$	$N-2$	$A-4$	Electron orbits change to that of daughter nucleus	Occurs in elements with a mass number greater than 150. Daughter products may undergo further decay by a variety of the processes mentioned below
Negatron emission	β^-	$Z+1$	$N-1$	–	Electron orbits change to that of daughter nucleus	Proton changes to neutron in nucleus. Negatron emitted from the nucleus with a spread of energies but the energy of the negatron plus the energy of the antineutrino is constant for a given nuclide. Daughter nucleus may further decay by prompt or delayed gamma-ray emission competing with internal conversion (IC)
Positron emission	β^+	$Z-1$	$N+1$	–	Electron orbits change to that of daughter nucleus	Neutron changes to proton in nucleus. The positron is emitted with a neutrino and the sum of their energies is constant for a given nuclide. The process only occurs if the energy loss by the parent nucleus can be greater than 1.02 MeV. Positron is annihilated by collision with electron and two photons of annihilation radiation, each of energy 0.511 MeV are produced. Daughter nucleus may decay by gamma radiation and/or IC
Gamma radiation	γ	–	–	–	No effect on the number of nucleons in the nucleus but the process may compete with IC	Produced by the quantum jump from excited state of the nucleus to a lower energy. Excited states of measurable half-life are defined as *metastable* and the transition is *isomeric*
Internal conversion	IC	–	–	–	Characteristic radiation and Auger electrons emitted	An inner orbital electron of the atom interacts with the nucleus and is ejected from the atom. The electron is given the excess nuclear energy. This creates a vacancy in the shell and results in the emission of characteristic radiation and Auger electrons
Electron capture	EC	$Z-1$	$N+1$	–	Characteristic radiation and Auger electrons of the daughter nucleus are emitted	An inner orbital electron is captured by the nucleus and changes a proton to a neutron. A neutrino is emitted, carrying energy changes of the nucleus. The nucleus may decay spontaneously by gamma-ray emission. The vacancy left in the electron orbit results in the emission of characteristic radiation and Auger electrons
Fission	f	Size and structure of the fragments may vary			Bonds may be broken or ionization caused by fragment	Fission may be spontaneous or neutron activated. The nucleus splits, producing two or more fragments, gamma-rays and neutrons. Controlled fission is used in nuclear reactors and the neutrons can be used to produce artificial radionuclides (see Ch. 37)

Chapter | 20 |

The exponential law

20.1 AIM

The aim of this chapter is to introduce the exponential law and consider its applications to radiographic science. The law is fundamental to an understanding of radioactive decay and the attenuation of certain electromagnetic radiations (e.g. X-rays and gamma-rays).

20.2 DESCRIPTION OF THE EXPONENTIAL LAW

Perhaps the best everyday example of the exponential law concerns money. If £100 is invested with a financial institution which gives a fixed interest rate of 5% per annum

then the growth of that money over a 25-year period is shown in Table 20.1 (See page 140).

Notice that the net increase per year is initially quite small (£5.00 in the first year) but the amount increases with time (£16.13 in the 25th year). This is an example of exponential growth in that as the time increases by *equal amounts* (1 year) the money increases by *equal fractions* (5%). If we draw a graph of the total money with the financial institution we get a smooth curve, as shown in Figure 20.1 (See page 140). This is the typical shape of an increasing exponential.

For a second example, consider a situation where we possess an initial sum of £100. If we consider a tax system where 5% of this money is removed each year as a tax, then the fate of the original £100 is shown in Table 20.2 (See page 141). Again we can note that the net decrease is greatest during the first year (£5.00) and is least during the 25th year (£1.46). The rate of decrease is, however, the same, at 5% per annum. This is an example of exponential decay in that as the time increases by *equal amounts* (1 year) the money left will decrease by 5% of that remaining, but will never reach zero (i.e. there will always be some money left). If we draw a graph of the total money left, we again get a smooth curve, as shown in Figure 20.2 (See page 141). This is the typical shape of a decaying exponential.

The common factor in these two examples is that the change each year is 5%. This is characteristic of all exponential change and may be expressed as follows:

Definition

A quantity *y* is said to vary *exponentially* with *x* if equal changes in *x* produce equal *fractional* (or percentage) changes in *y*.

The two major examples of the exponential law in radiographic science are radioactive decay and the attenuation of electromagnetic radiation by matter. Both of these are described in the following sections.

Table 20.1 Growth of £100 at 5% per annum

YEAR	INTEREST RATE (%)	MONEY AT END OF YEAR	NET INCREASE FOR YEAR
1	5	£105	£5.00
2	5	£110.25	£5.25
3	5	£115.76	£5.51
4	5	£121.55	£5.79
5	5	£127.63	£6.08
6	5	£134.01	£6.38
7	5	£140.71	£6.70
8	5	£147.74	£7.03
9	5	£155.13	£7.39
10	5	£162.90	£7.77
11	5	£171.03	£8.13
12	5	£179.59	£8.56
13	5	£188.56	£8.97
14	5	£197.99	£9.43
15	5	£207.89	£9.90
16	5	£218.29	£10.40
17	5	£229.90	£10.91
18	5	£240.66	£11.46
19	5	£252.70	£12.04
20	5	£265.33	£12.63
21	5	£278.60	£13.27
22	5	£292.53	£13.93
23	5	£307.15	£14.62
24	5	£322.51	£15.36
25	5	£338.64	£16.13

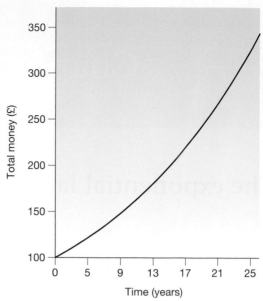

Figure 20.1 Growth of £100 at 5% per annum. Note that the rate of growth becomes greater with time. This is an example of *exponential growth*.

several forms, including the ejection of alpha-particles, beta-particles (both positive and negative) and gamma-rays from the nucleus. These and other modes of decay have been discussed more fully in Chapter 19. The particular mode of decay is, however, not important to our discussion in this section as the application of the exponential law is valid for all the modes. It can be stated as:

Definition

The *law of radioactive decay* states that the rate of decay of a particular nuclide (i.e. the number of nuclei decaying per second) is proportional to the number of such nuclei left in the sample (i.e. it is a fixed fraction of the number of nuclei left in the sample).

This is exactly analogous to the changes that occurred in the decaying exponential sum of money, in that a fixed fraction (or percentage) will decay each unit time (similar to the loss of money from the lump sum). Figure 20.3 shows a graph depicting the above situation. Note that the initial fall in number of atoms is steep but slows down as fewer and fewer of the original nuclei are left. Also note that the number of original nuclei never reaches zero. This is exactly the same as happened in the case of the lump sum of money and you should also note the similarities between Figure 20.3 (See page 141) and Figure 20.2.

20.3 RADIOACTIVE DECAY AND THE EXPONENTIAL LAW

Radionuclides are said to *decay* when they change from one nuclear configuration to another. This decay takes

Table 20.2 Decrease of £100 at 5% per annum

YEAR	TAX RATE (%)	MONEY AT END OF YEAR	NET DECREASE FOR YEAR
1	5	£95.00	£5.00
2	5	£90.25	£4.75
3	5	£85.74	£4.51
4	5	£81.45	£4.29
5	5	£77.38	£4.07
6	5	£73.51	£3.87
7	5	£69.83	£3.68
8	5	£66.34	£3.49
9	5	£63.02	£3.32
10	5	£59.87	£3.15
11	5	£56.88	£2.99
12	5	£54.04	£2.84
13	5	£51.33	£2.70
14	5	£48.77	£2.57
15	5	£46.33	£2.44
16	5	£44.01	£2.32
17	5	£41.81	£2.20
18	5	£39.72	£2.09
19	5	£37.74	£1.99
20	5	£35.85	£1.89
21	5	£34.06	£1.79
22	5	£32.35	£1.70
23	5	£30.74	£1.62
24	5	£29.20	£1.54
25	5	£27.74	£1.46

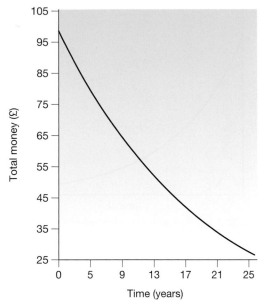

Figure 20.2 Decay of £100 at 5% tax per annum. Note that the rate of decay decreases with time and the amount of money left never reaches zero. This is an example of *exponential decay*.

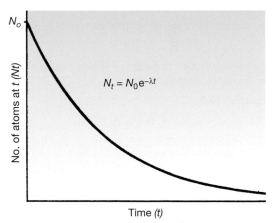

Figure 20.3 Exponential decay of the *number of atoms* of a particular radionuclide. (Note the similarity to Figure 19.2.)

the nuclear disintegrations by counting the number of gamma-rays (for example) emitted, using a suitable counter. In this way we may make an estimate of the total number of disintegrations per second occurring within the radioactive sample at any given time. This quantity is known as the *activity* of the sample and is measured in becquerels, where 1 Bq is 1 nuclear disintegration per second. We may now plot *activity* against *time* (Fig. 20.4) and we obtain exactly the same curve as in Figure 20.3. The equation for this curve is expressed as:

Equation 20.1

$$A_t = A_0 e^{-\lambda t}$$

20.4 MEASURES OF RADIOACTIVITY

In practice it would be extremely difficult to measure the number of nuclei remaining and draw a graph like Figure 20.3. What we can measure more easily is the *effects* of

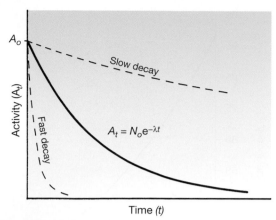

Figure 20.4 Exponential decay of the *radioactivity* of a particular radionuclide.

where A_t is the activity after a time t, A_0 is the initial activity, e is the exponential constant, λ is the decay constant and t is the time after the initial measurement.

Insight

In practice it is often easier to use Equation 20.1 in its logarithmic form. (For more information on logarithms, see Appendix A.) Consider Equation 20.1:

$$A_t = A_0 e^{-\lambda t}$$

If we take logarithms to the base e of both sides of the equation then we get:

Equation 20.2

$$\log_e A_t = \log_e A_0 - \lambda t$$

This equation and its use with logarithmic graph paper will be considered further at the end of this chapter.

Figure 20.4 shows the decay curves for radionuclides which have different rates of decay. As we cannot consider the time it will take a nuclide to reach zero as a measure of its rate of decay, a quantity called the *half-life* is used to describe the rate of decay. This is further considered in the next section.

20.5 HALF-LIFE AND DECAY CONSTANT

Definition

The *half-life* of a radionuclide is the time required for the activity of the radioactive sample to decay to one-half of its original value.

An illustration of the half-life of a particular radionuclide is shown in Figure 20.5 (See page 143). The activity of the sample when $t = 0$ is A_0. When the activity is reduced to $A_0/2$ then the radionuclide has undergone one half-life. This is indicated by the time $t_{1/2}$. If another half-life passes, then the activity is reduced by a further factor of 2 and is now $A_0/4$, and so on for further half-lives. Notice that, as in our monetary example (Fig. 20.2), the curve never reaches zero activity, so no radioactive source is ever completely 'dead'.

If we now consider Equation 20.1, we can use this to establish a relationship between the decay constant and the half-life:

$$A_t = A_0 e^{-\lambda t_{1/2}}$$

Now, by definition, at the half-life, $A_0/2 = A_0 e^{-\mu t_{1/2}}$. Thus the equation can be rewritten in the form:

Equation 20.3

$$\frac{A_0}{2} = A_0 e^{-\lambda t_{1/2}}$$
$$\frac{1}{2} = e^{-\lambda t_{1/2}}$$
$$2 = e^{\lambda t_{1/2}}$$
$$\log_e 2 = \lambda t_{1/2}$$
$$0.693 = \lambda t_{1/2}$$
$$\lambda = \frac{0.693}{t_{1/2}}$$

The decay constant is thus measured in time^{-1} since it is inversely related to the half-life. The decay constant is simply a *constant of proportionality* (see Appendix A).

Example

The half-life of $^{99}\text{Tc}^m$ is 6 h. What is its decay constant? From Equation 20.3:

$$\lambda = \frac{0.693}{t_{1/2}}$$
$$\lambda = \frac{0.693}{6} \text{h}^{-1}$$
$$= 0.1155 \text{ h}^{-1}$$

Because of this relationship between the half-life and the decay constant, we may also write Equation 20.1 as follows:

Equation 20.4

$$A_t = A_0 e^{-(0.693/t_{1/2})}$$

Another important point is that it does not matter from which time measurement of the half-life is begun. Figure 20.6 (See page 143) shows the decay of a radionuclide over a time of one half-life starting from an arbitrary

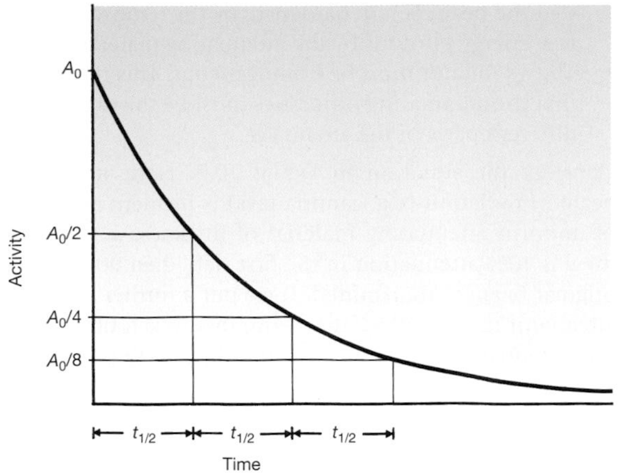

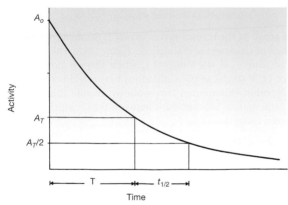

Figure 20.5 Half-life ($t_{1/2}$) and the radioactive decay. Note that each $t_{1/2}$ reduces the level of radioactivity by one-half.

Figure 20.6 The half-life ($t_{1/2}$) is measured from an arbitrary time, T. It is found that the value of $t_{1/2}$ so obtained does not depend on the value of T, so the half-life may be measured from any starting time.

time, T. Note that the value of $t_{1/2}$ shown in Figure 20.6 is exactly the same as the value shown in Figure 20.5. Thus, over an interval of $t_{1/2}$ the activity is reduced by a factor of 2, independent of the starting time, T.

This example at the top of the next column gives some clue as to the general method of solving such problems. Assuming n half-lives of decay, the decayed activity A_n can be calculated from the formula:

Equation 20.5

$$A_n = \frac{A_0}{2^n}$$

where A_0 is the original activity.

Similarly, we can use this equation to *look back* to consider how much original activity would be required on a certain date to give us the required activity at the time of

---

> ### Example
>
> A radioisotope of iodine, ^{131}I, has a half-life of 8 days. Its activity was measured as 14.4 MBq at 09:00 on 3 February. What will be its activity at 09:00 on 27 February?
>
> The time interval over which we are considering the decay of the nuclide is 24 days. With a half-life of 8 days, this represents decay through three half-lives.
>
> After one half-life the activity will be reduced by a factor of 2.
>
> After two half-lives the activity will be reduced by a factor of $(2 \times 2) = 4$.
>
> After three half-lives the activity will be reduced by a factor of $(4 \times 2) = 8$.
>
> So each successive half-life reduces the activity by a factor of 2.
>
> Thus the activity after three half-lives = 14.4/8 = 1.18 MBq.
>
> The activity at 09:00 on 27 February will therefore be 1.18 MBq.

use of the isotope. Here the unknown is A_0 and the equation can be rearranged as follows:

Equation 20.6

$$A_0 = 2^n \times A_n$$

> ### Example
>
> An activity of 36.5 MBq of $^{99}Tc^m$ is required at 17:00 on 22 March. The radionuclide has a half-life of 6 h. What activity of the isotope must be dispensed at 05:00 on 22 March to give the required activity?
>
> Using Equation 20.6:
>
> $$A_0 = 2^n \times A_n$$
> $$= 22 \times 36.5\ \text{MBq}$$
> $$= 146\ \text{MBq}$$

20.6 PHYSICAL HALF-LIFE, BIOLOGICAL HALF-LIFE AND EFFECTIVE HALF-LIFE

In all the considerations of radioactive decay so far we have considered the *physical half-life* of an isotope – the half-life as it would be measured using a quantity of isotope in the laboratory. In *nuclear medicine* there are two other types of half-life we need to consider:

1. The *biological half-life* is the time taken for the concentration of a certain chemical in an organ to be

reduced to half its original concentration. In this case, the concentration of the chemical is the important part and its activity is not important. This value is affected by the body's ability to excrete the chemical.

2. The *effective half-life* is the time taken for the activity of a certain radionuclide in a certain organ to be reduced to half of its original activity. This will be affected by the physical half-life and the biological half-life.

The three types of half-life are connected by the equation:

Equation 20.7

$$\frac{1}{t_{1/2_{(eff)}}} = \frac{1}{t_{1/2_{(phys)}}} + \frac{1}{t_{1/2_{(bio)}}}$$

20.7 ATTENUATION OF ELECTROMAGNETIC RADIATION BY MATTER

The attenuation of electromagnetic radiation by matter constitutes the other major application of the exponential law in radiography.

The types of interactions which electromagnetic radiation undergoes when it passes through matter are explained in Chapter 23. A detailed knowledge of these mechanisms is not required at this stage. If we consider a slab of material which has 100 units of radiation incident on it and the transmitted radiation measures 90 units, then we can say that the material *attenuates* 10 units of radiation (the differences between absorption and attenuation will be explained in Ch. 23).

For the exponential law to be applied, certain conditions must be satisfied:

• The radiation beam must be parallel. This means that it is not affected by the inverse square law.
• The radiation beam must be homogeneous (i.e. the photons must all have the same energy). This means

that the beam is not 'hardened' by the removal of low-energy photons by the attenuating material.
• The attenuator must be homogeneous. This means that the attenuating properties must be the same in different parts of the attenuator.

Consider the situation in Figure 20.7. Here, a parallel beam of radiation (e.g. gamma-rays) is incident on a slab of uniform attenuating material of thickness x. Suppose there is 10% attenuation in the first slab, then 90% of the original beam is transmitted. If we put a further identical attenuator in the path of the beam, then it is found that it also attenuates 10% of the radiation incident upon it and 81% (0.9 × 90%) will be transmitted. A third identical attenuator transmits 90% of this amount (72.9%), and so on for further attenuators. From this we can say that *equal changes in x produce equal fractional (or percentage) changes in the transmitted radiation intensity*. This is again an exponential relationship, so we can say that:

> *The attenuation of a monoenergetic parallel beam of electromagnetic radiation by a uniform attenuator will vary exponentially with the attenuator thickness.*

A graph of the transmitted intensity I_x through the attenuator of thickness x is shown in Figure 20.8. The incident radiation I_0 is the value of I_x when there is no attenuator ($x = 0$). Note the similarities between this curve and the other exponential curves shown in this chapter. The mathematical relationships between the quantities can be given using equation:

Equation 20.8

$$I_x = I_0 e^{-\mu x}$$

where μ (mu) is the *total linear attenuation coefficient* and so takes into account all the processes of attenuation. The equation therefore refers to variations of transmittance within linear distance, x.

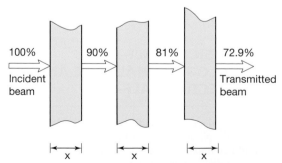

Figure 20.7 Exponential attenuation of a parallel beam of electromagnetic radiation by matter. Equal thickness (x) of the attenuator will transmit equal fractions (in this case 9/10) of the incident radiation.

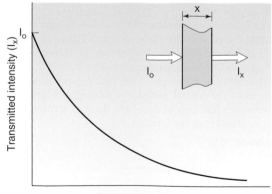

Figure 20.8 Graph showing changes in transmitted intensity due to exponential attenuation of radiation by a uniform attenuator. Note the similarity to Figure 20.3.

20.8 HALF-VALUE THICKNESS

If we consider Figure 20.9, we can see that successive half-value thicknesses (HVTs) reduce the intensity by factors of 2, and are therefore in a position to define HVT more precisely.

The HVT therefore depends on the attenuating properties of the substance itself and the penetrating power of the beam of electromagnetic radiation incident upon it. In diagnostic radiography, we might compare the penetrating properties of two beams using aluminium to the HVTs, whereas in therapeutic radiography we would do this using copper as our attenuator. This is because the photon energy is higher in therapeutic radiography so we need to use a material with a higher atomic number.

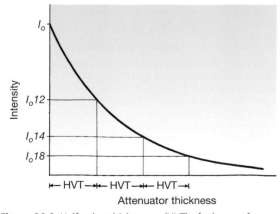

Figure 20.9 Half-value thicknesses (HVT) of a beam of electromagnetic radiation. Each HVT of the attenuator reduces the intensity by one-half. Note the similarity to Figure 20.5.

To complete the analogy with radioactive decay, Equation 20.3 is paralleled by:

Equation 20.9

$$\mu = \frac{0.693}{\text{HVT}}$$

Example

a. The HVT for a beam of radiation is found to be 2.8 mm of aluminium. What is the total linear attenuation coefficient of this beam in aluminium?
   From Equation 20.9:

$$\begin{aligned}
\mu &= \frac{0.693}{\text{HVT}} \\
&= \frac{0.693}{2.8}\,\text{mm}^{-1} \\
&= 0.2475\,\text{mm}^{-1}
\end{aligned}$$

b. The HVT for a particular beam of gamma-rays is 3 mm of lead. What thickness of lead must be placed in the beam such that only 0.1% of it is transmitted?

There are several ways of tackling this and similar problems. Below is one method.

One-hundred per cent of the beam is incident on the lead and 0.1 % is transmitted. This gives a reduction factor of 100/0.1 = 1000.

Now each HVT gives a reduction factor of 2 between the incident and the transmitted radiation, as shown in the table below:

NUMBER OF HVTS	INTENSITY REDUCTION FACTOR
1	2
2	4 (i.e. 2 × 2)
3	8
4	16
5	32
6	64
7	128
8	256
9	512
10	1024

This sort of table is very easy to check so there should be little chance of arithmetic errors.

After 10 HVTs, the intensity reduction factor is 1024, which is very close to the required factor of 1000.

Thus, 30 mm of lead (10 HVTs) must be used to reduce the transmitted intensity to 0.1% of the incident intensity.

As was the case with radioactive decay (see Equation 20.5), we can use a formula to calculate the intensity (I_n) after n HVTs:

Equation 20.10

$$I_n = \frac{I_0}{2^n}$$

20.9 TENTH-VALUE THICKNESS

It should be clear at this stage that values of absorber thickness other than the HVT will produce equal fractional changes in transmission and so it is possible to define a 'fifth-value thickness' or a 'tenth-value thickness' (TVT), etc. Although the HVT is a very common method of measuring the attenuation of electromagnetic radiation through matter, the TVT is also used when considering large amounts of attenuation. An example of this would be when designing the walls of a radiotherapy treatment room when a very high intensity of radiation from the treatment machine must not be allowed to penetrate through the wall in significant quantities. One TVT would reduce the intensity by a factor of 10; two would reduce the intensity by a factor of 100, and so on.

20.10 USE OF LOGARITHMIC FORM OF THE EXPONENTIAL LAW

Consider Equation 20.2, which is the logarithmic form of the exponential law:

$$\log_e A_t = \log_e A_0 - \lambda t$$

If we look at this equation, we see that it is in the form of $y = c - mx$ and so we would expect its graph to be in the form of a straight line. If we plot $\log_e$ of the activity on the y-axis and time on the x-axis, we get the graph shown in Figure 20.10.

The requirement to calculate the logarithm for each result and the antilogarithm for each reading from the graph is overcome by the use of logarithmic graph paper (for a fuller description, see Appendix A). Suitable graph paper in this case is log/linear graph paper, i.e. the y-axis is logarithmic and the x-axis is linear.

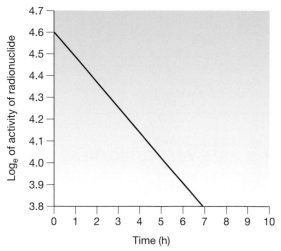

Figure 20.10 Graph of the logarithm to the base e of the activity of a radionuclide plotted against time. Note that the previous exponential curve (see Fig. 20.4) is now a *straight line*.

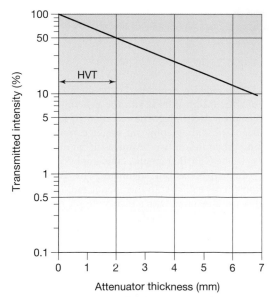

Figure 20.11 An example of the use of logarithmic graph paper to plot an exponential relationship. Note that the previous exponential curve (Fig. 20.8) has now has become a straight line. The half-value thickness (HVT) for the beam of radiation is 2 mm, as read from the graph. Half lives may also be determined in the same manner.

An example of such a graph for the attenuation of a beam of electromagnetic radiation is shown in Figure 20.11. Note that equal spaces on the log scale represent changes by factors of 10, and so the logarithmic scale never reaches zero. This type of paper allows us to plot the points directly on the paper and then draw the best straight line through them. Such a linear graph makes it easier to interpolate and to extrapolate (see Appendix A) information from the graph.

Summary

In this chapter, we have considered the following factors pertinent to the exponential law:
- The description of the exponential law (see Sect. 20.2).
- Radioactive decay and the exponential law (see Sect. 20.3).
- Measures which can be made of the activity of a radionuclide (see Sect. 20.4).
- The relationship between the half-life and the decay constant for a radionuclide (see Sect. 20.5).
- The relationships between the physical half-life, the biological half-life and the effective half-life (see Sect. 20.6).
- How the attenuation of electromagnetic radiation by matter obeys the exponential law (see Sect. 20.7).
- The HVT for a beam of radiation and a given attenuator (see Sect. 20.8).
- The use of the TVT (see Sect. 20.9).
- The use of the logarithmic form of the exponential law (see Sect. 20.10).

FURTHER READING

Radioactivity and the exponential law

Chapter 19 of the current text contains more information on this topic.

Ball, J.L., Moore, A.D., Turner, S., 2008. Ball and Moore's Essential Physics for Radiographers, fourth ed. Blackwell Scientific, London (Chapter 20).

Dendy, P.P., Heaton, B., 1999. Physics for Diagnostic Radiology, Institute of Physics, second ed. (Chapter 1).

Webb, S. (Ed.), 2000. The Physics of Medical Imaging, second ed. Institute of Physics, Bristol. (Chapter 6).

Exponential attenuation of radiation

Ball, J.L., Moore, A.D., Turner, S., 2008. Ball and Moore's Essential Physics for Radiographers, fourth ed. Blackwell Scientific, London (Chapter 17).

Bushong, S.C., 2009. Radiologic Science for Technologists: Physics, Biology and Protection, ninth ed. Mosby, New York (Chapter 4).

Dendy, P.P., Heaton, B., 1999. Physics for Diagnostic Radiology, Institute of Physics, second ed. (Chapter 3).

Part | 4 |

X-rays and matter

Chapter | 21 |

Production of X-rays

CHAPTER CONTENTS

21.1 AIM

The aim of this chapter is to consider the mechanisms by which X-rays are produced at the target of the X-ray tube. The concept of the X-ray spectrum will be introduced and this chapter will act as a foundation for Chapter 22 where the factors affecting the X-ray spectrum will be considered.

21.2 INTERACTIONS OF ELECTRONS WITH MATTER

In Chapter 30 we will discuss the construction of the X-ray tube and the functions of its various components.

In this chapter we will look in detail at the processes involved at subatomic level in the target of the X-ray tube to allow the production of X-rays.

Electrons are produced at the filament of the X-ray tube, accelerated towards the target of the tube and then made to collide with the target atoms. There are a number of ways in which high-energy electrons from the filament of the X-ray tube may lose their energy when they collide with the atoms of the target. These are shown in Figure 21.1:

* Electrons from the filament lose energy because of interactions between them and the outer electrons surrounding the atoms of the target material (see electron 1 in Fig. 21.1).
* Electrons from the filament lose energy because of interactions between them and the nuclei of the atoms of the target material (see electrons 2 and 3 in Fig. 21.1).
* Electrons from the filament lose energy because of interactions between them and individual inner electrons of the target atoms (see electron 4 in Fig. 21.1).

The interactions between electrons and target atoms may be elastic where there is conservation of kinetic energy or inelastic collisions in which kinetic energy is lost (see Section 3.3). It is also important to realise that an electron from the filament may experience many interactions (typically about 1000) before it is brought to rest within 0.25–0.5 mm of the target surface.

21.3 INTERACTIONS BETWEEN ELECTRONS FROM THE FILAMENT AND THE OUTER ELECTRONS OF THE TARGET ATOMS IN THE X-RAY TUBE

As you will see in Chapter 30, the main material of the X-ray tube target is tungsten, which has an atomic number

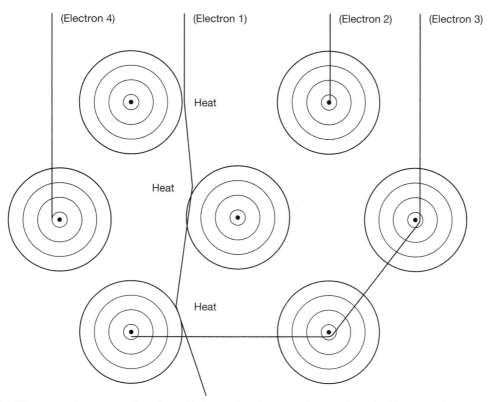

(Electron 4)   (Electron 1)   (Electron 2)   (Electron 3)

Heat

Heat

Heat

Figure 21.1 Diagrammatic representation of possible interactions between electrons from the filament and target atoms in an X-ray tube. An explanation of the interactions is given in the text.

of 74. Thus each target atom is surrounded by 74 electrons in various orbitals. These electrons have the effect of deflecting the approaching electron from the filament from their original path because of the electrostatic repulsion between them and the filament electron. Such deflections from the electron's original path are small and so the loss of kinetic energy is small. The kinetic energy lost by the electron is emitted as a photon of electromagnetic radiation. The energy of this photon is such that it falls into the infrared part of the spectrum and so heat is produced in the target material. If we consider the statistical probability of this process occurring rather than the other two processes identified in Section 21.2, we can see that it has a very high probability of occurring.

This is because the other two processes involve an interaction between either the incoming electron and the nucleus or the incoming electron and the inner orbital electrons. The area occupied by the nucleus and the inner electron orbitals is very small compared to the size of the whole tungsten atom and so an incoming electron has a much greater chance of interacting with the whole atom. For the above reasons, about 95–99% of the energy produced at the target of the X-ray tube is in the form of heat.

21.4 INTERACTIONS BETWEEN ELECTRONS FROM THE FILAMENT AND THE NUCLEI OF THE TARGET ATOMS IN THE X-RAY TUBE

As mentioned at the beginning of this chapter, the interactions of electrons from the filament with the nuclei of the target atoms can be elastic interactions or inelastic interactions. As each of these results in a different outcome, they will now be considered separately.

21.4.1 Elastic collisions with the nuclei

The electron has a relatively low mass and a negative charge while the tungsten nucleus has a larger mass (about 334 000 times that of the electron) and a positive charge (74 times that of the electron). Thus the electron is attracted to the more massive tungsten nucleus.

As shown in Figure 21.2, the closer the electron travels to the nucleus, the more it is deflected from its original path

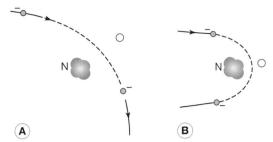

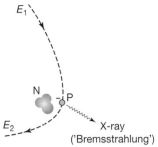

Figure 21.2 The deflection of an electron from the filament when it interacts with the nucleus of a target atom in the X-ray tube: (A) a small deflection; (B) a large deflection.

Figure 21.3 The production of Bremsstrahlung X-rays. An electron at point P suddenly loses energy by the emission of an X-ray photon. The electron continues with a reduced energy, E_2.

by the attraction of the positive nucleus. Because the mass of the electron is so tiny compared to that of the nucleus, the amount of energy it transfers to it is proportionately small.

These events therefore serve only to produce very tortuous paths for the electrons within the tungsten, without transferring much energy to the tungsten. The number of such events compared to the number of inelastic collisions discussed in the next section increases with the atomic number of the target material and so they are very frequent in tungsten.

21.4.2 Inelastic collisions with the nuclei – production of Bremsstrahlung radiation

Classical physics concluded that when a charged particle changed its velocity, this *always* resulted in the emission of electromagnetic radiation. However, we have already seen that this is not the case, as the electrons in the Bohr model of the atom are continuously changing their velocity (see Sect. 18.4). We have also seen in the previous section that electrons can undergo elastic collisions with the nucleus which result in no electromagnetic radiation being produced. As shown in Figure 21.2, the electron must accelerate towards the nucleus during its deflection but, despite this acceleration, a quantum of electromagnetic radiation is emitted in only a small percentage of cases. When such a quantum is emitted, the kinetic energy of the electron is suddenly reduced by an amount equal to the energy of the quantum, and so the electron is suddenly slowed down or *braked*.

This is an example of an inelastic interaction since the total kinetic energy of the electron and of the nucleus is not conserved because some energy is removed by the emission of the quantum of radiation. The energy of the quantum may be in the X-ray part of the electromagnetic spectrum and the radiation is known as *braking* or *Bremsstrahlung* radiation. The exact energy of this quantum will vary and may be very small if the electron does not lose much energy in its interaction with the nucleus

or it may be up to the total kinetic energy of the electron if it is involved in a direct collision with the nucleus (see electron 2 in Fig. 21.1).

Note that not every electron passing close to the nucleus will emit such a photon of radiation but only those which are able to undergo a sudden loss of energy by an inelastic interaction with the nucleus.

The Bremsstrahlung process is illustrated in Figure 21.3, where the X-ray photon is emitted at the point P and the electron continues with reduced energy on the pathway shown. The probability of Bremsstrahlung radiation being produced is very small (about 1–5% for diagnostic X-ray tubes). The intensity (I) of the radiation produced is related to the atomic number of the target material (Z) and the energy of the electron beam (E) by the equation:

Equation 21.1

$$I \propto ZE^2$$

In diagnostic X-ray tubes, tungsten is used as the target material as its high atomic number (74) leads to a higher intensity of X-ray production.

The effect on the X-ray spectrum of changing the energy of the electron beam will be discussed in more detail in Chapter 22, but it is worth noting at this stage that the higher electron energies used in linear accelerators mean that there is more efficient X-ray production and that a smaller percentage of the energy is converted into heat.

If the law of conservation of momentum (see Sect. 3.4) is applied, then, in order to conserve momentum, the greater the energy of the incident electrons, the more likely the Bremsstrahlung radiation is to be emitted in the same direction as the electrons. Thus, for low-electron-energy beams the X-rays are directed almost isotropically, in diagnostic X-ray tubes (medium-energy range) the central ray of the X-ray beam is at right angles to the electron beam, and in linear accelerators (high-energy) the useful X-ray beam is transmitted forward through the anode in the same direction as the electrons.

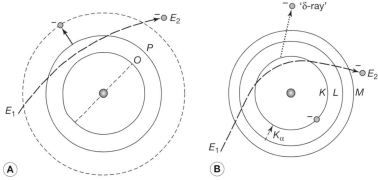

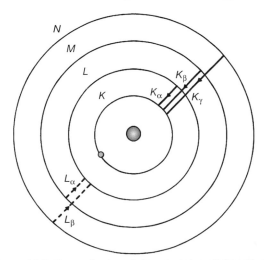

Figure 21.4 (A) Excitation and (B) ionization caused by the passage of an energetic electron through a tungsten atom. Both processes result in the production of heat and ionization produces characteristic radiation (K_α radiation is shown in the diagram). E_2 is less than E_1 in both diagrams. Note that, for clarity, only the electron orbitals which have a direct bearing on the interaction are shown.

21.5 INELASTIC COLLISIONS WITH THE ELECTRONS OF THE TARGET ATOMS – PRODUCTION OF CHARACTERISTIC RADIATION

As can be seen from Figure 21.1 (see route of electron 4), it is also possible for an electron from the filament to be involved in an inelastic collision with one of the orbital electrons of the target atoms. Such interactions are shown in more detail in Figure 21.4. Depending on the energy transferred to the orbital electron, such collisions may result either in excitation of the atom (Fig. 21.4A) or ionization of the atom (Fig. 21.4B). For excitation to occur the incident electron must be given sufficient energy to raise

Figure 21.5 The production of characteristic radiation. The K-lines are formed by quantum jumps down to the K-shell. Also note that the energy of the K_α-line must be less than the binding energy of the K-shell. (The significance of this fact is discussed when photoelectric absorption edges are considered in Sect. 23.5.)

it to its new orbital, whereas for ionization the incident electron must be given sufficient energy to overcome its binding energy and thus be liberated from the atom. In the case of ionization of the target atom, the electron is ejected from its orbital with a given kinetic energy and is often referred to as a delta-ray. This electron may have sufficient energy to excite or ionize other atoms in its path.

The process of ionization causes a vacancy in the electron shell involved – the K-shell in the atom shown in Figure 21.4B. This vacancy is quickly filled by one of the outer electrons undergoing a quantum jump downwards to fill the vacancy and emitting a quantum of electromagnetic radiation in the process. The energy of the quantum emitted is given by:

Equation 21.2

$$E = E_1 - E_2$$

where E_1 is the energy of the electron before the jump and E_2 is the energy of the electron after the jump. As this energy varies for the same transition in different materials, it is known as *characteristic radiation* as it is characteristic of the material emitting the radiation.

If we consider Figure 21.5 where a vacancy has been created in the K-shell of the atom, then the most probable jump is from the L-shell with the next probability being a jump from the M-shell followed by the probability of a jump from the N-shell. These are known as K_α, K_β, K_γ transitions and the radiation known as K_α- characteristic radiation, etc. If we assume that the vacancy in the K-shell has been filled by a transition from the L-shell, there will now be a vacancy in this shell which can be filled from the M-shell or the N-shell, etc., with the emission of L_α or L_β characteristic radiation. In this way, a cascade of electrons will occur with each one emitting a photon of energy given by Equation 21.2. In the diagnostic X-ray tube, only the K and L characteristic radiations are of any significance as the others are absorbed by the target material or the insert envelope.

As well as the characteristic radiation produced, both excitation and ionization result in the production of heat

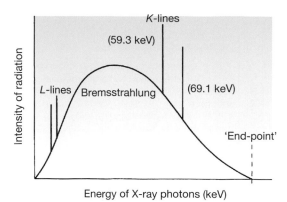

Figure 21.6 An X-ray spectrum as emitted at the anode of an X-ray tube with a tungsten target. For an explanation of this spectrum, see the text.

within the target. In *excitation*, this is by the absorption of energy by the target as the electron falls back to its original orbital and in *ionization* by the increased kinetic energy received by the tungsten atoms as they slow down the electrons ejected by the collision.

21.6 THE X-RAY SPECTRUM

So far in this chapter we have considered the production of X-ray quanta by two major mechanisms:

1. Energetic electrons from the filament interact with the nuclei of target atoms and are slowed down, thus giving off energy in the form of X-ray quanta – Bremsstrahlung radiation. As we mentioned earlier, the energy of the quantum may be very small if the interaction with the nucleus is small, or it may be up to the energy of the incoming electron if this electron is brought to rest by the nucleus. All energies between the two extremes are possible and so it can be seen that the Bremsstrahlung radiation will form a continuous spectrum (see Sect. 17.6).
2. Vacancies created in inner electron orbitals are filled by the electrons from orbitals further away from the nucleus making a quantum drop to fill the vacancy and giving off a photon of radiation in the process. This is the characteristic radiation from the atom. As the energy differences between specific orbitals is constant for an atom, this will take the form of a series of line spectra (see Sect. 17.6).

If the overall X-ray intensity is plotted against the energy of the radiation, a summation of the two effects known as the *X-ray spectrum* is produced. Such a spectrum produced at the tungsten target of an X-ray tube is shown in Figure 21.6.

Certain important features of this spectrum are worthy of further discussion:

- The energy of the Bremsstrahlung radiation is expressed in keV and lies somewhere between zero and a maximum value. This maximum photon energy

is achieved if an electron which has the maximum kinetic energy gives up all its energy to form a single photon. The value of this photon for a specific beam may be deduced as follows. Suppose the potential difference across the X-ray tube is 100 kVp. An electron accelerated across the tube when the peak voltage is applied would have achieved a kinetic energy of 100 keV at its point of contact with the anode. If it now gives up all this energy as a single photon, the energy of the photon will be 100 keV and this will be the maximum photon energy for a tube operating at this kVp. Similarly, for an X-ray tube operating at 50 kVp, the maximum photon energy will be 50 keV. Thus it can be seen that *the maximum photon energy is dependent on the potential difference across the tube (kVp) but is independent of the material of the target.*

- The Bremsstrahlung radiation is a continuous spectrum. The intensity of the low-energy photons within this spectrum is decreased because of absorption of these photons by the target material; as will be seen in Chapter 22, the intensity is further decreased by the filtration of the X-ray beam before it leaves the tube.
- The average energy of the X-ray beam is about one-third to one-half of its maximum energy – this is related to the quality of the X-ray beam (see Ch. 22).
- The total intensity of the beam – the *quantity* of the radiation – is given by the area under the curve.
- The energies of the K, L, M, etc. lines are always in the same position, although the energy of lines from M onwards is so small that it is likely to be totally absorbed in the X-ray tube. These discrete energies form a line spectrum – the exact energy of the line is determined by Equation 21.2.
- The line spectra will not be produced unless the energy of the electron beam from the filament exceeds the binding energy of the appropriate electron shell of the atom. To produce the K-characteristic lines at a tungsten target, electrons must have an energy ≥69 keV and to produce L-lines, electrons must have an energy ≥11 keV. In practice, this means that K-lines are not produced when the potential across the tube is less than 70 kVp.

In the spectrograph in Figure 21.6 we have considered the intensity of the radiation plotted against the photon energy. It is sometimes useful to calculate the wavelength of the radiation rather than know its photon energy. As you may remember from Section 17.3.2, the photon energy and its associated wavelength are related by Planck's equation (see Equation 17.6). From this we can see that the maximum photon energy corresponds to the minimum wavelength. Since the numerical value of the maximum photon energy is the same as the kVp, we can calculate the minimum wavelength from the equation:

Equation 21.3

$$\lambda_{min} = \frac{1.24}{kVp}$$

Insight

Although we have explained the maximum and minimum energies in the continuous spectrum, we have not explained the shape – the distribution of energies – of the spectrum. This is quite a complicated process and involves consideration of the chances of photons of various energies being produced, the direction of the radiation emitted and the chances of this radiation being absorbed or scattered within the target.

Consider an ultra-thin target, which is constructed in such a way that there are only a few layers of target atoms and so incoming electrons from the filament are only likely to have one interaction and there is negligible attenuation by the target of the radiation produced. In such circumstances, the number of photons of each energy produced will be related to the statistical chance of an electron losing that amount of energy in its Bremsstrahlung interaction with the nucleus. As the nucleus of the atom is relatively small compared to the whole atom, the chance of an electron from the filament colliding with it and so producing a maximum-energy photon is equally small. The chance of a filament electron getting close to the nucleus is statistically larger and so there should be more photons produced which have less than the maximum energy compared with the number which have the maximum energy. Thus, as we increase the diameter of the circle around the nucleus within which we consider electrons interacting to produce X-ray photons, so we increase the statistical possibility of producing photons with that energy – as these electrons are further from the nucleus of the atom, the energy of the photon produced would be smaller.

The production of lower-energy photons is further increased in a target with a finite thickness if we still ignore any radiation attenuation by the target. A target of finite thickness – normally a few millimetres – can really be considered as a series of ultra-thin targets one on top of the other. Because of this, the energy of the electrons reaching the second ultra-thin layer is less due to their energy loss in the first layer – this again favours the production of lower-energy X-ray photons. Thus, the deeper we go into the target, the lower the predicted energy of the photons produced.

Because of the two processes described, we would expect the number of photons produced to increase as the photon energy decreases. This is shown by the broken line in Figure 21.7.

In an X-ray tube, the target is just a few millimetres thick so we must consider X-rays being produced below the surface of the target. As these photons leave the target they are attenuated by the target atoms. Both scattering and absorption (see Ch. 23) favour attenuation of the lower-energy photons. Thus, lower-energy photons are heavily attenuated by the target atoms. The attenuation of the lower-energy photons is increased because they are more likely to be produced deeper in the target material and so have further to travel through the target. This attenuation of the photons produced by the target material produces a continuous spectrum similar to the solid line in Figure 21.7.

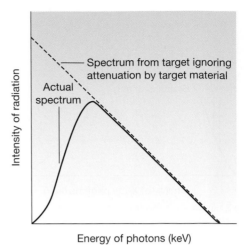

Figure 21.7 A comparison between the continuous spectrum produced if attenuation by the target material is ignored and the actual spectrum produced from a tube target.

The effect of various parameters on the spectrum of radiation emitted from the X-ray tube will form the material of the next chapter.

Summary

In this chapter, you should have learnt the following:
- The three major mechanisms by which electrons from the filament of the X-ray tube may lose energy when they interact with the atoms of the target (see Sect. 21.2).
- The result of interactions between electrons from the filament of the X-ray tube and the outer electrons around atoms of the target material (see Sect. 21.3).
- The result of elastic interactions between electrons from the filament and the nuclei of atoms of the tube target (see Sect. 21.4.1).
- How inelastic collisions between electrons from the filament and the nuclei of atoms of the target of the X-ray tube result in the production of Bremsstrahlung radiation (see Sect. 21.4.2).
- How inelastic collisions between electrons from the filament and the orbital electrons of target atoms may result in the production of characteristic radiation (see Sect. 21.5).
- The graphical representation of the X-ray spectrum and the significant features of this graph (see Sect. 21.6).

FURTHER READING

You will find that Chapter 22 of this text deals with further detail of the factors which affect the spectrum of X-rays from the X-ray tube. In addition, you may find that the chapters from the following texts provide useful further reading.

Ball, J.L., Moore, A.D., Turner, S., 2008. Ball and Moore's Essential Physics for Radiographers, fourth ed. Blackwell Scientific, London (Chapter 16).

Dowsett, D.J., Kenny, P.A., Johnston, R. E., 1998. The Physics of Diagnostic Imaging. Chapman & Hall Medical, London (Chapter 3).

Webb, S. (Ed.), 2000. The Physics of Medical Imaging. Institute of Physics, Bristol (Chapter 2).

Chapter | 22 |

Factors affecting X-ray beam quality and quantity

Definitions

The *quantity* of radiation in an X-ray beam is a measure of the number of photons in the beam. The terms *quantity* and *exposure* are often interchanged in radiography as the higher the quantity or amount of radiation, the greater the exposure to a structure. In fact, probably the simplest method of comparing the quantity of two beams of radiation is to compare the exposure received by a structure. As we shall see in Chapter 27, the exposure is measured using the unit of *air kerma*. As the quantity of radiation increases, so does the *intensity* of the beam.

The *quality* of a beam of X-rays is a measure of its penetrating power. As we saw in Section 21.6, the quality of the beam is related to its average photon energy. In Sections 20.7 and 20.8 we saw that a monochromatic beam of radiation is exponentially absorbed by a uniform medium and so the penetrating power of two beams may be compared by comparing their half-value thickness – the higher the value of the half-value thickness, the more penetrating the beam. Although the beam of X-rays from the tube is not monochromatic, but has a continuous spectrum over a wide range of energies, the half-value layer is a useful way of comparing the penetrating power of X-ray beams.

However, changing the quality of the radiation beam also affects the *intensity* of the beam. For a given quantity of radiation, the higher the quality of the radiation, the greater the intensity of the radiation beam.

The *intensity* of a beam of X radiation is defined as the total amount of energy – measured at right angles to the direction of the beam – passing through unit area in unit time. Although measured in units of joules per metre squared per second, in radiography we tend to use one of its effects – the ionization of air or of *air kerma* – as a measurement of radiation beam intensity.

As can be seen from the definitions of quantity and quality, any factors which change the quantity or the quality of the radiation beam will bring about a change in the beam's intensity.

22.1 AIM

The aim of this chapter is to consider the various factors which have an influence on the quantity and/or the quality of the beam of radiation from the X-ray tube.

22.2 INTRODUCTION

In Chapter 21 we considered the mechanisms by which X-rays were produced at the anode of the X-ray tube. In this chapter we will consider the various factors which influence the *quantity* and/or the *quality* of the X-ray beam and hence its *intensity* at a given point. Before we look at this

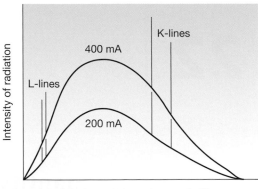

Figure 22.1 The effect of the mA on the X-ray spectrum. Note that the quantity of the radiation changes – as shown by the alteration of the area under each curve – but the quality of the radiation is unaltered – as shown by the maximum photon energy and the peak photon energy being at the same energy for each graph. Thus we can say that the mA selected for an exposure affects the quantity of the X-ray beam but does not affect the quality of the beam – an increase in the mA will produce an increase in the quantity of radiation from the target.

in any more detail, it is first important to ensure that we understand the meaning of the terms *quantity*, *quality* and *intensity* as applied to a beam of X radiation.

22.3 THE EFFECT OF mA ON THE X-RAY BEAM

If the current through the X-ray tube (mA) is, for example, doubled, the number of electrons flowing across the tube in unit time is doubled. If all the other factors remain unchanged, each electron will have the same chance of creating X-ray photons and so the number of photons of each energy produced per unit time will be doubled. If the mA is halved, the same argument can be used to show that the number of X-ray photons of each energy is also halved. Thus we can say that the quantity of the X-ray beam per unit time (or the beam intensity) is directly proportional to the mA through the tube.

Equation 22.1

$$I \propto mA$$

The effect on the X-ray beam of altering the mA is shown in Figure 22.1. Note that the area under the graph for 200 mA is half the area under the graph for 400 mA. The maximum photon energy and the minimum photon energy are the same in each case and the average photon energy remains unaltered.

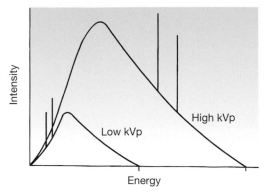

Figure 22.2 The effect of kVp on the X-ray spectrum. Note that the kVp affects both the quantity and the quality of the radiation beam. Also note that the lower of the two curves is unable to produce *K*-characteristic radiation, although both curves can produce *L*-lines.

22.4 THE EFFECT OF kVp ON THE X-RAY BEAM

The kVp across the X-ray tube influences the force of attraction experienced by an electron released by the filament as it moves towards the anode. Thus, if the kVp is increased, then the kinetic energy of the electron at the point when it starts to interact with the target will be increased. As we saw in Section 21.4.2, the efficiency of X-ray production by Bremsstrahlung is proportional to E^2 and so this improved efficiency means that:

Equation 22.2

$$I \propto kVp^2$$

As we already discussed in Section 21.4.2, increasing the kVp will also increase the energy of the maximum-energy photons in the beam – if the kVp is 50, then the maximum photon energy is 50 keV and if the kVp is 100, then the maximum photon energy is 100 keV. As the average photon energy is approximately 30–50% of the maximum photon energy, increasing the maximum photon energy will also increase the average photon energy.

As mentioned earlier, increasing the kVp will increase the kinetic energy of the electrons from the filament when they reach the target and so this may mean that characteristic radiation is seen on the higher kVp spectrum but not at the lower value – at 100 kVp the electrons reaching the target have energies up to 100 keV and so can displace *K*-shell electrons in tungsten, whereas at 50 kVp the 50-keV electrons have insufficient energy to displace a *K*-shell electron from the tungsten atom.

The spectrum produced at 100 kVp and at 50 kVp is shown in Figure 22.2 where the changes mentioned above can be identified.

Thus we can say that the kVp selected for an exposure affects both the quantity and the quality of the X-ray beam

Table 22.1 Comparison of the characteristic radiation energies produced from a tungsten target and a molybdenum target

	ENERGY OF K_α CHARACTERISTIC RADIATION (KeV)	ENERGY OF L_α CHARACTERISTIC RADIATION (KeV)
Tungsten	59.32	8.39
Molybdenum	17.48	2.22

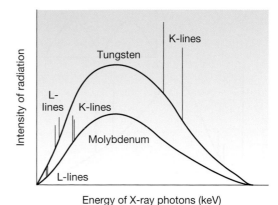

Figure 22.3 The effect of the target material on the X-ray spectrum. Note that the lower atomic number of molybdenum means that there is a reduction in the quantity of the radiation but the quality of the Bremsstrahlung radiation is not affected. The characteristic radiation is at a lower photon energy for the target with the lower atomic number.

produced – an increase in kVp will produce an increase in the quantity and the quality of the radiation from the target.

22.5 THE EFFECT OF THE TARGET MATERIAL ON THE X-RAY BEAM

As mentioned in Section 21.4.2, the atomic number of the target material has an effect on the X-ray beam from the tube. The higher the atomic number of the target material, the more positive the nucleus of the target atom and so the more it attracts the electrons from the filament which pass close to it. Thus the production of X-rays by the Bremsstrahlung process is more efficient and the intensity of the beam is increased. The maximum and minimum photon energies in the beam are not affected by the target material.

The target material also affects the characteristic radiation produced. The energies of the characteristic radiations from a tungsten and a molybdenum target are shown in Table 22.1. Thus, although the target material does not affect the quality of the Bremsstrahlung radiation, it does affect the energy of the characteristic radiation and this does have some effect on the overall quality of the X-ray beam – this effect may be enhanced by filtering the radiation with the same material as the target (this will be considered further in Ch. 23 when absorption mechanisms are discussed).

The radiation spectra from a tungsten and a molybdenum target are shown in Figure 22.3.

22.6 THE EFFECT OF RECTIFICATION ON THE X-RAY BEAM

The type of high-tension rectification of the X-ray generator affects the spectrum of radiation produced at the target of the X-ray tube. This is because of the changing energy of the electron beam striking the target each half-cycle. If we consider full-wave rectification with no capacitor smoothing,

as produced by the two-pulse generator in many dental X-ray units, then the potential across the tube varies from zero to the kVp each half-cycle. Thus the energy of the electrons striking the target varies from zero to a keV with a numerical value equal to that of the kVp. The maximum photon energy at differing stages in the half-cycle will vary across the same range as the electron energies.

We can see how this affects the spectrum produced if we consider Figure 22.4A (see page 162) and consider the spectra produced at point B in the voltage waveform and at point C. The time-averaged spectrum for full-wave rectification is shown in Figure 22.4B. Now consider a constant potential, similar to the voltage waveform from the medium-frequency generator, being applied to the X-ray tube during the entire exposure. This would be the same as if voltage B is applied for the whole exposure, and so the spectrum for voltage B is labelled in Figure 22.4B as the spectrum from a constant-potential unit. Note that for constant potential, the area under the graph is increased and the value of the photon energy of the average photon is also increased.

Thus we can say that the rectification – or the type of X-ray generator – affects both the quantity and the quality of the X-ray beam produced – the nearer the voltage across the tube is to a constant potential, the higher the quantity and the quality of the radiation produced at the target.

22.7 THE EFFECT OF FILTRATION ON THE X-RAY BEAM

In all the discussion so far we have considered the beam of X radiation produced at the target of the X-ray tube.

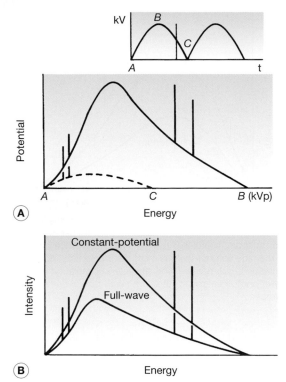

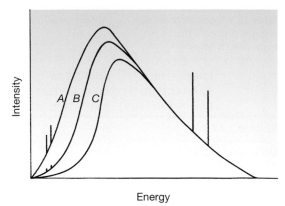

Figure 22.5 The effect of filtration on the X-ray spectrum. Line *A* represents the spectrum produced at the target of the X-ray tube; line *B* shows how this spectrum is modified because of the inherent filtration of the tube; and line *C* shows how the spectrum is modified because of the total filtration. Note that filtration causes a reduction in the *quantity* of the radiation but an increase in the *quality*.

Figure 22.4 (A) The spectrum of radiation produced with a single-phase two-pulse rectified waveform as kVp values *B* and *C* are applied across the X-ray tube. (B) The effect of rectification on the X-ray spectrum where the constant potential generator produces radiation of higher *quantity* and higher *quality*.

Before this radiation can be utilized in radiography or radiotherapy, it must first leave the tube. In leaving the tube, the radiation beam must first pass through the glass of the tube insert, the oil in the housing and finally the window of the housing – plus any additional filtration – and it is filtered at each stage of this process. Thus, to consider the beam which will interact with the patient, we need to consider the effect of filtration on the spectrum of radiation produced at the tube target.

Spectrum *A* in Figure 22.5 shows the distribution of energies emitted from the tube target. This would be the spectrum of the radiation before it leaves the glass envelope of the tube. As we will discuss in Chapter 23, when a beam of radiation passes through any medium, the beam is attenuated by the processes of absorption and scattering. We will see that the lower the photon energy, the higher the chance of it being absorbed or scattered. So the passage of the X-ray beam through the glass envelope, the oil and the exit window of the shield results in selective attenuation of the lower-energy photons. Since this filtration is inherent to the tube construction, it is known as the *inherent filtration* of the X-ray tube. The spectrum emitted after the inherent filtration is shown as spectrum *B* in Figure 22.5.

This beam still contains a significant number of low-energy photons. If these were allowed to interact with the tissues of a patient, they would be absorbed by superficial tissues and so would contribute to the

Insight

Aluminium has a low atomic number (13) and so is able to absorb many of the low-energy X-ray photons in a beam of diagnostic energy, by photoelectric absorption (see Ch. 23). High-energy X-ray photons have a low probability of being absorbed or scattered by the aluminium and so are relatively unaffected by the filtration. This makes aluminium the ideal material for filtration of diagnostic energy X-ray beams.

The radiation beam from the therapy X-ray tube has a much higher average energy than the diagnostic beam. This beam is often hardened – low-energy radiations are removed – by the use of a composite filter. An example of this is when the beam is first filtered through copper ($Z = 29$) and then is further filtered through an aluminium filter. The copper is responsible for the initial filtration but transmits some low-energy radiation due to the photoelectric absorption edge of copper. The copper also produces low-energy characteristic radiation as a result of photoelectric absorption in the copper atoms. The function of the aluminium filter is to absorb the radiation transmitted through the copper because of the *K*-shell photoelectric absorption edge of copper and also to remove the characteristic radiation produced by the photoelectric absorption in the copper. These concepts will be further discussed in the next chapter.

Table 22.2 Factors affecting the quantity and quality of the X-ray beam

FACTOR	EFFECT ON THE QUANTITY OF THE X-RAY BEAM	EFFECT ON THE QUALITY OF THE X-RAY BEAM
Increase in the X-ray tube current (mA)	Produces an increase in the quantity of radiation directly proportional to the increase in mA	The quality of the radiation from the tube is unaffected by an increase in the tube current
Increase in the potential difference (kVp) across the X-ray tube	An increase in the kVp produces an increase in the quantity of radiation produced at the target proportional to the kVp^2	An increase in the kVp produces an increase in the average energy of the photons in the X-ray beam and so produces an increase in the quality of the beam
Target material	An increase in the atomic number of the target material will produce an increase in the quantity of radiation produced which is proportional to the increase in the atomic number	A change in the atomic number of the target material will produce no change in the quality of the beam produced by the Bremsstrahlung process. A higher atomic number will produce characteristic radiation of higher energy and, if this is in significant amounts, it will increase the quality of the overall spectrum
Rectification	The closer the voltage across the X-ray tube is to a constant potential, the greater the quantity of radiation produced	The closer the voltage across the X-ray tube is to a constant potential, the greater the quality of radiation produced
Filtration	Filtration reduces the quantity of radiation emerging from the X-ray tube. The reduction is related to the thickness and the atomic number of the filter	Filtration improves the quality of the radiation from an X-ray tube by selective removal of the low-energy photons

patient dose but would make no contribution to the radiograph – or to the tumour treatment in the case of radiotherapy. The amount of low-energy photons in the spectrum can be significantly reduced by incorporating additional filtration into the beam, near the exit port of the tube, before it interacts with the patient's tissues. Such a spectrum is shown as line C in Figure 22.5. The inherent filtration of diagnostic X-ray tubes is usually expressed in *millimetres of aluminium equivalent,* i.e. the inherent filtration is equivalent to the filtration of the beam achieved by the stated number of millimetres of aluminium. The inherent filtration of most diagnostic X-ray tubes is between 0.5 and 1.0 mm of aluminium equivalent. The total filtration in the beam is the sum of the inherent filtration and the additional filtration. This total filtration is between 1.5 and 2.5 mm depending upon the maximum kVp at which the tube is designed to operate.

As can be seen from Figure 22.5, filtration affects both the quantity and the quality of the X-ray beam – the greater the thickness of the filtration in the X-ray beam, the less the quantity but the greater the quality of the X-ray beam emerging from the X-ray tube.

22.8 SUMMARY OF THE FACTORS AFFECTING THE QUANTITY, QUALITY AND INTENSITY OF THE X-RAY BEAM

The factors which affect the quantity and/or quality of the beam of X-radiation emerging from an X-ray tube are summarized in Table 22.2.

Summary

In this chapter, you should have learnt the following:
- The meaning of the terms *quantity* and *quality* as applied to the X-ray beam (see Sect. 22.2).
- The effect of the current through the X-ray tube (mA) on the quantity of the X-ray beam produced (see Sect. 22.3).
- The effect of the potential difference across the X-ray tube (kVp) on the quantity and the quality of the X-ray beam produced (see Sect. 22.4).

(Continued)

- The effect of the atomic number of the target material on the quantity of the radiation produced and on the characteristic radiation from the target (see Sect. 22.5).
- The effect of the voltage waveform applied to the X-ray tube (rectification) on the quantity and the quality of the X-ray beam produced (see Sect. 22.6).

- The effect of filtration on the quantity and the quality of the radiation beam emerging from the X-ray tube (see Sect. 22.7).

FURTHER READING

Ball, J.L., Moore, A.D., Turner, S., 2008. Ball and Moore's Essential Physics for Radiographers, fourth ed. Blackwell Scientific, London (Chapter 16).

Carter, P.R., Hyatt, A.P., Pirrie, J.R., Milne, A., 1994. Chesneys' Equipment for Student Radiographers. Blackwell Scientific, London (Chapters 2 and 3).

Webb, S. (Ed.), 2000. The Physics of Medical Imaging. Institute of Physics, Bristol (Chapter 2).

Chapter | **23** |

Interactions of X-rays with matter

CHAPTER CONTENTS

23.1 AIM

The aim of this chapter is to introduce the reader to the interaction processes which may occur when radiation photons interact with matter. The factors which influence such interaction processes will be discussed. An understanding of the processes is important both for consideration of the production of the radiograph and in the consideration of the biological effects of radiation on tissue.

23.2 OUTLINE OF POSSIBLE INTERACTIONS

When a beam of X-rays interacts with a medium, e.g. a volume of patient tissue, there are a number of possible interactions between the photons and the atoms of the medium. These are outlined in Figure 23.1 (see page 166). If we consider photon A, we can see that this interacts with an atom of the medium and is deflected from its path – this deflection may or may not be accompanied by a loss of photon energy. This process is known as *scattering*. Photon B, on the other hand, interacts with an atom of the medium and loses all of its energy to the atom. This process is known as *absorption*. The third photon, photon C, passes through the material without interacting with any of the atoms. If we measure the intensity of the radiation in a given area before it interacts with the medium and again in a similar area after the interactions, we find that there is a lower intensity of radiation after passing through the medium – *the beam of radiation has been attenuated* (see Sect. 20.7).

Thus we can say:

> When a beam of radiation passes through a medium, it is attenuated by the processes of absorption and scattering.

The reactions considered above involve an interaction between a photon and an orbiting electron rather than between a photon and the nucleus of the atom (this will be discussed in more detail in the rest of this chapter) and so, for an interaction to occur, a photon must pass close to the electron orbiting the atom with which it is capable of interacting. Thus we can consider the atoms in

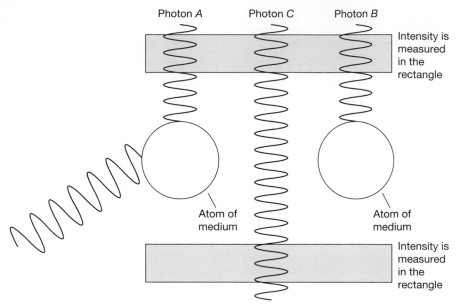

Figure 23.1 Mechanisms of interaction of X-ray photons with matter. Photon A is scattered, photon B is absorbed and photon C is transmitted. Note that the number of photons passing through the lower rectangle is less than the number passing through the upper rectangle and so attenuation has taken place.

a medium as targets which, if hit, will attenuate a photon from the primary radiation beam.

Note: For the purposes of this discussion, we are considering a parallel beam of radiation so that reduction in intensity only occurs here because of the attenuation processes and no reduction in intensity occurs because of the inverse square law.

23.2.1 Probability and cross-sections

The probability of an X-ray photon interacting with a particular atom is low, but the very large number of atoms even in a small volume of a solid substance makes the probability of a photon interacting with some atom much greater. In Figure 23.2, a beam of X-rays of area A is incident upon a medium whose atoms appear to the beam to have an area of a. This area is called the cross-section of the atom to a particular type of radiation, a typical area being $1.5 \times 10^{-28}\,\text{m}^2$. If an X-ray photon hits one of the atoms, it is either absorbed or scattered from the primary beam.

Note that the area a is not the true size of the atom but is the apparent area of the atom likely to interact with the X-ray beam. The value of a depends on a number of things, including the atomic number of the material and the energy of the X-ray photon.

The probability of an interaction occurring can be predicted by dividing the total area of the atoms within the irradiated area by the size of this area. If we consider Figure 23.2 and take it that there are N atoms per unit

volume of the material, then the number of atoms in the irradiated cylinder of cross-sectional area A is $N \times A \times x$. Thus the total area of the atoms in the irradiated area is $a(N \times Ax)$ or $aNAx$.

The probability of an interaction:

Equation 23.1

$$\begin{aligned} &= \frac{aNAx}{A} \\ &= aNx \end{aligned}$$

23.2.2 The total linear attenuation coefficient (μ)

As we discussed in Section 20.7, a parallel beam of monoenergetic radiation – radiation where all the photons have the same energy – will undergo exponential attenuation as it passes through a uniform medium. The intensity of the incident beam (I_0) and the intensity after a thickness x are given by the equation:

Equation 23.2

$$I_x = I_0 e^{-\mu x}$$

where μ is the total linear attenuation coefficient. If we now consider Equations 23.1 and 23.2, it can be seen that as the probability of an interaction increases (aNx), the linear attenuation coefficient μ will also increase. The total linear coefficient may be defined:

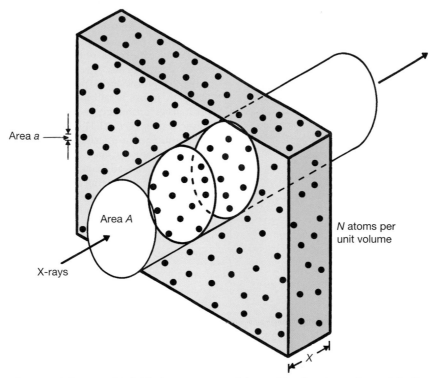

Figure 23.2 Consideration of the area of individual atoms as part of the total irradiated area. If any of the X-ray photons passing through area A hits an atom (area a) then the photon is removed from the beam. As fewer photons will exit from the medium than entered the same area, the beam is said to be attenuated. For further explanation, see the text.

Definition
The total linear attenuation coefficient, μ, is the fraction of the X-rays removed from a beam per unit thickness of the attenuating medium.

Definition
The total mass attenuation coefficient, μ/ρ, is the fraction of the X-rays removed from a beam of unit cross-sectional area by unit mass of the medium.

23.2.3 The total mass attenuation coefficient (μ/ρ)

As we have seen from Equation 23.1, the probability of an interaction between an X-ray photon and a medium containing N atoms is proportional to N. If we consider the medium shown in Figure 23.2 and take a situation where it is heated until it has expanded to a thickness of $2x$, then the number of atoms in the thickness x will be $N/2$ and the linear attenuation coefficient (μ) will also be halved. As the number of atoms per unit volume has halved, the density of the material (ρ) will also have halved. However, the ratio μ/ρ will be the same in both cases. This ratio μ/ρ is known as the total mass attenuation coefficient and is defined:

If we wish to calculate the amount of radiation which would pass through a given *length* of a material, then we would use the linear attenuation coefficient. In most other cases the mass attenuation coefficient would be used as this is unaffected by the state of the medium; it may be solid, liquid or gas as long as the changes in density are taken into account. Thus, if we wish to consider the effect of a change, for instance, of photon energy on the transmitted beam, this type of calculation would be undertaken using the mass attenuation coefficient.

The following sections of this chapter will consider the effect on the mass attenuation coefficient of the different types of X-ray interactions and of different attenuating materials. An understanding of these is fundamental to consideration of the formation of the radiograph (see Ch. 25).

of the processes, energy is transferred from the photons in the X-ray beam to the atoms of the medium and so *absorption* is said to have taken place. Thus, an absorption process must involve the transfer of energy from the photons to the atoms of the material.

In other processes, the photon is deflected from its original path and so is said to be scattered. This may involve no transfer of energy to the medium (see coherent or elastic scatter, Sect. 23.4) or it may involve deflection of the photon and a transfer of energy to the medium (see Compton scattering, Sect. 23.6).

As we have already noted, attenuation consists of both absorption and scattering and the contribution of each of the individual processes to the whole is shown in Table 23.1. As can be seen from the table, the total mass absorption coefficient will be composed of the mass absorption coefficients from each of the attenuation processes. This may be defined as follows:

23.3 ATTENUATION AND ABSORPTION

The four interaction processes described in the rest of this chapter involve *attenuation* since the intensity of the primary X-ray beam is reduced as a result of each process. In some

23.4 ELASTIC (COHERENT) SCATTERING

When the energy of a photon is considerably less than the binding energies of orbiting electrons of the atoms of the attenuator, the photon may be deflected from its path

Table 23.1 Contribution of each of the attenuation processes to absorption and scatter

PROCESS	CONTRIBUTION TO ABSORPTION COEFFICIENT	CONTRIBUTION TO SCATTER
Elastic (coherent) scattering	No contribution to absorption as no energy is permanently absorbed by the medium	Makes only a very small contribution to the total scatter in medical radiography
Photoelectric absorption	Usually the energy of the photon is absorbed and so this process makes a contribution to the total absorption coefficient	No scattering of the photon occurs as part of the photoelectric process
Compton scattering	Some of the energy of the photon is transferred to the medium during the scattering process and so it contributes to the absorption coefficient	This is the major source of scatter in medical radiography
Pair production	Depending on the energy of the photon, this process produces partial or complete absorption	This process produces no scattering of the primary beam photons

with no loss of energy after it has interacted with one of the electrons. This process is known as elastic scattering or coherent scattering (sometimes also known as *classical scattering* or *Rayleigh scattering*).

In this process the incoming photon interacts with an electron and raises its energy but does not give it sufficient energy to become excited or ionized. The electron then returns to its previous energy level by the emission of a photon which is equal in energy to the incoming photon but is in a different direction; hence scattering has occurred. The photon is scattered predominantly in the forward direction, because elastic scattering cannot occur if the recoil experienced by the atom as a whole during the scattering process is sufficient to produce excitation or ionization. There is no absorption since no energy has been given permanently to the material and the attenuation, although present, is small since the majority of the photons are only scattered through a small angle. This is particularly so if the energy of the photon is higher than 100 eV and the atomic number of the attenuator is relatively low. The factors affecting the mass attenuation coefficient due to elastic scattering are shown in Equation 23.5:

Equation 23.5

$$\frac{\sigma_{coh}}{\rho} \propto \frac{Z^2}{E}$$

where σ_{coh}/ρ is the mass attenuation coefficient due to elastic scattering, Z is the atomic number of the attenuator and E is the photon energy.

In medical radiography, the effect of elastic scattering can be largely ignored since the average atomic number of tissue is low (approximately 7.4) and the photon energy is too high to allow significant elastic scatter.

Elastic scattering may occur as a result of a photon interacting with the nucleus of an atom of the attenuator but the effect is even less and so may safely be ignored in medical radiography.

23.5 PHOTOELECTRIC ABSORPTION

The previous section has shown that elastic scattering has little significance for radiography except at extremely low photon energies. The process of photoelectric absorption, which

we will now discuss, is important even at very low energies and continues to be important at the photon energies found in the typical X-ray spectrum for diagnostic radiography.

In photoelectric absorption, the X-ray photon is involved in an *inelastic* collision with an orbiting electron of an atom of the absorber. The photon gives up all its energy to the electron (and thus disappears) and the electron is ejected from the atom. As ejection of the electron from the atom is a necessary part of the process, photoelectric absorption can only take place if the photon energy is equal to, or greater than, the binding energy of the electron.

The process of photoelectric absorption is shown schematically in Figure 23.3, where it is assumed that the X-ray photon of energy $h\nu$ ejects an electron from the K-shell of the atom. Some of the energy of the photon is used in overcoming the binding energy of the electron and the rest is given to the electron as kinetic energy. If we assume that the electron has a binding energy of B, then the kinetic energy after ejection (it is then referred to as a *photoelectron*) is $(h\nu - B)$. The vacancy thus created in the K-shell will be filled by electrons in orbitals further from the nucleus performing a series of quantum jumps downwards, producing characteristic radiation (see Sect. 21.5) and the possible emission of Auger electrons (see Sect. 19.6.3) from orbitals further out from the nucleus. As you may remember from Section 21.5, the energy of the characteristic radiation is equal to the difference in energy of the electron before and after the quantum jump. In the case of X-ray photons interacting with atoms of body tissue, this energy difference is very small (normally between 1.2×10^{-2} eV and 1.8×10^{-2} eV) and so is in the infrared part of the electromagnetic spectrum.

The probability of a photoelectric interaction occurring at a particular shell depends on the binding energy of the electrons in the shell and the energy of the incoming

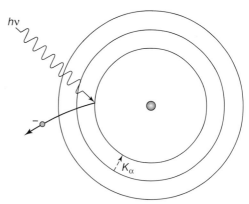

Figure 23.3 The process of photoelectric absorption and the subsequent emission of a quantum of characteristic radiation. The incoming photon ($h\nu$) is absorbed by the K-shell electron which is then displaced from that shell. The vacancy is filled from the L-shell with the emission of K_α characteristic radiation.

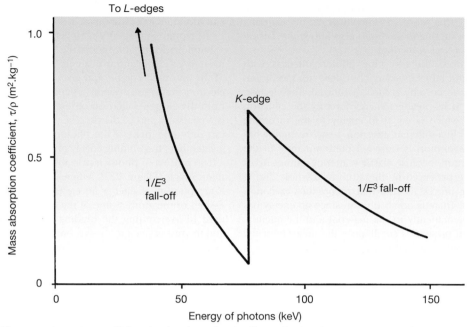

Figure 23.4 The mass absorption coefficient for the photoelectric effect in lead and its variation with photon energy.

photon. The probability is zero when the energy of the photon is less than the binding energy of the electron; it is greatest when the photon energy is equal to the binding energy and thereafter decreases rapidly with increasing photon energy. A graph of the mass absorption coefficient for photoelectric absorption in lead is shown in Figure 23.4 to illustrate these points.

The outer orbital shells of the atom are affected by the lower photon energies, only to have a reducing absorption as the photon energy increases. When the photon energy reaches the binding energy of the orbital then electrons in that orbital can take part in photoelectric absorption, thus producing a sudden increase in the amount of absorption. Such an increase is shown for the K-shell electrons of the lead atom in Figure 23.4. This sudden increase is known as an absorption edge and so Figure 23.4 shows the K absorption edge for the lead atom. Between the absorption edges, the mass attenuation coefficient due to the photoelectric effect (τ/ρ) is approximately proportional to $1/E^3$.

23.5.1 Photoelectric absorption, attenuation and absorption coefficients

The mass attenuation coefficient for the photoelectric effect (τ/ρ) is related to the atomic number (Z) of the absorber and the photon energy of the radiation (E).

A very approximate guide to this relationship is given by the equation:

Equation 23.6

$$\frac{\tau}{\rho} = \frac{Z^3}{E^3}$$

This equation applies to energies up to about 200 keV. At higher energies, the E^3 term approximates to E^2 and eventually to E.

In photoelectric absorption, the X-ray beam is both attenuated and absorbed since individual photons are removed from the beam (attenuation) and energy is imparted to the absorbing medium (absorption). The absorbed energy is composed of the following parts:

- Kinetic energy of the ejected photoelectron.
- Energy of recoil of the absorbing atom.
- Energy of the photons of characteristic radiation and Auger electrons

The ejected photoelectron is quickly brought to rest by the surrounding atoms and delivers its energy to them in the process. A similar thing happens with the Auger electrons. It is possible, however, for the characteristic radiation to escape from the absorber, especially if the energy of the characteristic radiation is high and it is produced near the surface of the absorber. In such cases, the *mass absorption coefficient* is slightly less than the *mass attenuation coefficient* since not all of the energy of the original photon has been absorbed by the medium. For this difference to be significant, the characteristic radiation must have high photon energy. The effect is thus only important in materials with high atomic numbers. As most of the atoms which make up body tissues have low atomic numbers, it may be considered that the mass absorption coefficient and the mass attenuation coefficient are equal for photoelectric absorption in practical radiography.

When we consider the absorption of X-ray photons to produce a radiographic image, we need to look at the linear attenuation coefficient. From Equation 23.6 we can see that, for the photoelectric effect at a given photon energy, this is proportional to the density of the absorber and its atomic number cubed. Bone is approximately twice as dense as soft tissue and its atomic number is also approximately twice that of soft tissue. For these reasons, the linear attenuation coefficient for photoelectric absorption for bone is approximately 16 times that of soft tissue. As the blackening on a radiograph is proportional to the radiation dose it receives, this explains why bones appear lighter than the same thickness of soft tissue. This process is the main one responsible for the contrast of the radiographic image.

23.6 COMPTON SCATTERING

In the case of the photoelectric effect, the X-ray photon has an energy close to or just above the binding energy of the electron. If the energy of the X-ray photon is very much higher than the binding energy of the electron, the electron may be regarded as a *free electron*. The reaction between an X-ray photon and a free electron is known as *Compton scattering* and results in the partial absorption of the energy of an X-ray photon which undergoes such scatter. Because the interaction is between a photon and a free electron, the electron density of the material is important in determining the probability of Compton scatter occurring.

The Compton scattering process is shown diagrammatically in Figure 23.5. The incident X-ray photon has an energy $E_1(=h\nu_1)$ and collides with the electron, which recoils, thus taking some of the photon energy. The energy remaining, $E_2(=h\nu_2)$, is the energy of the deflected (or scattered) photon. Since E_2 is less than E_1, then the wavelength of the scattered photon must be greater than the wavelength of the incident photon, as shown in Figure 23.5 (see Sect. 17.3.2 for the relationship between photon energy and wavelength). Compton scattering interactions are termed *inelastic* in that the photon energy is not conserved, although the total energy of the interaction is conserved.

After a Compton scattering process, the photon may travel in any direction but the electron can only travel in a forward direction relative to the incident photon. Thus, in Figure 23.5, θ may be any value, while Φ lies between $1° \pm 90°$ relative to the direction of the incident photon. The division of the energy of the original photon between the electron and the scattered photon depends

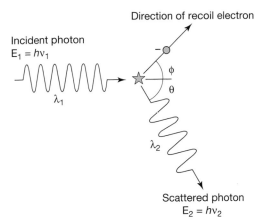

Figure 23.5 The process of Compton scattering. The scattered photon has less energy than the incident photon and may be scattered through any angle. The recoil electron is always scattered in a 'forward' direction.

on the original photon energy (E_1) and the angle through which it has been scattered. It may be shown that in order to preserve both energy and momentum, the following equation must be obeyed:

Equation 23.7

$$\lambda_2 - \lambda_1 = \frac{(h(1 - \cos\theta))}{mc}$$

where the quantity $\lambda_2 - \lambda_1$ is called the Compton wavelength shift, h is Planck's constant, m is the mass of the electron and c is the velocity of electromagnetic radiation.

Two important conclusions may be drawn from Equation 23.7:

1. $\lambda_2 - \lambda_1$ depends only on h, m, c and θ and so is not dependent on the wavelength of the incident photon or the composition of the attenuating material.

2. For a given value of scattering angle, θ, the value of $\lambda_2 - \lambda_1$ is constant. Low-energy photons have longer wavelengths, so that the wavelength change represents a smaller *fractional* change in λ and hence only a slight reduction in the energy of the scattered photons. By applying the same argument, high-energy photons scattered through the same angle will experience a much larger fractional change in their wavelength and energy.

Equation 23.7 shows what happens to the photon wavelengths when scattered through an angle of θ. It does not give any information on the relative probability of a photon actually being scattered through that angle. Mathematical predictions based on quantum mechanics, and practical measurements, have shown that low-energy photons (up to about 100 eV) are scattered in all directions with almost equal probability. High-energy photons (greater than 1 MeV) are scattered predominantly in a forward direction, i.e. they have small scattering angles.

An alternative way of writing Equation 23.7 using the photon energy change instead of the wavelength change is:

Equation 23.8

$$\frac{1}{E_2} - \frac{1}{E_1} = \frac{(1 - \cos\theta)}{511}$$

where E_1 and E_2 are in keV.

23.6.1 Compton attenuation, absorption and scatter coefficients

The mass attenuation coefficient for Compton scattering (σ/ρ) is given by the equation:

Equation 23.9

$$\frac{\sigma}{\rho} = \frac{\text{electron density}}{E}$$

As shown in the above equation, the probability of Compton scattering occurring in unit mass is inversely proportional to the energy of the photon – the amount of Compton scattering occurring in unit mass decreases as the photon energy increases.

It can also be seen from the above equation that the probability is also directly proportional to the electron density. As we saw in Section 3.6, it is possible to use Avogadro's number to calculate the number of atoms per mole of an element ($N_a = 6 \times 10^{23}\,\text{mol}^{-1}$). We can therefore calculate the number of atoms per unit mass by simply dividing this by the mass number (A) for the element:

Equation 23.10

$$\text{number of atoms per unit mass} = \frac{N_a}{A}$$

The number of electrons in a normal atom is the same as the number of protons and is given by Z – the atomic number (see Sect. 18.3). The electron density is the number of electrons per unit mass and is given by the equation:

Equation 23.11

$$\text{electron density} = N_a \times \frac{Z}{A}$$

If we assume that most elements in tissue have approximately equal numbers of protons and neutrons in the atomic nucleus, then the value of Z/A is 0.5. The exception to this rule is hydrogen which contains no neutron in its nucleus and so $Z/A = 1$. Thus hydrogen contains 6×10^{23} electrons per gram (or 6×10^{26} electrons per kilogram) whereas all other substances contain approximately half this value (between 2.5 and 3.5×10^{23} electrons per gram). The lower values are for the heavier elements which have a larger neutron-to-proton ratio.

Thus we can see from Equation 23.9 that, at a given photon energy, the mass attenuation coefficient due to

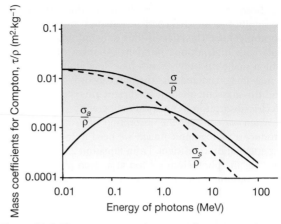

Figure 23.6 The mass attenuation, mass absorption and mass scattering coefficients for Compton scattering. As the energy increases, the absorbed energy (σ_a/ρ) becomes an increasing proportion of the total energy of the interaction (σ/ρ). See text for further details.

Compton scattering is very similar for all elements except hydrogen where it is twice as large.

The *mass absorption coefficient* for Compton scattering (σ_a/ρ) represents the average energy transferred to the electron (and hence the medium) as a fraction of the total energy in the beam. As shown in the previous section, the higher the energy of the photon, the higher the average energy lost by the photon as a result of Compton scattering. This means that the electron takes more energy in the recoil process as the photon energy increases. As a result of this, the values for the mass absorption coefficient (σ_a/ρ) and the mass attenuation coefficient (σ/ρ) are closer to the same value at higher photon energies than they are at lower photon energies. This situation is shown in Figure 23.6.

As we have already noted in Equation 23.9, the *mass attenuation coefficient* (σ/ρ) is *inversely* proportional to the photon energy and so we would expect σ/ρ to decrease as the photon energy increases. This is also shown in Figure 23.6.

Also shown in Figure 23.6 (represented by the broken line) is the *mass scattering coefficient* (σ_s/ρ). This represents the fraction of the total beam energy left to the photons after a Compton scattering event. At the point where the two curves cross (approximately 1.5 MeV), the electrons and the photons share equal amounts of energy. Below this energy, the scattered photon carries more energy than the electron, and above the energy, the reverse is true.

When considering the coefficients, it is important to remember that the mass attenuation coefficient is a measure of the *total* energy removed from the primary beam, whereas the absorption coefficient and the scattering coefficient are a measure of the proportion of energy removed from the beam by the electron and scattered photon respectively.

Since the sum of the energies of the electron and the scattered photon must equal the energy of the incident photon, then we can say:

Equation 23.12

$$\sigma = \sigma_a + \sigma_s$$
$$\text{and } \frac{\sigma}{\rho} = \frac{\sigma_a}{\rho} + \frac{\sigma_s}{\rho}$$

In diagnostic radiography, many consider that the Compton process produces scatter which degrades the radiograph so makes no contribution to contrast. However, it should be remembered that linear absorption is also affected by the density of the medium and so the Compton process is responsible for the differences in absorption (and hence contrast) which we get between soft tissue and air or contrast agents and air in high kV radiography.

23.7 PAIR PRODUCTION

Pair production resulting in the formation of two charged particles from a single high-energy photon can only occur at photon energies of 1.02 MeV or above. (Because of this high photon energy requirement, this is not a process encountered in diagnostic radiograph but is encountered in therapeutic radiography and in positron emission tomography (PET) scanning.) This is because this value represents the energy equivalent of the masses of two electrons. One of these, the negatron, has a negative charge, just like a normal electron, while the other particle, the positron, has an equal and opposite positive charge. The total charge present as a result of the interaction is therefore zero and equal to the uncharged photon creating the interaction. The process is illustrated in Figure 23.7.

The interaction, which occurs as the photon interacts with the electrical field of the nucleus, is an example of mass–energy equivalence (see Sect. 16.4.1) as the energy from the photon is converted into mass. Any photon energy remaining after the interaction is passed to the particles as kinetic energy. This can be stated using the following equation:

$$E = (m_0c^2 + T_1) + (m_0c^2 + T_2)$$

where E is the energy of the photon, m_0 is the rest mass of positron or electron, c is the velocity of electromagnetic radiation, T_1 is the kinetic energy of the electron and T_2 is the kinetic energy of the positron.

This equation can be further simplified to give:

$$E = 2m_0c^2 + T_1 + T_2$$

If we consider the rest mass of the electron and positron pair then we can calculate that $2m_0c^2$ is equal to 1.02 MeV. This explains why pair production will not take place if

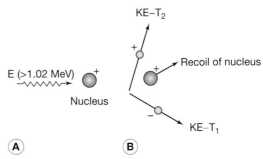

Figure 23.7 The mechanism of pair production. (A) A photon of energy (E) ≥1.02 MeV approaches the nucleus of an atom of the attenuating material. When the photon passes close to the nucleus, it produces a positron and a negatron, as shown in (B). KE, kinetic energy.

the photon energy is less than 1.02 MeV as this amount of energy is required to create the electron and positron pair. The equation may now be written in the form:

Equation 23.13

$$E \text{ (MeV)} = 1.02 + T_1 + T_2$$

This shows that 1.02 MeV of the energy of the photon is used to create the electron and positron pair and the rest is given to the two particles in kinetic energy.

23.7.1 Attenuation, absorption and scatter coefficients for pair production

The linear attenuation for pair production is usually given the symbol π so that the mass attenuation coefficient is π/ρ. This is related both to the photon energy and the atomic number, as shown by Equation 23.14:

Equation 23.14

$$\frac{\pi}{\rho} \propto (E - 1.02)Z$$

where E is the photon energy in MeV and Z is the atomic number of the attenuation material. (Note that this is the only process where the amount of attenuation increases with an increase in the photon energy.)

The kinetic energies of the electron and positron pair are absorbed by the medium as the particles slow down in it. Thus the energy absorbed by the medium is less than the energy of the original photon and is equal to ($E - 1.02$) MeV from Equation 23.14. The electron will eventually lose all its kinetic energy and come to rest. However, the positron will eventually collide with an electron and both will disappear with the emission of two photons of annihilation radiation where each photon has an energy of 0.51 MeV. This is the conversion of matter into energy, sometimes termed annihilation, and it is the reverse of pair production. If the two photons of annihilation radiation produced by this reaction are completely absorbed by the material, then the total energy absorbed is given by the relationship $(E - 1.02) + (2 \times 0.51) = E$, i.e. the whole of the energy of the original photon which caused the pair production.

There is, however, no certainty that this will happen. In such cases, the absorption coefficient (π_a) is less than the attenuation coefficient (π) by a fraction: $(E - 1.02)/E$. This can be rewritten as $1 - (1.02/E)$ and so we have:

Equation 23.15

$$\pi_a \propto \frac{\pi(1 - 1.02)}{E}$$

By analogy with the absorption and scatter coefficient for Compton scatter (see Equation 23.12), in the case of pair production, we may write:

Equation 23.16

$$\pi = \pi_a + \pi_s$$
$$\frac{\pi}{\rho} = \frac{\pi_a}{\rho} + \frac{\pi_s}{\rho}$$

where π_s is the fraction of the energy carried by the two annihilation photons each of energy 0.51 MeV, so $\pi_s = 1.02/E$.

However, in all but the most accurate work, it is usual to ignore the scattering coefficient, π_s, since it is usually very small at the photon energies used in therapeutic radiography and so the more exact Equation 23.16 is replaced by more approximate relationships which assume that $\pi_s = 0$:

Equation 23.17

$$\pi = \pi_a$$
$$\frac{\pi}{\rho} = \frac{\pi_a}{\rho}$$

23.8 RELATIVE IMPORTANCE OF THE ATTENUATION PROCESSES IN RADIOGRAPHY

As we have already established in Equations 23.3 and 23.4, at a particular photon energy, some or all of the above processes may be competing to remove photons from the radiation beam. Thus the total linear attenuation coefficient, μ, is the sum of the linear attenuation coefficients due to photoelectric absorption, Compton scattering and pair production. Thus, the relationship $I_x = I_0 e^{-\mu x}$ can be rewritten as:

Equation 23.18

$$I_x = I_0 e^{-(\tau + \sigma + \pi)x}$$

where τ is the linear attenuation coefficient due to photoelectric absorption, σ is the linear attenuation coefficient due to Compton scattering and π is the linear attenuation coefficient due to pair production. From the above equation we can also deduce the relationships given in Equations 23.3 and 23.4:

Equation 23.19

$$\mu = \tau + \sigma + \pi$$
$$\frac{\mu}{\rho} = \frac{\tau}{\rho} + \frac{\sigma}{\rho} + \frac{\pi}{\rho}$$

By applying the same argument to absorption, we can arrive at very similar equations:

Equation 23.20

$$\mu_a = \tau_a + \sigma_a + \pi_a$$
$$\frac{\mu_a}{\rho} = \frac{\tau_a}{\rho} + \frac{\sigma_a}{\rho} + \frac{\pi_a}{\rho}$$

Similarly, for scatter, we can write equations:

Equation 23.21

$$\mu_s = \sigma_s$$
$$\frac{\mu_s}{\rho} = \frac{\sigma_s}{\rho}$$

where the contribution to the scattering from pair production is ignored. It should also be remembered that photoelectric absorption contributes to energy absorption but not to scatter.

These points are illustrated in Figures 23.8 and 23.9 (see page 175) where the mass attenuation coefficients for photoelectric absorption (τ/ρ), Compton scattering (σ/ρ) and pair production (π/ρ) are shown for air and for lead. The total mass attenuation coefficients (μ/ρ) are shown as thick lines and the total mass absorption coefficients (μ_a/ρ) are shown as broken lines.

The following important points about the attenuation processes should be noted from the graphs:

- Photoelectric absorption dominates at low energies (up to 50–500 keV depending on the atomic number of the absorber).
- The absorption edges become more pronounced as the atomic number of the absorber increases.
- Compton scattering dominates over a wide range of energies ($\approx$50 keV to 5 MeV) in all materials.
- The Compton region is almost identical in all attenuating materials (except hydrogen) because of the similarity of electron density of all materials. Thus the shape of the Compton curve is independent of the attenuator (the curve for σ/ρ is the same shape for both air and lead).
- Only photoelectric absorption and Compton scattering are important to diagnostic radiography.
- Pair production is only significant for high energies ($\geq$1.02 MeV) and for attenuating materials of high atomic number.

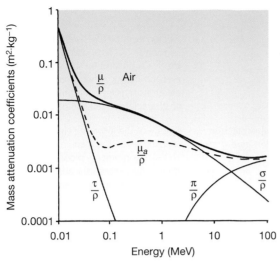

Figure 23.8 Mass attenuation coefficients for air – μ/ρ is the total mass attenuation coefficient, τ/ρ is the mass attenuation coefficient due to photoelectric absorption, σ/ρ is the mass attenuation coefficient due to Compton scattering and π/ρ is the mass attenuation coefficient due to pair production. Also shown (broken line) is the total mass absorption coefficient (μ_a/ρ).

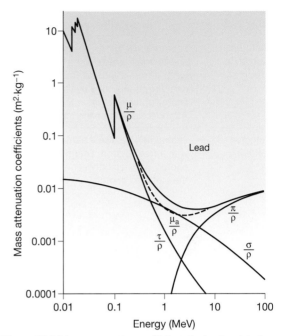

Figure 23.9 Mass attenuation coefficients for lead – μ/ρ is the total mass attenuation coefficient, τ/ρ is the mass attenuation coefficient due to photoelectric absorption, σ/ρ is the mass attenuation coefficient due to Compton scattering and π/ρ is the mass attenuation coefficient due to pair production. Also shown (broken line) is the total mass absorption coefficient (μ_a/ρ).

- The significance of the contribution of pair production increases as the photon energy increases above 1.02 MeV. This is the opposite to the effect on the other processes of increasing the photon energy.
- Pair production is an important absorption mechanism in therapeutic radiography and in PET scanning.

23.9 CONCLUSION

As can be seen from the above, the attenuation of an X-ray beam as it passes through a patient's tissues is a complicated affair depending on the energy of the photons, the tissue thickness and the atomic number of the tissue through which the beam passes. In both radiography and radiotherapy, we are able to alter the photon energy and this has important consequences for the absorption pattern and the intensity pattern of the beam emerging from the patient. These will be discussed in more detail in Chapter 25 when the formation of the radiographic image is considered.

The significance of the high absorption of materials with high atomic numbers (as shown by the graph for lead in Fig. 23.9) will also be considered in Chapter 27, which considers the topic of radiation protection.

A summary of the interaction processes, which may be useful in subsequent chapters of this text, is given in Table 23.2.

Table 23.2 Summary of the interaction processes

PROCESS	DESCRIPTION OF INTERACTIONS	EFFECT OF Z, E	COMMENTS
Elastic scattering	Photon interacts with bound atomic electron. Photon energy is less than the electron binding energy. Photon is re-radiated from the material with no energy loss	$\sigma_{coh}/\rho \propto Z^2/E$	No energy absorption in the medium. Photon scattered in the forward direction. Effect is negligible in biological tissues because of low Z

(Continued)

Table 23.2 Summary of the interaction processes (Continued)

Photoelectric absorption	Photon of energy $\geq$ the binding energy of an electron interacts with bound electron and ejects it from its orbital. Photon disappears as all its energy is absorbed by the electron. Kinetic energy of the electron $= E -$ binding energy. Atom recoils, conserving momentum	$\tau/\rho \propto Z^3/E^3$	Ejected electron loses velocity to surrounding atoms. giving energy to them; i.e. absorption takes place. The electron vacancy created is filled by electrons making quantum jumps and so characteristic radiation is emitted
Compton scattering	Photon behaves like a particle and collides with a free electron. Energy of the incident photon is shared between the electron and the scattered photon	$\sigma/\rho \propto$ electron density/E	Energy of the displaced electron is absorbed by the medium, so Compton process produces attenuation and partial absorption. Electron densities of all materials except hydrogen are similar and so σ/ρ values are largely independent of the type of attenuator
Pair production	Photon of energy ≥ 1.02 MeV may spontaneously disappear in the vicinity of the nucleus of an attenuator atom, producing an electron and a positron. Atom recoils and preserves momentum. Positron eventually annihilated with an electron to form two photons of annihilation radiation, each with energy of 0.51 MeV	$\pi/\rho \propto (E - 1.02)Z$	Probability of pair production increases with E above 1.02 MeV. Contribution of π_s is very small compared to π and is often ignored

Summary

In this chapter, you should have learnt the following:

- The meaning of the terms *attenuation*, *absorption* and *scattering* as applied to a beam of radiation passing through matter (see Sect. 23.2).
- The factors which control the probability of an interaction taking place between the X-ray photon and an atom of the attenuator (see Sect. 23.2.1).
- The meaning of the terms *total linear attenuation coefficient* and *total mass attenuation coefficient* and where it is appropriate to use each (see Sects 23.2.2 and 23.2.3).
- The interrelationships between attenuation and absorption (see Sect. 23.3).
- The mechanism of elastic (coherent) scattering and the factors affecting it (see Sect. 23.4).
- The mechanism of photoelectric absorption and the factors affecting it (see Sect. 23.5).
- The mechanism of Compton scattering and the factors affecting it (see Sect. 23.6).
- The mechanism of pair production and the factors affecting it (see Sect. 23.7).
- The relative importance of each of the attenuation processes in radiography (see Sect. 23.8).

FURTHER READING

Ball, J.L., Moore, A.D., Turner, S., 2008. Ball and Moore's Essential Physics for Radiographers, fourth ed. Blackwell Scientific, London (Chapter 17).

Curry, T.S., Thomas, S., Dowdey, J.C., et al., 1990. Christensen's Physics of Diagnostic Radiology. Lea & Febiger, London (Chapters 4 and 5).

Webb, S. (Ed.), 2000. The Physics of Medical Imaging. Institute of Physics, Bristol. (Chapter 2).

Chapter | 24 |

Luminescence and photostimulation

24.1 AIM

The aim of this chapter is to introduce the topics of luminescence, fluorescence, phosphorescence, thermoluminescence and photostimulation. In the case of each of the processes, the relevance to radiographic imaging will be briefly discussed.

24.2 INTRODUCTION

If we irradiate a material with high-energy photons and this causes the material to emit photons of lower energy, the material is exhibiting the property of luminescence. Within the strict laws of physics, provided that the energy is lower than that of the original radiation beam, the emitted radiation can be in any part of the electromagnetic spectrum. In radiography we are more interested in luminescence when the radiation emitted falls in the visible part of the spectrum. Before we can discuss the process in detail, we need to define some basic terms.

24.3 LUMINESCENCE, FLUORESCENCE AND PHOSPHORESCENCE

As mentioned above, if we irradiate a material and it emits visible light, then that material is said to exhibit *luminescence.*

Fluorescence occurs when the light emission ceases almost immediately after the irradiation has stopped (the time interval is about 10^{-8} s), then it can be seen that we require materials that exhibit fluorescence as this allows us to remove the image receptor from the cassette and process it immediately after the X-ray exposure has taken place.

Phosphorescence occurs if the material continues to emit light for a significant time after the initial period of radiation. For this reason, phosphorescence is often referred to as *afterglow.* Such a phenomenon is generally not desirable in radiography – if we had significant afterglow then we would have to wait before cassettes could be emptied and refilled. Afterglow can also cause image lag in fluoroscopy.

From the above we can say that luminescence occurs when we irradiate a material and the substance produces light. If the production of light ceases within 10^{-8} s of the end of the irradiation, then the process is one of fluorescence; if it continues beyond this point, then we have phosphorescence.

24.3.1 Mechanism of fluorescence

The mechanism of fluorescence can be explained by reference to the electron band theory. Fluorescence is caused by an electron in a high-energy state dropping to a lower-energy state and thereby emitting a quantum of radiation (Fig. 24.1). If the wavelength of the emitted quantum is in the range 400–700 nm, this will form part of the visible spectrum. If we consider a phosphor used in radiography being irradiated with X-ray photons, then the first process necessary is that some of the electrons of the phosphor atoms are involved in photoelectric interactions with the X-ray photons raising the energy of the electrons. As already mentioned, the overall efficiency of a phosphor may be improved by the addition of activators. These impurities encourage the formation of luminescent centres within the phosphor; the efficiency of lanthanum oxybromide will be increased by the addition of terbium as an activator. The activators possess discrete electron energy levels which are different from that of the phosphor crystal and these are used to form the luminescent centre.

This is shown diagrammatically in Figure 24.1. Part A shows the electron energy level arrangement in a pure crystal and part B the arrangement in a crystal with a luminescent centre. These centres will produce fluorescence more efficiently than the pure crystal. The sequence of events occurring within the crystal is as follows:

- An X-ray photon undergoes a photoelectric interaction with an electron of one of the crystal atoms.
- The photoelectric interaction liberates the electron and gives it some kinetic energy so that it is free to move within the conduction band, leaving a 'hole' in the valence band.
- The energetic electron, on passing close to other atoms, excites and ionizes these atoms and so more electrons are raised into the conduction band (leaving more holes in the valence band).
- Some of the electrons so liberated will lose small amounts of energy which will allow them to adjust their energy to the energy level of the luminescent centres.
- At the same time, some of the holes in the valence band will have their energy raised to allow them to reach the lower energy level of the luminescent centre.
- Some of the electrons at the upper level of the luminescent centre will perform a quantum jump to neutralize the holes at the lower level of the centre. This is shown diagrammatically in Figure 24.1B where the energy of the emitted photon is $E_l = hv^1$, where v_1 is the frequency of the emitted photon and h is Planck's constant.
- The difference in energy between the upper and lower levels in the luminescent centre controls the photon energy E_l and the colour of the emitted (fluorescent) light.

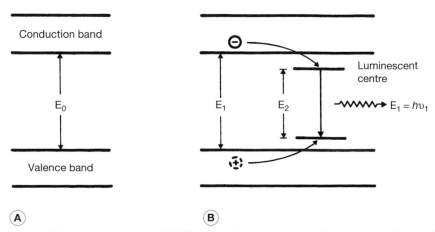

Figure 24.1 Mechanism of fluorescence in a crystal. (A) The outer electron structure of a pure crystal; (B) the effect of an impurity atom on the electron levels. Such impurities enhance fluorescence by forming luminescent centres. These impurities are known as activators. The explanation of the fluorescent process will be found in the text.

Table 24.1 Measures of the efficiency of two phosphors used in radiography (the energy of the incident radiation was 60 keV)

PHOSPHOR	QUANTUM DETECTION EFFICIENCY (%)	QUANTUM CONVERSION EFFICIENCY (%)	SCINTILLATION EFFICIENCY (%)
Calcium tungstate	13	5	0.65
Gadolinium oxysulphide	51	20	10.2

- As more electrons enter the luminescent centres than are involved in the initial photoelectric interactions, the number of fluorescent photons is greater than the number of absorbed photons.

As can be seen from the above, the process of fluorescence occurs as a number of stages and inefficiency at any one stage can affect the efficiency of the whole process. This allows us to compare the operation of different phosphors by comparing efficiency at each of the stages

The *quantum detection efficiency* (QDE) is a measure of the percentage of the quanta (e.g. X-rays) incident on the phosphor which are stopped by the phosphor.

The *quantum conversion efficiency* (QCE) is a measure of the percentage of the quantal energy stopped by the phosphor which is converted into light photons.

The *scintillation efficiency* (ScE) is a measure of the percentage of the quantal energy incident on the phosphor which is converted into useful light photons.

As the ScE is a measure of the overall process, it is affected by changes in the QDE or QCE: if the QDE is 50% and the QCE is 20%, then the ScE will be 10% (ScE = QDE × QCE). These measures of efficiency are shown in Table 24.1 for two phosphors used in radiography.

24.3.2 Mechanism of phosphorescence

Phosphorescence is caused by the presence of electron traps within the crystal structure of the phosphor. The mechanism is as follows:

- An X-ray photon undergoes a photoelectric interaction with an electron of one of the crystal atoms.
- The photoelectric interaction liberates the electron and gives it some kinetic energy so that it is free to move within the conduction band, leaving a 'hole' in the valence band.
- The energetic electron, on passing close to other atoms, excites and ionizes these atoms and so more electrons are raised into the conduction band (leaving more holes in the valence band).
- Some of the electrons so liberated will lose small amounts of energy which will cause them to fall into the electron traps.

- The electrons remain in the traps until they are released as a result of interatomic vibrations. If the traps are sufficiently near the conduction band, this may happen without the application of additional energy (see trap A in Fig. 24.2).
- Some of these released electrons will find luminescent centres and light will be produced by the process described for fluorescence.

Because there is a measurable length of time when the electron is 'stuck' in the electron trap, the luminescence will occur after the irradiation of the material has ceased. This is phosphorescence or *afterglow*.

The phenomenon diminishes exponentially (see Ch. 20) from the time of cessation of the irradiation. Such a process is generally regarded as a nuisance in radiography, especially for image intensifier and monitor phosphors, since the phosphor may still 'remember' the previous image when a new one is being produced.

24.3.3 Mechanism of thermoluminescence

If we refer to Figure 24.2, we can see that trap B is too 'deep' below the conduction band for the electrons in it

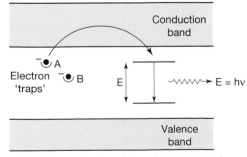

Figure 24.2 The production of phosphorescence and thermoluminescence. An electron enters trap A as a result of energy absorbed from the radiation beam striking the phosphor. After the exposure, this electron can subsequently enter the conduction band as a result of interatomic vibration and hence produce fluorescent photons (phosphorescence) as shown. The electron in trap B will only be released if the material is heated (thermoluminescence), as discussed in the text.

to leave and enter the conduction band. This is a typical arrangement for a thermoluminescent material, e.g. lithium fluoride, as the material contains energy gaps between the valence and conduction bands. The mechanism of thermoluminescence is as follows:

- An X-ray photon undergoes a photoelectric interaction with an electron of one of the crystal atoms.
- The photoelectric interaction liberates the electron and gives it some kinetic energy so that it is free to move within the conduction band, leaving a 'hole' in the valence band.
- The energetic electron, on passing close to other atoms, excites and ionizes these atoms and so more electrons are raised into the conduction band (leaving more holes in the valence band).
- Some of the electrons so liberated will lose small amounts of energy which will cause them to fall into the electron traps.
- These electrons get stuck in the traps (see trap B in Fig. 24.2), however the traps are too deep in the forbidden energy gap for normal interatomic vibration to release them. If more energy is applied to the substance by heating it, the electrons will gain energy as a result of the increased interatomic vibrations and can move up into the conduction band.
- Some of these electrons will find luminescent centres and light will be produced by the process described for fluorescence.
- Thus, the intensity of the light emitted from the thermoluminescent material is directly proportional to the amount of radiation incident on the material. This is the basis of thermoluminescent dosimetry, which will be discussed in Chapter 27.

24.3.4 Fluorescent screens in radiography

Fluorescent screens, with film as a recording medium, were once the most common image receptors used in radiography. They have now been replaced by photostimulable plates and other image receptors (see Ch. 34 for more information).

24.3.5 Further examples of fluorescence

Four further examples of fluorescence applicable to radiographic imaging will now be briefly considered (more detailed descriptions may be found in specialist textbooks on X-ray equipment):

1. If we use an image intensifier in fluoroscopy, then this contains an input phosphor and an output phosphor. The input phosphor is usually made of caesium iodide and absorbs X-ray photons and re-emits the energy as light photons. The light photons fall on a photocathode which will emit electrons when bombarded by light. The electrons are accelerated and focused on to an output phosphor where their energy is used to create light photons by the fluorescent effect. The net result of this is that the image is intensified by about 5000 times between the input phosphor and the output phosphor.

2. In the television monitor, the phosphor on the face of the monitor is bombarded by electrons. Such high-energy electrons are capable of causing the phosphor to fluoresce, producing the image on the television monitor.

3. Scintillation counters made of sodium iodide crystals coupled with photomultiplier tubes or solid-state devices can be used to detect small amounts of X-rays and gamma-rays. The intensity of the fluorescence from the crystals is proportional to the intensity of the radiation hitting the crystal. Such devices are used in nuclear medicine, computed tomographic scanners and osteoporosis scanners

4. Radiographic departments are lit by fluorescent lighting. An electrical discharge in the gas in the tube causes the emission of ultraviolet radiation. This is absorbed by a suitable phosphor coated onto the inside of the tubes which then emits visible light.

24.4 PHOTOSTIMULATION

Photostimulated luminescence is said to have been discovered in the mid 19th century by Becquerel, but its practical application was not developed until the early 1970s.

The basic structure of a photostimulable plate is shown in Figure 24.3. The process of photostimulation is very similar to the process of thermoluminescence (Sect 24.3.3). A suitable phosphor (e.g. europium activated barium fluorohalide (BaF(BrI):Eu^2)) is irradiated and the following process takes place:

- An X-ray photon undergoes a photoelectric interaction with an electron of one of the phosphor atoms.

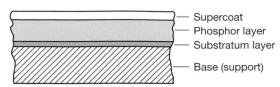

— Supercoat
— Phosphor layer
— Substratum layer
— Base (support)

Figure 24.3 Section (not to scale) through a photostimulable plate. The function of the transparent supercoat is to protect the phosphor layer from mechanical damage, while the substratum layer binds the phosphor layer to the base, which provides a firm support to the plate.

- The interaction liberates an electron, giving it kinetic energy so that it is free to move to the conduction band, leaving a 'hole' in the valence band.
- The energetic electron, on passing close to other atoms, excites and ionizes these atoms, liberating more electrons and raising them into the conduction band and leaving more holes in the valence band.
- A few electrons with sufficient energy find luminescent centres and light in the blue–green range (550 nm) of the spectrum will be produced by the process described for fluorescence.
- The majority of the liberated electrons lose small amounts of energy, causing them to fall into the electron traps (also called colour centres) in the forbidden gap between the valence and conduction bands.
- The 'trapped' electrons do not have sufficient energy to 'escape' from the traps and remain there.
- At a later time, the imaging plate is scanned in an image reader by a red laser beam. This process 'pumps' energy into the phosphor giving energy to the trapped electrons. They can then leave the electron traps and move into the conduction band.
- These liberated electrons will find luminescent centres in the conduction band and light in the blue–green range (550 nm) of the spectrum will be produced by the process described for fluorescence.
- The intensity of the light emitted from each area of the phosphor is proportional to the amount of radiation each area received.
- The emitted light is detected and channeled to a photomultiplier where it is converted into an electrical signal; the signal may be passed into a computer system (or less commonly be used to operate a laser printer to produce 'hard copy').
- Finally, the plate is exposed to an intense white light. This imparts more energy to the phosphor, releasing all 'trapped' electrons and preparing the plate for another exposure to X radiation. Unlike film which can only be used once, photostimulable plates can be reused for about 1000 cycles.

This process is the basis of photostimulable plates which are used in computed radiography imaging systems (see Ch. 34).

Summary

In this chapter, you should have learnt the following:
- The meaning of the terms *luminescence*, *fluorescence* and *phosphorescence* (see Sect. 24.3).
- The mechanism of fluorescence (see Sect. 24.3.1).
- The meaning of the terms *quantum detection efficiency*, *quantum conversion efficiency* and *scintillation efficiency* (see Sect. 24.3.1).
- The mechanism of phosphorescence (see Sect. 24.3.2).
- The mechanism of thermoluminescence (see Sect. 24.3.3).
- Other uses of fluorescence in radiography (see Sect. 24.3.5).
- The mechanism of photostimulation radiography (see Sect. 24.4).

FURTHER READING

Curry III, T.S., Dowdey Jr., J.E., Murry, R.C., 1990. Christensen's Physics of Diagnostic Radiography, fourth ed. Lee & Febiger, London (Chapter 2).

Roberts, D.P., Smith, N.L., Gunn, C., 1994. Radiographic Imaging: a Practical Approach. Churchill Livingstone, Edinburgh (Chapters 2 and 5).

Webb, S. (Ed.), 2000. The Physics of Medical Imaging, second ed.. Institute of Physics, Bristol (Chapter 2).

Chapter | 25 |

The radiographic image

25.1 AIM

The aim of this chapter is to consider the major factors involved in the production of a radiographic image. The chapter will first consider the attenuation patterns in a patient that will produce an X-ray image and will then consider how this reacts with a recording medium to produce a radiograph. The chapter also summarizes how the selection of exposure factors affects the quality of the radiographic image produced.

25.2 INTRODUCTION

The quality of the radiographic image is affected by a number of geometrical factors that determine the magnification of the image and the amount of geometrical unsharpness produced. The radiographic image depends on more than geometrical considerations. This chapter considers the other factors which contribute to the image quality. To understand this, it is necessary to understand the contribution of photoelectric absorption and Compton scattering to the final radiographic image (see Ch. 23).

It is easier to understand the final image quality if we consider image formation as a two-stage process:

1. The production of an X-ray image pattern as the beam of radiation is attenuated by the patient.
2. The production of a radiographic image as this radiation pattern interacts with a recording medium.

Therefore, this chapter will consist of two halves, each looking at one of these stages.

25.3 THE X-RAY IMAGE PATTERN

25.3.1 Attenuation of the X-ray beam by the body

We will assume, for simplicity, that the radiation beam from the X-ray tube striking the body is of uniform intensity across the beam. When this beam interacts with the body substance, different structures will cause different amounts of attenuation and a 'pattern' of radiation intensities is transmitted to the imaging device. If all structures in the beam attenuated the radiation by the same amount, there would be no pattern and no image of any structures would be seen on the radiograph. A simple example of such differential absorption is shown

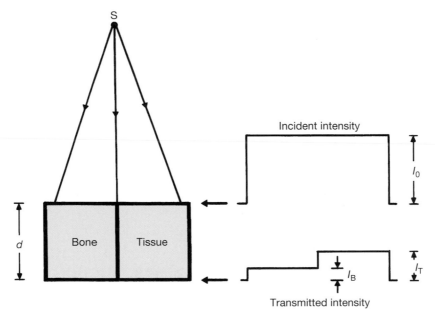

Figure 25.1 A comparison of the attenuation of an X-ray beam by an equal thickness of bone and soft tissue. Note that the attenuation of X-rays by bone is greater than that by soft tissue.

in Figure 25.1, where two separate rectangular blocks of bone and soft tissue are shown interacting with the X-ray beam. The profiles of the incident (I_0) and the transmitted (I_T) radiation intensifies are also shown. If again we assume, for simplicity, that the attenuation of the radiation beam is exponential, then:

Equation 25.1

$$I_B = I_0 e^{-\mu(B)d}$$
$$I_T = I_0 e^{-\mu(T)d}$$

where I_0 is the intensity of the X-ray beam before it enters the patient, $\mu(B)$ is the total linear attenuation coefficient for bone and $\mu(T)$ is the total linear attenuation coefficient for soft tissue. I_B is the intensity of the radiation transmitted through a thickness d of bone and I_T is the intensity transmitted through a similar thickness of soft tissue. As can be seen from Figure 25.1, I_B is less than I_T. This is because $\mu(B)$ is greater than $\mu(T)$. There are two physical reasons for this:

1. The density of bone is approximately twice that of soft tissue ($\rho_B = 1.8$; $\rho_T = 1.0$).
2. The average atomic number of bone is approximately twice that of soft tissue ($Z_B = 14$; $Z_T = 7.5$).

The total linear attenuation coefficient is proportional to the number of atoms present in unit volume and the density of the medium. As the density of bone is twice that of soft tissue, then there must be twice as many atoms in unit volume and so, all other things being equal, the linear attenuation coefficient for bone would be twice that for soft tissue.

To appreciate the importance of the difference in atomic number, we must consider the attenuation process occurring. The equations for each process are summarized below:

Equation 25.2

$$\tau \propto \rho \times \frac{Z^3}{E^3}$$
$$\sigma \propto \rho \frac{(\text{electron density})}{E}$$

where τ is the linear attenuation coefficient for the photoelectric effect, σ is the linear attenuation coefficient for Compton scattering, ρ is the density of the attenuator, Z is its atomic number and E is the photon energy. The higher atomic number of bone means that it will greatly attenuate suitable radiation by the photoelectric effect.

As the total attenuation is a combination of both the photoelectric effect and Compton scattering, in the diagnostic energy ranges, a given thickness of bone will attenuate radiation approximately 12 times the level of an equal thickness of soft tissue.

The findings are summarized in Table 25.1. The process of photostimulation is (See page 185). The essential points to be taken from the table are that in the diagnostic range of photon energies, the higher atomic number of bone results in photoelectric absorption being the main attenuation process, whereas the lower atomic number of soft tissue means that Compton scattering is the main attenuation process. (In the therapy range of photon energies, the dominant attenuation processes are Compton scattering and pair production, both of which are less dependent on the atomic number of the attenuator.)

Table 25.1 Comparison of linear attenuation in bone and soft tissue

ATTENUATOR	PHOTOELECTRIC $\tau \propto$ $\rho \times Z^3/E^3$	COMPTON SCATTERING $\sigma \propto \rho$ (ELECTRON DENSITY)/E	TOTAL ATTENUATION $\mu = \tau + \sigma$
Bone $Z = 14$ $\rho = 1.8$	Photoelectric absorption is high when photon energy is low: 12–16 times greater than soft tissue	Predominates at high photon energies 500 keV to 5 MeV	Mainly photoelectric absorption at diagnostic energies
Soft tissue $Z = 7.5$ $\rho = 1.0$	Significant at low photon energies <25 keV	predominates at photon energies > 30 keV	Compton scattering is the dominant process if the average photon energy is greater than about 30 keV

A more realistic example of attenuation is given in Figure 25.2. This simulates the presence of a piece of bone surrounded by soft tissue. A profile of the transmitted radiation intensity is also shown and it can be seen that its minimum corresponds to the maximum thickness of the bone (point A in the figure).

The *fraction* of the incident radiation transmitted through the thickness $D - d$ of soft tissue is $e^{-\mu(T)(D-d)}$. The total fraction can be found by *adding* the two fractions so that:

Equation 25.3

$$\frac{I_2}{I_0} = e^{-\mu(B)d} + e^{-\mu(T)(D-d)}$$
$$\text{so } I_2 = I_0 e^{-\mu(B)d} + e^{-\mu(T)(D-d)}$$
$$\text{or } I_2 = I_0 e^{-\mu(T)D - [-\mu(B)-\mu(T)]d}$$
$$\text{and } I_1 = I_0 e^{-\mu(T)D}$$

The difference between I_2 and I_1 is responsible for the contrast on the radiograph.

25.3.2 Scatter and the radiographic image

So far, the sections of this chapter have been oversimplified in that the emerging radiation beam is assumed to be composed only of transmitted primary beam. If only photoelectric absorption took place this would be true, but it is not true in the case of Compton scatter where only partial absorption of the photon energy occurs. This scattered radiation may escape from the patient and reach the image recording medium. Unfortunately, such scatter will form an image on the medium, *but the image formed by the scatter forms an overall fog and so is not a useful image.* Unless this scatter can be limited, serious image degradation can occur.

Scatter to the radiograph may be limited in two ways:

1. Limiting the amount of scatter formed.
2. Stopping any scatter formed from reaching the image recording medium.

Each of these will now be considered in turn.

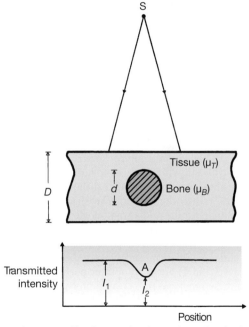

Figure 25.2 A profile of transmitted X-ray intensity obtained from a bone embedded in soft tissue.

25.3.2.1 Limiting scattered radiation formation

The amount of scatter formed in the patient depends on the number of atoms involved in scattering interactions. Thus, scatter formation is volume dependent, i.e. *the greater the volume of patient irradiated, the greater the quantity of scatter formed.* One of the major ways the operator can limit scatter formation is to reduce the volume of tissue irradiated. This can be done by collimation using a light-beam diaphragm or cones or, in some cases, by tissue displacement. Both these methods will not only produce an improvement in image quality but also reduce the radiation dose to the patient and others by limiting the scatter formation.

Insight

Most operators know from experience that the scattered radiation to the radiograph is increased as kVp is increased. This process is a somewhat complicated one. If the kVp is increased then photon energy is increased, and σ/ρ is proportional to $1/E$. Thus, with higher-energy photons there are fewer scattering events within a given volume of tissue. With higher photon energy, the angle of scatter is smaller and consequently the scatter has a higher energy and is more likely to leave the body. We have more scatter leaving the patient and the scatter is in a more forward direction and so is more likely to hit the image receptor.

25.3.2.2 Stopping scatter from reaching the image receptor

Once formed, the most common way of stopping scatter from reaching the image receptor is to use a secondary radiation grid. Such a grid can remove about 90% of the scatter from the beam. A secondary radiation grid consists of strips of high-atomic-number material (e.g. lead) interspaced with strips of low-atomic-number material (e.g. carbon fibre). A section through such a grid is shown in Figure 25.3 where the lead strips are shaded. Primary radiation should hit the grid at right angles to its surface (or nearly right angles to it), so that it will easily pass between the lead strips (see ray 2 primary radiation (ray 1). may strike a lead strip and be absorbed. Because scatter (rays 3 and 4) are at an oblique angle to the primary beam these rays have an increased probability of striking a lead strip and being absorbed may strike a lead strip and be absorbed, if the angle is very small sees (ray 4) such scatter may' miss' the lead strip and strike the image receptor. Because scatter is at an oblique angle to the

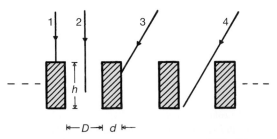

Figure 25.3 The principle of action of a secondary radiation grid. Scattered rays (3 and 4 in the diagram) are more likely to strike the lead and be absorbed by the lead than the primary rays (1 and 2 in the diagram).

primary beam it has an increased probability of striking a lead strip and being absorbed. The fraction of the primary beam stopped is given by the ratio $d/(D + d)$, since this is the fraction of the grid covered by lead; in practice this means the exposure must be increased when using a grid. Because scattered radiation is at an oblique angle to the primary beam, it has an increased probability of striking a lead strip and being absorbed. If the angle is very small, such scatter may be able to pass between the strips and reach the image receptor, but such rays do not contribute as much to image degradation as the more oblique rays.

Various factors of grid design may be chosen to optimize the performance of a secondary radiation grid for a particular application:

- The *grid ratio* (*r*) is the height of the strips (*h*) to the width between them (*D*):

Equation 25.4

$$r = \frac{h}{D}$$

It can be appreciated from Figure 25.3 that increasing the height of the lead strips or reducing the space between them (i.e. increasing the grid ratio) will increase the efficiency of the grid in absorbing scattered radiation with a relatively small scatter angle

- The *grid lattice* or *lattice density* is a measure of the number of lines of absorber per centimetre. If we consider that the space between each strip is controlled by the grid ratio, then the number of lines per centimetre will affect the thickness of the individual lines. Grids with a high lattice density (i.e. 30–40 lines per centimetre) will have very fine lines and so do not degrade the image. If grid lattice density is low, the grid lines are visible which detract from image quality. A solution to this problem is to move the grid during the exposure so that the grid lines are blurred out. Such a device is known as a *Potter–Bucky diaphragm* or, more commonly, as a Bucky.
- As mentioned earlier, the grid will absorb some of the primary radiation and so it is necessary to increase the exposure when using a grid to compensate for this. The amount by which the exposure must be increased is known as the grid factor.

Equation 25.5

$$\text{grid factor} = \frac{\text{exposure with grid}}{\text{exposure without grid}}$$

Note: This equation is only accurate if the kVp used for the exposure remains constant. A change of kVp will result in a change in the amount and type of scatter produced (see Insight, Sect. 25.3.2.1). It will also change the contrast range of the image (see Sect. 25.3.3). For most grids encountered in a diagnostic department, the grid factor will be between 2 and 6.

25.3.3 Effect of kVp on the X-ray image

The effect of a change of kVp on the spectrum of radiation produced by the X-ray tube has been discussed in Section 22.4 and, as can be seen from Figure 22.2, the average energy for a single-phase two-pulse generator is about one-third to one-half of the maximum photon energy. This means that if 90 kVp was applied across the X-ray tube, the maximum photon energy would be 90 keV, but the *average* photon energy would be approximately 40 keV. We can apply the various scattering and attenuation coefficients to a beam of radiation generated at 90 kVp that we would apply to a monoenergetic beam of photon energy of 40 keV. The effect of increasing kVp is to increase the average photon energy and reduce the linear attenuation coefficients of both bone and soft tissue. The radiation beam is more penetrating.

From Equation 25.2, it can be seen that increasing photon energy will reduce the amount of photoelectric absorption (τ) more than it will reduce Compton scattering (σ) because the photoelectric effect is proportional to $1/E^3$. Because of less photoelectric absorption, there is less differentiation in absorption between bone and soft tissue – there is less contrast between the densities in the radiographic image. As already mentioned, an increase in kVp will also result in more scatter reaching the image receptor, further reducing contrast. Increasing kVp degrades image contrast in the ways mentioned above. There are practical advantages in using a high kVp. These are:

- It increases the intensity of the radiation beam, allowing a reduction in exposure time.
- It results in a higher percentage of the radiation beam being transmitted through the patient, again allowing a reduction in the exposure time.
- Because a higher percentage of the incident beam is transmitted through the patient, the absorbed radiation dose received by the patient is reduced.

Insight

The 'best' image is the one that most clearly demonstrates the structures we wish to see! There are some situations in which a low kVp is used to produce a high contrast between tissues of almost the same density (e.g. mammography) and others where we may wish to use a high kVp to demonstrate structures of very different radiopacity in the same image (e.g. high kV chest radiography).

25.4 THE RADIOIGRAPHIC IMAGE PATTERN

The X-ray image pattern discussed so far in this chapter may be used to form an image on a number of different image receptors, for instance on a visual display unit (VDU), a photostimulable imaging plate (PSP) or even a film-intensifying screen combination, although the latter is very rarely used today.

When the image is displayed on a VDU, the light intensity is directly proportional to the radiation intensity, while a PSP has a similar linear response. This is not so when the radiation image is transferred to a photographic emulsion using intensifying screens. The intensifying screen produces light in proportion to the intensity of the X-ray image pattern. This light produces a latent image in the film. Processing then converts the invisible latent image into a permanent one. This blackening effect is *not linear*. An instrument called a *densitometer*, which is calibrated to measure optical density, can be used to assess the density or amount of blackening produced. Density is defined as $\log_{10}(I_0/I_t)$, where I_0 is the intensity of the light on the processed film and I_t is the intensity of the light transmitted through it. Examination of a processed image will show that the darker the image, the less light transmitted through it and the higher the optical density. When plotting the density of the film at different exposures, it is usual to plot density against the logarithm of the relative exposure to accommodate the wide range of exposures to which the emulsion can respond. A graph of these densities can be produced; this is known as the *characteristic curve* of that emulsion. Figure 25.4 shows a typical characteristic curve.

Features of this graph will now be discussed (see Figure 25.4 page 188):

- Even when the relative exposure is zero, the emulsion will show some density. This is referred to as *base plus fog*. It results from the small amount of fog produced by the chemical activity of the developing process and any tint that may be present in the base material of the film. The density of this region is normally less than 0.2.
- There follows an initial horizontal portion where an increase in exposure produces no increase in density. This is often referred to as the *threshold* of the curve.
- The *toe* of the curve is the point at which the emulsion is becoming increasingly responsive to differences in exposure.
- There follows a region where an increase in exposure produces a linear increase in density. We aim to set X-ray exposure factors so that the exposure to the film falls in this part of the characteristic curve.
- The linear increase 'flattens' off at the shoulder. This usually occurs at densities between 3 and 4. We can only see contrasts between densities of just over 2 with the unaided eye; densities above this are seen as black. Industrial radiography makes use of this region.

In contrast, the PSP has a linear response over the entire exposure range, giving it a very high bit depth (see Ch. 34). Image processing software permits the selection of the range of the bit depth of the displayed image and also compensates for both over- and underexposure, although with gross underexposure, image pixelation is more noticeable.

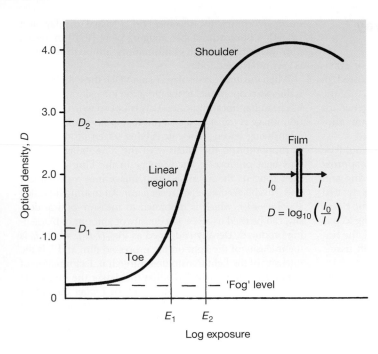

Figure 25.4 Response of a film screen combination obtained by plotting density against the log of the relative exposure.

25.5 PRACTICAL CONSIDERATIONS IN EXPOSURE SELECTION

Where anatomical exposure selection in not available, the interrelationships between the various factors that affect image quality are complex and require considerable skill to master. There is a strong subjective element in selecting the 'best' image but no absolute rules can be laid down for exposure factors. The wide degree of variability in shape and size of the patients themselves, together with other practical difficulties (e.g. patients who are unable to keep still during the exposure), would provide so many exceptions that it is impossible to adhere to a strict set of rules. The operator's experience is therefore critical in producing images of consistently high quality under all conditions. The following paragraphs should be considered with these general comments in mind.

In Chapter 22 we saw that, broadly speaking, the quality of the radiation in an X-ray beam depends on the kVp across the X-ray tube and the quantity of radiation produced on the mAs that flows through the X-ray tube during the exposure. If the kVp selected is too low, denser body structures (e.g. the bony skeleton) will not be penetrated by the X-ray beam resulting in excessive contrast and an increase in radiation dose to the patient. On the other hand, too high a kV reduces the contrast between structures and can produce significant amounts of scattered radiation. Unless this scatter is prevented from reaching the image receptor by the use of a secondary grid, image degradation can occur.

Image manipulation software can compensate for excessive density if too high an mAs is selected, but the operator may not be aware of their error and the patient will receive an excessive dose of radiation as a result. The exposure index shown on the monitor screen is an indicator of this. If the mAs selected is excessively low, image manipulation software can often produce an acceptable image, although pixelation may be present.

Summary

In this chapter, you should have learnt the following:
- How the X-ray beam is attenuated by bone and soft tissue (see Sect. 25.3.1).
- The effect of scattered radiation on the X-ray image and subsequently on the radiograph (Sect. 25.3.2).
- Methods of limiting the amount of scattered radiation formed (see Sect. 25.3.2.1).
- Methods of reducing the amount of scatter reaching the image receptor, including factors that affect the efficiency of a secondary radiation grid (see Sect. 25.3.2.2).
- The effect of a change of kVp on the X-ray image pattern (see Sect. 25.3.3).
- How the X-ray image pattern is changed into the radiographic image (see Sect. 25.4).
- What is meant by the characteristic curve of an emulsion (see Sect. 25.4).
- Practical considerations in the choice of exposure factors (see Sect. 25.5).

FURTHER READING

Ball, J.L., Moore, A.D., Turner, S., 2008. Ball and Moore's Essential Physics for Radiographers, fourth ed. Blackwell Scientific, London (Chapter 16).

Curry III, T.S., Dowdey Jr., J.E., Murry, R.C., 1990. Christensen's Physics of Diagnostic Radiography, fourth ed. Lee & Febiger, London (Chapter 2).

Fauber, T., 2005. Radiographic Imaging and Exposure, second ed. Mosby, New York (Chapters 3 and 4).

Gunn, C., 2002. Radiographic Imaging – A Practical Approach, third ed. Churchill Livingstone, Edinburgh (Chapters 4, 5 and 8).

Webb, S. (Ed.), 2000. The physics of medical imaging, second ed. Institute of Physics, Bristol (Chapter 2).

Chapter | 26 |

The inverse square law

26.1 AIM

The aim of this chapter is to introduce the reader to the inverse square law and to explore its applications in radiography.

26.2 INTENSITY OF RADIATION

To understand the inverse square law we must first understand what is meant by the term *intensity*.

As we have seen in Chapter 17, electromagnetic radiation is composed of quanta, each of which has an energy. If we draw a square of unit area at right angles to the path of a uniform beam of electromagnetic radiation (such as X-rays), then the total per energy second from all the quanta passing through the square is defined as the *intensity* of the beam, so that:

Definition

The intensity of a beam of electromagnetic radiation at a point is the total energy per second flowing past that point when normalized to a unit area.

It is not necessary at this stage to understand the units of energy or exposure to allow us to apply the inverse square law; these will be dealt with in other chapters.

26.3 STATEMENT OF THE INVERSE SQUARE LAW

The intensity of the radiation emitted from a small isotropic source is inversely proportional to the square of the distance from the source, provided there is negligible absorption or scattering of the radiation by the medium through which it passes.

Note: This statement of the inverse square law also gives the conditions under which the law may be directly applied:

- *Small source* – in practice this means small compared to the distance from the source to the point of measurement.
- *Isotropic source* – this means that it emits radiation in all directions. This is necessary in order that the intensity of the radiation is independent of the *direction* from the source.
- *No absorption or scattering of radiation* – this ensures that the radiation passing through an area is not affected by the medium through which the radiation passes. It is important to remember that back scattering of the beam from objects beyond the point

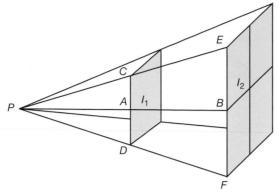

Figure 26.1 Similar-triangles proof of the inverse square law. Note that the radiation at I_2 is spread over four times the area of I_1 and so the intensity at I_2 is a quarter of the intensity at I_1.

Table 26.1 Relationships between distance and intensity

DISTANCE	AREA	INTENSITY	1/(DISTANCE)²
X	1	I_x	$1/X^2$
$2X$	4	$I_x/4$	$1/4X^2$
$3X$	9	$I_x/9$	$1/9X^2$
$4X$	16	$I_x/16$	$1/16X^2$
$5X$	25	$I_x/25$	$1/25X^2$
$10X$	100	$I_x/100$	$1/100X^2$

of measurement must also be eliminated, as this would produce an increase in the intensity.

As we will see, it is not possible to meet all of these conditions in many situations in radiography. In such cases, the law must be applied with caution or even with appropriate correction factors (e.g. absorption due to air may be important when we consider low-energy beams of X-rays).

Insight

A situation where the inverse square law does not apply is in the case of a laser beam. Because the light is essentially parallel, the intensity is constant and does not depend on distance from the source.

26.4 SIMILAR-TRIANGLES PROOF OF THE INVERSE SQUARE LAW

Consider the situation shown in Figure 26.1. The radiation is produced at a point P and is allowed to fall on the square of side CD and the square of side EF. PB is twice the length of PA. Because the triangles are similar, we can say that EF must be twice the length of CD. So the area of the square of side EF is four times the area of the square of side CD.

Remembering that the intensity is the total energy per unit time divided by the area, we can calculate that I_1 must be four times the value of I_2.

By doubling the distance between the point and the source of radiation, we can see that the intensity of the radiation is reduced to one quarter.

Stated mathematically, this is:

Equation 26.1

$$\frac{I_1}{I_2} = \frac{d_2^{\,2}}{d_1^{\,2}}$$

Using the relationship established by Equation 26.1, we can produce a table of intensities at given distances (see Table 26.1).

26.5 THE INVERSE SQUARE LAW AND THE X-RAY BEAM

If we consider the three conditions listed earlier for the inverse square law to be applied, we can see that, strictly speaking, the X-ray beam does not satisfy these conditions because:

- X-rays are not emitted from a true point source as the focal spot has a finite size
- they are not emitted equally in all directions as the anode heel effect (see Ch. 30) causes the intensity to vary across the beam
- absorption and scattering of the X-ray beam occur as it passes through air.

Because the effects are small for X-ray beams generated above 50 kVp, the inverse square law can be applied to such beams.

26.6 mAs AND THE INVERSE SQUARE LAW

In radiography, if the kVp is unaltered, the radiation output from the tube is altered by altering the mAs – if the mAs is doubled, then the output will be doubled. We can

Examples

a. The absorbed dose rate in air at a distance of 60 cm from the focal spot of an X-ray tube is $0.5\,\text{mGy.s}^{-1}$ (do not worry about the unit, as this does not affect the calculation!). What is the absorbed dose rate at 75 cm from the focus?

Using Equation 26.1 we can say that:

$$\frac{I_1}{I_2} = \frac{d_2^2}{d_1^2}$$

where $I_1 = 0.5\,\text{mGy.s}^{-1}$, $d_1 = 60\,\text{cm}$ and $d_2 = 75\,\text{cm}$. I_2 is what we need to calculate.

The equation can be rearranged thus:

$$I_2 = \frac{I_1 \times d_1^2}{d_2^2}$$

(If you are unable to follow this, look at Section A.4 on cross-multiplication in Appendix A.)

$$= \frac{0.5 \times (60)^2}{(75)^2}\,\text{mGy.s}^{-1}$$
$$= 0.32\,\text{mGy.s}^{-1}$$

The absorbed dose rate at 75 cm will be $0.32\,\text{mGy.s}^{-1}$.

b. In the above example, at what distance would the exposure rate be $26.0\,\text{mGy.s}^{-1}$?

Again, starting with Equation 26.1:

$$\frac{I_1}{I_2} = \frac{d_2^2}{d_1^2}$$

where $I_1 = 0.5\,\text{mGy.s}^{-1}$, $d = 60\,\text{cm}$ and $I_2 = 26.0\,\text{mGy.s}^{-1}$. (This time d_2 is unknown).

The equation can be arranged in terms of d_2:

$$d_2^2 = \frac{I_1 \times d_1^2}{I_2}$$
$$= \frac{0.5 \times (60)^2}{2.0}$$
$$= \frac{(60)^2}{4}$$
$$d_2 = \sqrt{\frac{(60)^2}{4}}\,\text{cm}$$
$$= 30\,\text{cm}$$

The absorbed dose rate will therefore be $26.0\,\text{mGy.s}^{-1}$ at a distance of 30 cm from the tube focus.

(*Note:* By the inverse square law, if we halve the distance, the intensity will increase by a factor of four, so the calculation is correct.)

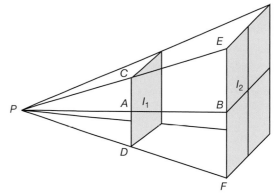

Figure 26.2 Radiographs taken at different focus to film distances. If we wish to get the same intensity of radiation on both radiographs then the mAs for *PB* must be four times the mAs required for *PA*.

see how this is affected by the inverse square law from the following discussion.

Suppose a given setting of mAs produces a satisfactory radiograph at a given focus to film distance (FFD). How will this setting of mAs have to be altered for a different value of FFD?

Consider the situation shown in Figure 26.2. If a radiograph was taken using an FFD of *PA* and the image produced was satisfactory, then this means that the image receptor has received the correct amount of radiation. If the receptor was repositioned for an FFD of *PB* and the exposure factors remained unaltered, then the amount of radiation received by the receptor would be one-quarter of the correct exposure (the distance has been doubled and so the intensity is quartered). This second radiograph would be too light or *underexposed*. In order that the receptor at *B* receives the same exposure as the original film at *A*, the amount of radiation leaving the tube must be increased by a factor of four. This means that both these radiographs would have the same *exposure index*.

From the above we can see that:

The mAs required to produce radiographs of the same exposure index at different FFDs is proportional to the FFD squared.

This can be expressed mathematically as:

Equation 26.2

$$\frac{\text{mAs}_1}{\text{mAs}_2} = \frac{\text{FFD}_1^2}{\text{FFD}_2^2}$$

It is important to form a mental picture of the difference between the straightforward measurement of the intensity of the radiation at a point where the amount of radiation leaving the source is constant (this involves applying the inverse square law) and this second case where the amount of radiation at a point is kept constant by altering the output from the X-ray tube (this involves using Equation 26.2).

193

Example

A chest radiograph was produced at an FFD of 2 m and required the following exposure factors: 65 kVp and 16 mAs. If this radiograph is repeated some time later at an FFD of 1 m at the same kVp, what mAs will be required?

Using Equation 26.2, we can say that:

$$\frac{mAs_1}{mAs_2} = \frac{FFD_1^2}{FFD_2^2}$$

where mAs = 16 mAs, FFD_1 = 2 m and FFD_2 = 1 m. mAs_2 is unknown.

The equation can be arranged in terms of mAs_2 thus:

$$mAs_2 = \frac{mAs_1 FFD_2^2}{FFD_1^2}$$

$$= \frac{16 \times (1)^2}{(2)^2} \ mAs$$

$$= 4 \ mAs$$

Note: By the inverse square law, if we halve the distance then we will have four times the intensity. If we want to have the same intensity to the film, then we need one-quarter of the original mAs. Therefore, the answer is correct.

Summary

In this chapter, you should have learnt the following:
- The definition of radiation intensity (see Sect. 26.2).
- The inverse square law and its use in calculating the intensity of radiation at a given distance from a source (see Sects 26.3–26.5).
- How the mAs given for a radiograph is influenced by the FFD used because of the inverse square law (see Sect. 26.6).

FURTHER READING

Intensity of radiation

Ball, J.L., Moore, A.D., Turner, S., 2008. Ball and Moore's essential physics for radiographers, fourth ed. Blackwell Scientific, London (Chapter 15).

Inverse square law

Ball, J.L., Moore, A.D., Turner, S., 2008. Ball and Moore's essential physics for radiographers, fourth ed. Blackwell Scientific, London (Chapter 14).

mAs and the inverse square law

Fauber, T., 2005. Radiographic imaging and exposure, second ed. Mosby, New York (Chapter 10).

Part | 5 |

Radiation dosimetry

Chapter | 27 |

Principles of radiation dosimetry

27.1 AIM

The aim of this chapter is to introduce the reader to the concepts of exposure, absorbed dose and dose equivalent. It then goes on to consider methods of absolute measurement of radiation dose and different relative methods of dose measurement.

27.2 INTRODUCTION

As we saw in Chapter 1 of this book, we live in an environment where we are continuously subjected to ionizing radiation from natural causes such as cosmic rays and naturally occurring radionuclides. In fact, about 90% of the average UK radiation dose comes from natural sources. In addition, there are artificial contributions to the radiation dose because of fallout from weapons testing, leakage from nuclear power plants, manufacture of radionuclides and medical exposure to radiation. All ionizing radiations, whether natural or artificial, constitute a hazard. It is assumed that the greater the radiation dose to which the population is exposed, the greater the hazard. The accurate measurement of radiation dose received by the population is therefore important in trying to quantify the hazard. As can be seen from Figure 1.4, medical radiation constitutes the largest single contribution of the artificial radiation exposure to the population in the UK and so it is important to minimize this radiation dose and hence the total population dose. However, the hazards associated with medical irradiation must be considered against the benefits of diagnosis and treatment. This risk–benefit concept will be discussed in Chapter 44.

27.3 UNITS OF EXPOSURE AND DOSE

When an X-ray beam passes through air, it produces excitation and ionization of the air molecules. The electrons ejected in this first interaction (e.g. during photoelectric absorption) can have sufficient energy to ionize other atoms and so produce more electrons – the delta rays. Delta rays are responsible for the great majority of ionizations, often referred to as secondary ionizations. The net effect on the air is:

- the formation of electrical charges in the air by ionization

- the absorption of energy by the air as the electrical charges are slowed down by collision with the air molecules (thus producing further ionization)
- the consequent production of heat energy because of the transfer of energy to the air molecules.

The traditional measure of exposure concerns the first of these effects only and is a measure of the amount of ionization that occurs in air. The unit of exposure is defined as:

Definition
The exposure at a particular point in a beam of X or gamma radiation is the ratio Q/m, where Q is the total electrical charge of one sign produced in a small volume of air of mass m.

The units of exposure are coulombs per kilogram ($C.kg^{-1}$) of air. It is important to remember that exposure can only be defined for air and only for X or gamma radiation.

Exposure rate ($C.kg^{-1}.s^{-1}$) is a measure of the intensity of a beam of given quality since the greater the number of photons at a given energy passing through unit area, the greater the amount of ionization of air in unit time.

In air, the proportions of ionization and heat produced by the absorption of radiation are approximately constant and therefore do not depend on the energy of the radiation. The total amount of ionization produced in air is proportional to the energy absorbed from the beam, e.g. the average energy required to produce ionization in air is about 33 eV, so an X-ray photon of energy 33 keV which is fully absorbed in air produces about 1000 primary ionizations.

The atomic number of air is 7.64, which is close to that of muscle at 7.42. For this reason, the mass absorption coefficients of air and muscle are very similar. This means that the energy absorbed from an X-ray beam by a given *mass* of air is very similar to the energy absorbed from the beam by the same *mass* of muscle. The energy absorbed by both air and muscle is thus proportional to the exposure measured in air. This is the main reason for the importance of air as a medium in radiation dosimetry as it allows the dose in tissue to be calculated from knowledge of the air exposure.

27.3.1 Exposure and air kerma

In recent years, the term 'exposure' has fallen out of common usage and has been replaced by *absorbed dose in air* or *air kerma* (the initials of kerma stand for kinetic energy released per unit mass of absorber); for instance, the maximum permissible radiation leakage rate from the X-ray tube is now quoted in air kerma. The main reason for this is that it is much easier to calculate the absorbed dose in a structure from the air kerma.

27.3.2 Absorbed dose and kerma

The measurement of the quantity of electrical *charge* produced in air by ionization is not the same as the measurement of the *energy* actually absorbed, although the two quantities are proportional to each other. The energy absorbed by unit mass of the medium is stated as the *absorbed dose* and is defined thus:

Definition
The *absorbed dose* in a medium is in the ratio E/m, where E is the energy absorbed by the medium due to a beam of ionizing radiation being directed at a small mass m.

The unit of absorbed dose is the *gray* (Gy) and so we can say that l gray = 1 joule per kilogram ($1\,Gy = 1\,J.kg^{-1}$).

Note that *exposure* is defined in terms of X and gamma radiation only, while *absorbed dose* is defined in terms of any ionizing radiation. Therefore, the absorbed dose from alpha-particles, beta-particles and neutrons are all measured in grays. However, ultraviolet radiation is only capable of excitation rather than ionization of the atoms of the medium and so is outside the scope of the definition of absorbed dose.

If all the electrons produced by the primary and secondary ionizations within a medium are stopped within it, then it can be seen that the energy *removed* from the beam of ionizing radiation is the same as the energy *absorbed* by the medium (this makes the assumption that all the fluorescent or characteristic radiation is absorbed, as is the case in body tissues). This does not necessarily apply to a very small volume within the medium – such a volume may be removing energy from the beam but the absorbed energy may be deposited *outside* the volume (but still within the body) due to the distance travelled by the electrons before coming to rest. Electrons with an energy of 1 MeV travel for about 5 mm in tissue before coming to rest.

This effect is illustrated in Figure 27.1 (See page 199). Here an incoming X-ray beam of high energy interacts with a volume element *V* within the medium. Because of the high energy of the beam, the electrons produced by Compton scatter are scattered in a forward direction, so much of their energy is absorbed outside the volume *V*. There will also be secondary ionizations resulting in the production of delta rays, but for simplicity these are not shown in the figure. In general, if the secondary electrons produced within the volume deposit a total energy E within the medium, and E_{IN} and E_{OUT} are the total energies of the electrons entering and escaping from the volume, then the absorbed dose in grays is given by:

Equation 27.1

$$\text{absorbed dose} = \frac{(E + E_{IN} - E_{OUT})}{m}$$

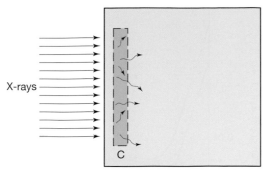

Figure 27.1 X-rays interacting with atoms in volume V produce electrons that may travel outside V.

where m is the mass of the particular small volume considered. If a larger volume is considered, then this formula can be used to calculate the average absorbed dose in that volume.

Electronic equilibrium is said to occur if $E_{IN} = E_{OUT}$, since there is no net loss or gain of the electrons over the small volume being considered. If $E_{IN} = E_{OUT}$ is a constant value not equal to zero, there is said to be *quasielectronic equilibrium*. If the intensity of the radiation is varied, the net loss or gain of electrons will vary in proportion. An example of electronic equilibrium occurs in the free-air ionization chamber, which will be discussed later in Section 27.5.2.

The absorbed dose expresses the quantity of energy absorbed in the medium due to a beam of ionizing radiation passing through it. As stated at the beginning of this section, the site of the attenuating events (e.g. photoelectric absorption) may be at some distance from the absorption process because of the distance travelled by the ejected electrons before coming to rest. The quantity which measures the amount of attenuation in a small volume is called the kerma (see Sect. 27.3.1).

Kerma is also measured in grays and may differ significantly from the absorbed dose at any particular position within the medium.

The absorbed dose and kerma along the axis of a beam of X radiation are shown in Figure 27.2. Figure 27.2A shows the case where an X-ray beam generated at 100 kVp is incident upon soft tissue: this type of situation might occur in diagnostic radiography. The electrons released in the primary and secondary ionizations are of relatively low energy and so are absorbed close to the site of the initial attenuating interactions. The kerma and absorbed dose at any particular point along the beam axis are essentially the same and the curves are coincident in the figure. This is not the case if the X-ray beam has high photon energy, since electrons produced by the initial ionization have considerable energy and so deposit their energy some distance from the point of the original attenuation process. As can be seen in Figure 27.2B, the kerma and the absorbed dose due to 4 MeV X-rays interacting with

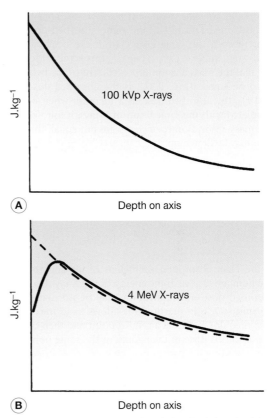

Figure 27.2 Kerma (dashed line) and absorbed dose for (A) 100 kVp diagnostic beam and (B) 4 MeV therapy beam. In (A) the two curves are coincident, but they are different in (B) because of the increased energy – and hence range – of the secondary electrons produced.

tissue are not the same. It may be easier to understand these curves if it is remembered that:

- the *kerma* is a measure of the *attenuation* – the number of photoelectric and Compton events
- the *absorbed dose* is a measure of the *energy deposited* in the medium by the primary and secondary electrons being brought to rest.

27.3.3 Effects of different media

Instruments that are used to measure absorbed dose or absorbed dose rate are called *dosimeters* and *dose-rate meters* respectively. Some of these instruments are described in more detail in later sections of this chapter (see Sect. 27.5 onwards). It is common practice to calibrate these meters to read the absorbed dose or dose rate in air through which the X- or gamma-rays are passing. Such a dosimeter may read 0.5 mGy as the total absorbed dose in air at a point within an X-ray beam. *It must not be inferred, however, that this is the absorbed dose that would be received by any other medium if placed in the same position.* For two media to receive the same absorbed dose, each must absorb the same energy from the beam per unit mass (remember, $1\,Gy = 1\,J.kg^{-1}$). This is the same as saying that the mass absorption coefficient of the two media must be equal. Thus, if D_{air} is the absorbed dose in air and D_m the absorbed dose in a medium when both are irradiated with the same beam of X-rays, it follows that if the mass absorption coefficients are not equal, this equation may by drawn up:

Equation 27.2

$$\frac{D_m}{D_{air}} = \frac{(\mu_a/\rho)_m}{(\mu_a/\rho)_{air}}$$

$$\text{or } D_m = D_{air} \times \frac{(\mu_a/\rho)_m}{(\mu_a/\rho)_{air}}$$

If the mass absorption coefficient of air and the given medium are known at the energy of the X-ray quanta, the absorbed dose in the medium may be calculated using Equation 27.2. In practice, this allows us to measure the absorbed dose in air at a certain point and then calculate the absorbed dose in the patient at the same point without subjecting the patient to a great degree of discomfort.

The mass absorption coefficients of both air and bone vary with photon energy. These variations of the two coefficients are shown in Figure 27.3A and the variations in the ratio of the two coefficients are shown in Figure 27.3B. As can be seen from the graphs, at low photon energies (50 keV is shown with the broken line in Figure 27.3A), the mass absorption coefficient of bone is considerably higher than that of air. This is because at low energies the photoelectric effect predominates ($\tau/\rho \propto Z^3/E^3$) and the atomic number of bone ($Z = 14$) is approximately double that of air ($Z = 7.64$). For this reason and because of the large difference in density, we get a high level of contrast between bone and air on a radiograph (this can be seen on the chest radiograph or on radiographs of the paranasal sinuses). At an energy of about 1 MeV, however, the two graphs are very close and the ratio of the two coefficients approaches 1. This is because of the dominance of Compton scatter in this region ($\sigma/\rho \propto$ electron density and the electron density for bone and air is approximately the same). This means that there would be a low level of contrast between the two if they were radiographed using 1-MeV photons. At above about 10 MeV the curves again diverge owing to the greater amount of pair production in bone compared to air ($\pi/\rho \propto Z$). Thus, it is clear that an instrument calibrated to read absorbed dose in air must be used with caution when calculating the absorbed dose in another medium as the relationships between the absorption coefficients vary with the photon energies. This is particularly the case in the diagnostic range of energies where absorption is principally by the photoelectric effect, which is very sensitive to both atomic number and photon energy.

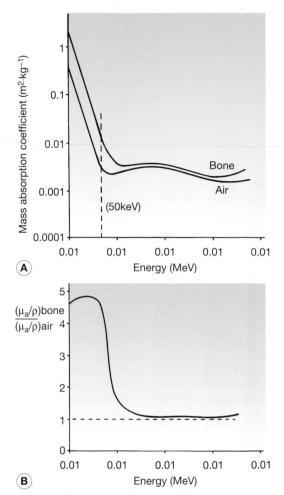

Figure 27.3 The variation of energy of (A) the mass attenuation coefficients of air and bone and (B) the ratio of the two coefficients.

27.4 QUALITY FACTOR AND DOSE EQUIVALENT

As described in the previous section, the *absorbed dose* measures the energy absorbed per unit mass of the medium when it is subjected to any type of ionizing radiation. The *biological effects* of the radiation on tissue, for instance, do not depend solely on the absorbed dose, but also on the *type of radiation* and on the *absorbed dose rate*. It is found that alpha-particles will cause considerably more damage (about 20 times as much) in a biological specimen compared to the same absorbed dose of X-rays. It is also found that radiation delivered as a single large dose will generally cause more biological damage than the same dose fractionated into multiple small doses and delivered over a period of time.

The differences in biological effects of different types of ionizing radiations are due to the different densities of ionizations they produce in a sample. Radiation which causes large numbers of ionization per unit length of track through a material will cause large amounts of biological damage. You may remember, when an atom is ionized (e.g. by a photoelectric interaction), an electron (negative ion) is released and the atom now becomes a positive ion – an ion pair has been formed. X rays and beta-particles do not produce ion pairs as close together as do the more massive protons or alpha-particles of the same energy. Protons or alpha-particles are brought to rest quickly within the medium by losing their kinetic energy in the production of many ions over a short distance – an alpha particle of energy 1 MeV will only travel 5×10^{-3} mm in tissue, protons will travel 3×10^{-2} mm and beta-particles will travel 5 mm before being brought to rest. Because of this, the larger particles break chemical bonds, which are very close together, and so the chance of repair is reduced. This means that they have a greater biological effect on the specimen. It is also found that neutrons will produce dense ionization by the ejection of protons from the nuclei or by nuclear recoil. The absorbed dose in grays is thus not an accurate measure of the biological effects of different types of radiation owing to the very different patterns of ionization produced. The unit used to measure the overall biological effects of different types of radiation is called the *unit of dose equivalent* and is measured in sieverts (Sv). The absorbed dose in grays and the dose equivalent in sieverts are related to each other, as shown in Equation 27.3:

Equation 27.3

dose equivalent (Sv) $= Q \times$ absorbed dose (Gy) $\times N$

where Q is known as the *quality factor* for the radiation and is related to the number of ion pairs produced per unit length by the radiation. N includes other factors that may affect the biological process, such as the *dose rate*. In many cases, the value of N is 1 and so the equation is frequently quoted without the factor N appearing.

Table 27.1 shows the value of the quality factor for different types of radiation. Note that Q is unity for X-rays and gamma-rays so the absorbed dose is the same as the dose equivalent for these radiations. The biological effect of particulate radiations is therefore compared to that of X-rays or gamma-rays by means of the value of Q. As can be seen from Table 27.1, electrons also have a quality factor of unity. This is because an external beam of electrons will produce secondary electrons with the same election density as X-rays and gamma-rays. However, alpha-particles have a Q of 20, indicating that the same absorbed dose will produce 20 times as much biological damage as the same absorbed dose of X-rays.

Since Q is a comparative number, the sievert has the same units as the gray (J.kg^{-1}). The quality factor may be considered a scaling factor relating the biological effect of absorbed dose to the same dose of X-rays or gamma-rays.

Table 27.1 Quality factors for different ionizing radiations

TYPE OF IONIZING RADIATION	QUALITY FACTOR
X-rays or gamma-rays	1
Electrons or beta-particles	1
Thermal neutrons	2.3
Fast neutrons (or neutrons of high energy)	10
Protons	10
Alpha-particles	20
Recoil nuclei (e.g. in alpha decay)	20
Fission fragments	20

Dose equivalent in sieverts has a vital role to play in radiation protection, where it is required to consider the sum of the effects of exposure to different types of radiation.

Insight

The dose equivalent is too crude a unit for use in radiobiology as it considers the *average* effect(s) on a group of cells. In radiobiology, we wish to look more precisely at individual effects on cells, e.g. impairment of cell reproduction. For this, we use a more precise scaling factor – the *relative biological effectiveness* (RBE). The RBE compares the absorbed doses of different ionizing radiations required to produce the same biological effect. As with the quality factor (Q), these are usually compared to the same dose of X or gamma radiation.

The remainder of this chapter is concerned with a brief overview of some of the methods used to measure exposure and absorbed doses.

27.5 ABSOLUTE MEASUREMENT OF ABSORBED DOSE

The absolute measurement of absorbed dose in air due to a beam of X-rays requires very careful techniques and very specialized equipment. It is more suited to a specialized laboratory than to a hospital or university department environment. In the UK, the National Physics Laboratory and in the USA, the National Bureau of Standards calibrates and checks specialized dosimeters under carefully controlled conditions. Such dosimeters are termed *absolute standards*. Dosimeters used in hospitals and universities are sent to such centres on a regular basis to be calibrated against the absolute standards: such dosimeters are then known as *secondary standards*. Further dosimeters are calibrated against these secondary standards. Such dosimeters are known as *substandards*. This initial section considers the manner in which an *absolute measurement* of absorbed dose may be made and the following section (Sect. 27.6) is an overview of the most common of the *relative methods* of assessing absorbed dose.

27.5.1 Calorimetry

A beam of X-rays or gamma-rays will be attenuated as it passes through a medium and the attenuation processes (see Ch. 23) will produce many ionizations within the medium. The atoms of the medium eventually absorb the kinetic energy of the electron ejected from their atoms. This results in these atoms having an increase in their kinetic energy – heat will be produced in the medium. The medium will experience a temperature rise that is proportional to the heat energy absorbed by the medium and therefore the absorbed dose. In Section 5.3.2, we have shown that:

$$Q = mc(T_2 - T_1)$$

where Q is the heat energy, m is the mass of the body, c is its specific heat capacity and $(T_2 - T_1)$ is the temperature rise experienced by the body.

We also know from the earlier sections of this chapter (see Sect. 27.3.2) that absorbed dose (D) is energy per unit mass of the medium and so:

$$D = \frac{Q}{m}$$

Thus, we can produce the equation:

Equation 27.4

$$D = c(T_2 - T_1)$$

Using the above equation, if we know the specific heat capacity of the medium, the absorbed dose may be calculated from the temperature rise produced in an irradiated medium. This is known as the calorimetric method of absorbed dose measurement. However, the temperature rise produced is very small: 1 Gy will produce a temperature rise of about $2 \times 10^{-4}\,°C$ and so the process needs very controlled conditions and is most appropriate when measuring very large absorbed doses of radiation. A more sensitive method is to collect the charge produced in an ionization chamber: this is described below.

27.5.2 The free-air ionization chamber

The free-air ionization chamber shown in Figure 27.4 uses ions produced by the absorption of an X-ray beam in air collected by oppositely charged plates situated in the air. The liberated electrons are attracted towards the positive plate and the positive ions are attracted towards the negative plate. Thus charge, whose magnitude is proportional to the exposure in coulombs per kilogram and the absorbed dose in grays, flows through the chamber. Certain precautions are necessary, however, to achieve accurate results:

- As shown in Figure 27.4 below, the central lower disc is surrounded by an annulus which is at earth potential. As Figure 27.4 is a vertical section through such a chamber, the annulus appears as if it were two separate plates. This construction enables an accurate estimation of the volume of air from which the ion pairs are collected, as it ensures that the lines of electrical force are at right angles to both the collecting

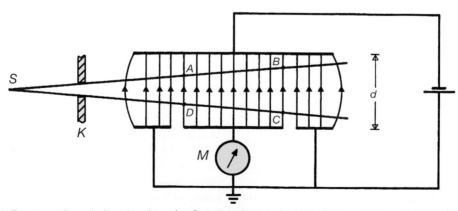

Figure 27.4 A diagrammatic vertical section through a free-air ionization chamber. *S* is the radiation source and *K* is a collimator. The electrons resulting from the ionization that takes place in the area *ABCD* are collected on the collecting plate *CD* which is connected to the meter *M*. This measure the negative charge produced as a result of the radiation.

plates. Note that this is not the case at the outer edge of the annulus, where the lines of electrical force are bowed outwards, thus including an unknown quantity of air beyond the edge of the plates. The volume of air from which the ion pairs are collected may be calculated by knowing the geometry of *ABCDI*. Ion pairs produced outside this volume are still collected by the annulus but do not pass through the meter *M* and its associated electronic amplifier and do not contribute to the current indicated by the meter.

- Some electrons produced by ionization in the region *ABCD* will escape and produce further ionizations over the annulus rather than the central disc. This suggests that the current measured by the meter, *M*, is too low, but this is not the case because on average the same number of electrons are gained by the volume under consideration. This is a case of electron equilibrium, described earlier (Sect. 27.3.2).
- The potential difference across the plates must be sufficiently high to collect all the ion pairs produced in the air. If we irradiate a free-air ionization chamber with a steady beam of radiation, the current flowing through the chamber will vary with the potential difference across the plates, as shown in Figure 27.5.
- Below the saturation voltage, some of the positive and negative ions recombine by mutual attraction (or germinal recombination) and so not all ions are collected. Above saturation voltage, the electrical field strength between the plates is large enough to ensure that all the ions move to the appropriately charged plate for collection. The actual voltage depends on the separation on the plates, but typically this is in the region of a few hundred volts.
- The separation of the plates, *d*, shown in Figure 27.4, must be sufficiently large to enable the production of all the secondary ionizations in air. No electron produced during the ionization process must reach the plates before it produces all the ion pairs of which it is capable. If *d* is too small, then the current

measured by the meter, *M*, will be too low since there are too few ion pairs produced in the air volume and hence the estimate of the exposure or absorbed dose will be too low. The required plate separation depends on the energy of the X- or gamma-ray beam, since photons with high energies will produce electrons with correspondingly high energies that will travel further in air. Typical values vary from about 20 cm for photon energies up to 250 keV to several metres for photons of energy above 1 MeV. From this it can be seen that the greater the energy of the beam, the more cumbersome the measurement, due to the necessity for greater separation of the plates.

- The total charge in coulombs measured by the free-air ionization chamber is a direct measure of the exposure in C.kg^{-1} and is proportional to the absorbed dose in grays (J.kg^{-1}). The mass of the air irradiated depends on the temperature and the pressure of air and must be corrected for the effects of these variations. If ρ_0 is the density of air at a known temperature and pressure, then the mass of the air m_0 in the irradiated volume, v can be calculated as $m_0 = \rho_0 v$ At a new temperature and pressure (T_1 and P_1), the density changes to $\rho_0 T_0 P_1 / T_1 P_0$ so the mass of the air, m', being irradiated is given by:

Equation 27.5

$$m' = m_0 \times \frac{T_0}{T_1} \times \frac{P_1}{P_0}$$

The exposure (in C.kg^{-1}) is the ratio of the total charge collected to the mass of air irradiated (m'). The absorbed dose (in grays) is calculated from the energy absorbed divided by m' – the energy absorbed can be calculated from the charge collected since it takes about 33 eV to produce one ion pair in air.

The ionization method is not suitable for use with liquids owing to the very rapid germinal recombination of the ions and the relatively high current which flows through many liquids, even when they are not being irradiated. A semiconductor (see Sect. 27.6.6) may, however, be used to collect the ion pairs produced by irradiation.

From the above it can be seen that the free-air ionization chamber is suitable for the absolute measurement of exposure and absorbed dose in air. The absorbed dose, which would have occurred in another medium, placed in the same beam of radiation may be calculated from the mass absorption coefficients, as explained earlier in Section 27.3.3.

27.5.3 Chemical methods of dose measurement

We have already established that radiation affects the chemical bonds between atoms of a material through which it passes by both ionization and excitation of electrons. Research by Fricke has shown that ionizing

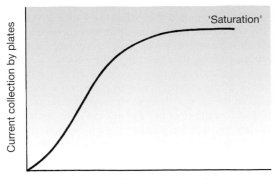

Figure 27.5 The variation of current flowing through the meter *M* in Figure 27.4 with the applied potential across the plates.

radiation is able to transform a dilute solution of ferrous sulphate, $FeSO_4$, to ferric sulphate, $Fe_2(SO_4)_3$, by rearrangement of the chemical bonds. The number of ferric ions so produced is proportional to the absorbed dose – 100 eV of absorbed dose will produce about 15 ferric ions. A chemical measurement of the concentration of the ferric ions produced at a given energy of a given radiation beam may used as a measure of the absorbed dose in water.

Such a chemical dosimeter may be calibrated against either of the two preceding methods of absorbed dose measure. It is included in this section on absolute methods of dose measurement because once the conversion factor between quantity of ferric ions is known, no further calibration is necessary. The process of calibration is similar to the calculation of absorbed dose in the free-air ionization chamber from the knowledge of the energy required to produce an ion pair in air.

The above method of dose measurement is known as the *Fricke dosimeter*, but it is only suitable for the estimation of very large doses, in excess of 20 Gy. This is because of chemical impurities present in the solution, the rapid rate of germinal recombination of the ions produced and relatively insensitive methods of chemical estimation of the quantity of ferric produced. However, it is particularly suitable for use with high-energy radiation beams and for irregular shapes of irradiated volumes The advent of conformational radiotherapy treatment and the requirement under the Ionizing Radiations (Medical Exposure) Regulations (IR(ME)R: see Ch. 44) to optimize radiation dose to the patient have resulted in the development of a number of polymer gels. These are tissue equivalent with a density of $0.99\,g.cm^{-1}$ and show a linear response to high-energy photons from 300 keV to in excess of 8 MeV. Ionizing radiation also has a polymerization effect on the gel supporting the ferrous sulphate atoms; this reduces germinal recombination and prevents migration of the ferric sulphate atoms formed outside the beam area. Magnetic resonance spectrometry is used to estimate the number of ferric sulphate atoms present. If placed (in a suitable container) in an amorphic phantom, such dosimeters may be used to confirm the steep dose gradients that are an essential feature of conformational therapy treatments.

27.6 TYPES OF DETECTORS AND DOSIMETERS

So far in this chapter we have considered the measurement of absorbed dose by *absolute* methods. These form a standard against which other types of dosimeter can be compared or calibrated. There are many such *relative* methods by which absorbed dose may be estimated, each with some advantages and disadvantages. The most common of these methods are briefly outlined in the following pages.

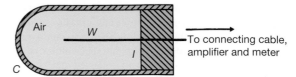

Figure 27.6 Construction of a thimble ionization chamber. *C*, cap; *I*, insulator; *W*, central wire.

27.6.1 The thimble ionization chamber

The size and configuration of the free-air ionization chamber discussed so far make it a suitable instrument for the standardization of radiation dose measurement but totally unsuitable for routine dose measurement in a hospital environment – a plate separation of 5 metres would be required if we needed to measure the dose rate at a patient's skin from a cobalt-60 source!

The thimble ionization chamber shown in Figure 27.6 circumvents some of these difficulties by, as it were, 'condensing' the air into a solid medium surrounding the central electrode. The cap of the thimble chamber is said to be *air equivalent*, i.e. it is made of a material that has the same atomic number as air (e.g. graphite, bakelite, plastic) and so its absorption properties are the same as the *same mass of air*. The central aluminium electrode has a fixed amount of positive charge put on it from an external source. When the chamber is irradiated, some of the more energetic electrons liberated in the cap will penetrate into the air of the chamber and be attracted to the central electrode. Thus, the central electrode will lose some of its positive charge. By the choice of suitable materials, the thimble chamber can be made to have the same absorbing properties as the same mass of air. Such a device is calibrated for several photon energies against a standard chamber, such as the free-air chamber described earlier in this chapter, and a correction factor is used to convert the indicated loss of charge from the central electrode to true absorbed dose. The choice of wall thickness of the cap is one of the factors that influence the applied correction, since a thin 'cap' may not produce sufficient electrons entering the chamber, while too thick a cap will absorb more radiation than it needs to. Note that the vast majority of the electrons used to measure the change in charge or the current through the chamber are produced in the wall of the chamber and not in the air cavity of the chamber, but it is the passage of such electrons into the air cavity that enables the change in charge or the current to be measured. Corrections for variations in the temperature and pressure of the air must be made, as is the case for the free-air chamber.

Thimble-type chambers are still extensively used in radiation measurements in hospitals. For example, the calibration of the radiation output from a teletherapy machine is usually accomplished by the use of a thimble chamber connected to an electronic amplification system, which measures and displays the charge produced in the chamber during irradiation. However, in order to relate the reading obtained because of a given exposure to the radiation output of the machine (usually expressed in $cGy.min^{-1}$), certain correction factors need to be applied. These include the following:

- The reading must be corrected for temperature and pressure.
- The reading must be corrected by a factor which relates the reading of this *substandard unit* to a *secondary standard unit* calibrated by a national body (e.g. the Health Protection Agency) – this correction factor depends on the energy of the radiation.
- The correction which requires to be applied to the secondary standard to compare it with the absolute standard – this is again related to the energy of the radiation and a factor to convert exposure to absorbed dose at the appropriate radiation energy.

In addition, there may be some machine-dependent correction factors, such as correction for 'switch-on' and 'switch-off' errors.

27.6.2 The Geiger–Müller counter

The thimble chamber described in the previous section is an example of an ionization chamber where the charge collected on the electrodes is proportional to the energy absorbed from the X-ray beam. The Geiger–Müller counter works on the principle of gas multiplication and gives the same magnitude of electrical pulse per absorption event whatever the energy of the absorbed radiation. The structure of a typical Geiger–Müller tube is shown in Figure 27.7A below.

The glass envelope contains an inert gas (argon) at low pressure and two electrodes – a positively charged central electrode and a negatively charged mesh cylinder. Ionization is caused in the gas by the entry of a photon or by the entry of particulate radiation (if the window is sufficiently thin to allow particles to enter the envelope). The ions are attracted to the appropriate electrode and, as they pass through the gas, they gain sufficient energy to eject electrons from the gas atoms if the potential difference between the electrodes is sufficiently great. The electrons so produced continue this process and rapid gas multiplication takes place, especially near the central electrode, since the field strength is great in this region. The effect of gas multiplication is such that well in excess of 1 million electrons are collected by the central electrode for every single ion produced in the primary absorption process. These 'electron avalanches' form the pulses, which allow the system to count the number of initial ionization events. The presence of a small quantity of alcohol vapour in the gas helps to quench the gas multiplication process so that it does not become continuous. It does this by absorbing the kinetic energy of the positive ions in the gas so that they are prevented from striking the mesh with sufficient energy to release further electrons and so keep the process going indefinitely. Alternatively, the potential difference between the electrodes may be momentarily reduced after an electron avalanche, thus terminating the gas multiplication. In either case, there is *a dead time* after each pulse, where another absorption event, if present, is not recorded. A typical dead time is $5\,\mu s$ and so the differences between the observed count rates and the real count rates are negligible except at high count rates – at an observed count rate of 1000 per second, the true count rate is 1005, whereas at an observed count rate of 100 000 per second, the true count rate is 200 000! The correct potential difference to be applied to a Geiger–Müller tube is determined in practice by plotting a graph of the count rate obtained when a small radioactive source is placed near the tube against the applied voltage. Such a graph is shown in Figure 27.7B. Three distinct regions of such a graph exist:

1. The *proportional region*, where some gas multiplication takes place and the sizes of the electrical pulses are

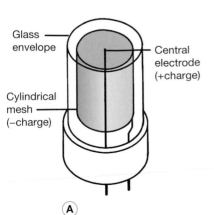

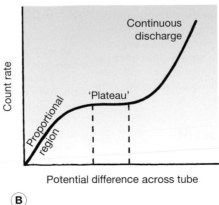

Figure 27.7 (A) Basic construction of the Geiger–Müller tube. (B) A graph of the operating characteristics of such a tube, which is operated on its plateau region.

proportional to the energy deposited in the gas by the radiation.

2. The *plateau region*, where maximum gas amplification takes place and all electrical pulses have the same size, irrespective of the energy of the radiation.

3. The *continuous-discharge region*, where the electrical field strength is sufficient to ionize the gas atoms and so produce continuous unwanted gas multiplication. The plateau is usually between 100 and 1500 V, depending on the size of the Geiger–Müller tube.

As can be seen, the Geiger–Müller tube is suitable for detecting the presence of radiation rather than for an accurate estimation of absorbed doses, since the pulses bear no relationship to the energy of the radiation causing them. For this reason it is often used as a contamination monitor for radioactive spillage or as a method of determining whether radiation is present in a specific area.

27.6.3 Scintillation detectors

The operation of a scintillation detector employing a sodium iodide crystal and a photomultiplier tube is described in Chapter 37, which considers radionuclide imaging and nuclear medicine in more detail.

Any suitable scintillating material can be used, whether solid or liquid, and the principle of operation is that the size of the electrical pulse produced by the photomultiplier is proportional to the energy deposited in the scintillator. Scintillation plastics have been produced which have an atomic number close to that of air and tissue. These can be termed as being *air equivalent* and so have similar variations of absorption to air, with variations in photon energy. They are useful in estimating absorbed dose in air. Sodium iodide has a much higher atomic number than air and will show a marked variation in absorption with photon energy, especially near its absorption edges (see Sect. 23.5). This requires correction factors to be applied for different photon energies if an accurate estimation of the absorbed dose in air is to be made. This is particularly so for thin crystals, which show a more marked variation in absorption with photon energy compared with thick crystals.

Scintillation counters are very sensitive devices and are used in many applications in radiography and radionuclide imaging, e.g. for the detection of radioactive contamination, for estimation of in-vitro radioactivity, as radiation detectors on computed tomography and osteoporosis scanners and as the detection mechanism in gamma cameras.

27.6.4 Thermoluminescent dosimetry (TLD)

The basic physics of thermoluminesce has already been described (see Sect. 24.5). Thermoluminescence may be used to estimate radiation doses by the use of lithium fluoride in the form of powder, extruded chips or impregnated Teflon discs or rods. The impurities in the lithium fluoride generate electron traps and the number of electrons which are 'stuck' in these traps is proportional to the absorbed dose in the lithium fluoride. The average atomic number of lithium fluoride is 8.2 so it is close to soft tissue ($Z = 7.5$). Both have similar absorption variations with photon energy. The small discs do not show up on radiographs and so may be strapped to the part of the body where we wish to measure the absorbed dose. After irradiation, the discs are heated and the amount of light emitted is compared to a standard dosimeter to which a known dose has been given. The dose to the disc can then be calculated by direct proportion. The discs are then annealed and may be reused.

The fact that the discs have radiolucency similar to tissue allows us to use them to estimate radiation dose without interfering with the radiograph or radiotherapy treatment. The discs are small, measuring only a few millimetres across, and so may be used to estimate the dose to different structures in the body during a diagnostic or therapeutic procedure. An additional advantage is that they can be used to monitor radiation dose ranging from 1 μGy to 1 KGy.

The role of TLD in personnel monitoring will be considered in Chapter 44.

27.6.5 Photographic film

Photographic film will produce an increase in optical density when it is irradiated and processed. The response, however, is not in linear proportion to the absorbed dose of the emulsion. A calibration graph for the particular film at known radiation doses and specific processing conditions must be produced. This is a major disadvantage if it is to be used as a method of dose estimation. It is also true that the film emulsion has a higher atomic number than tissue (AgBr has an average atomic number of 41) and so has significantly higher photoelectric absorption at low energies. For these reasons, the use of photographic film has largely been replaced by TLD dosimetry.

27.6.6 Semiconductor detectors

As we saw in Chapter 15, electrons in a semiconductor can readily have their energy raised to that of the conduction band and so can take part in electrical conduction. The absorption of energy from an X-ray photon (by either photoelectric absorption or Compton scattering) can raise an electron to the conduction band energies. This electron causes secondary electrons from the atoms of the material to be raised to the conduction band, by imparting some of its energy to them. If a potential difference is placed across the semiconductor, then these electrons are collected before they have time to recombine. Thus there is a current pulse whose magnitude is proportional to the number of electrons and hence the absorbed dose within the semiconductor. This is similar to the current through an irradiated ionization chamber and the semiconductor detector can be thought of as a solid-state ionization chamber. It has the great advantage over the air ionization chamber that it produces 10 times as many ion pairs for a given dose of radiation and so is much more sensitive to small doses. This is because only 3 eV is required to produce an ion pair in a semiconductor, compared to 33 eV to produce an ion pair in air. The electrical signal obtained from the semiconductor device is more accurate – it has a smaller statistical uncertainty – and may, for example, be used to produce very accurate gamma-ray spectra.

Semiconductor detectors may be calibrated against a thimble chamber, for example, for a given energy of radiation.

Semiconductor detectors tend to be used for more specialized forms of radiation detection, e.g. a small semiconductor detector may be inserted into the rectum to measure rectal dose.

Summary

In this chapter, you should have learnt the following:
- The definition of exposure and the relationship between exposure and absorbed dose (see Sect. 27.3).
- The definition of and the relationship between absorbed dose and kerma (see Sect. 27.2).
- The effects of different media on the absorbed dose (see Sect. 27.3.3).
- The meaning of the terms *quality factor* and *dose equivalent* and how their values vary for different types of radiation (see Sect. 27.4).
- Measurement of radiation exposure and absorbed dose by the free-air ionization chamber (see Sect. 27.5.2).
- Measurement of radiation exposure and absorbed dose by chemical dosimeters (see Sect. 27.5).
- Measurement of radiation exposure and absorbed dose by the thimble ionization chamber (see Sect. 27.6.1).
- Detection of the presence of radiation by the Geiger–Müller counter (see Sect. 27.6.2),
- Measurement of radiation exposure and absorbed dose by scintillation detectors (see Sect. 27.6.3),
- Measurement of radiation exposure and absorbed dose by thermoluminescent dosimetry (see Sect. 27.6.4).
- The use of photographic film in dosimetry (see Sect. 27.6.5).
- Measurement of radiation exposure and absorbed dose by semiconductor detectors (see Sect. 27.6.6).

FURTHER READING

Ball, J.L., Moore, A.D., Turner, S., 2008. Ball and Moore's Essential Physics for Radiographers, fourth ed. Blackwell Scientific, London (Chapter 16).

Part | 6 |

Equipment for X-ray production

Chapter | 28 |

Rectification

28.1 AIM

The aim of this chapter is to consider the various aspects of rectification as it applies to the X-ray generator. There is some initial discussion regarding the need for rectification and the ideal voltage waveform to apply to the X-ray tube, followed by a description of the rectification system in use today.

28.2 INTRODUCTION

In Chapters 10 and 14, it was seen that it is convenient to use an alternating current (AC) supply for diagnostic and therapeutic X-ray generators and linear accelerators because of the ease with which the potential can be stepped up or down. Both X-ray tubes and linear accelerators require a high potential difference across them in order to produce X-rays of the required energy. The voltage is stepped up using the high-tension transformer. However, the filament requires a potential of about 10 volts and a current of several amperes to heat it to a temperature sufficient for thermionic emission to occur, so the filament transformer (a step-down transformer) is used.

As shown in Chapters 21 and 30, the X-ray tube is designed to emit radiation when the cathode is negative and the anode is positive. The nearer the voltage across the tube is to a constant voltage, the more efficient the production of X-rays from the tube. This means that ideally we would like to change the alternating voltage supplied from the high-tension transformer to be turned into a *constant unidirectional voltage*. This process of converting an AC supply into a constant unidirectional supply, or a pulsating unidirectional supply, is called *rectification*. We will now consider different types of rectification in current use.

28.3 FOUR-DIODE FULL-WAVE RECTIFICATION

In order to utilize both halves of the AC cycle, full-wave rectification making use of four diodes arranged in a *Gratz bridge circuit* (Fig. 28.1) (see page 212) is used. Note that the diodes are arranged in two pairs and that the bar (or arrow) in the diode symbol *always* points away from the negative side of the output. D_1 and D_4 rectify one half cycle, while diodes D_2 and D_3 rectify the other half cycle. The arrows in Figure 28.1A show the direction of electron movement. It can be seen that electron movement across the X-ray tube is in the same direction in both half-cycles and that, although the potential varies, the anode never becomes negative. The circuit converts a 50-Hz AC supply into a pulsatile DC supply with 100 pulses per second.

28.4 CAPACITOR SMOOTHING

Capacitor smoothing of a pulsating unidirectional voltage has already been discussed in Section 16.11.3. This is

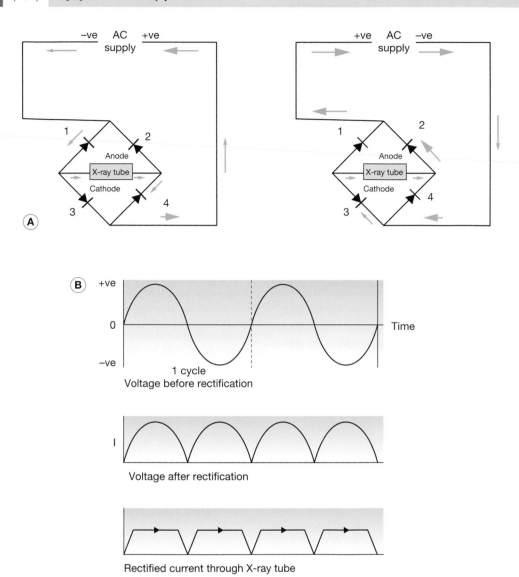

Figure 28.1 (A) Full-wave rectification circuit showing electron movement in both halves of the AC cycle (shown by the blue arrows). (B) Voltage waveforms before and after rectification and current flow through the X-ray tube after rectification.

illustrated in Figure 28.2 (see page 213). The similarities between the resultant waveform and that in Figure 13.6 should be noted.

The capacitors charge up quickly when the exposure starts but discharge more slowly through the X-ray tube. This produces a reduction in the voltage ripple across the X-ray tube. Note that the amount of smoothing depends on the capacitance of the capacitor selected and the value of mA selected. A larger capacitor will store more charge (at a given voltage) than a smaller one. If the current through the X-ray tube is large, the capacitor will discharge more quickly and its potential will fall more rapidly. The high-tension cables used to connect the high-tension transformer to the X-ray tube also possess

capacitance but it is quite small, so it only has a significant smoothing effect when the current is very small, e.g. during fluoroscopy. The result is that, although this voltage is smoother with less ripple, it is still not a constant potential. Note the amount of smoothing depends on the capacitance of the capacitor and the value of the mA selected.

Four-diode full-wave rectification (or the Gratz bridge circuit) was once the most commonly used rectification system. Today it is only used on its own in mobile X-ray units and dental and outpatient units. The Gratz bridge circuit is still found in modern generators where it forms an important part of the medium-frequency rectification system.

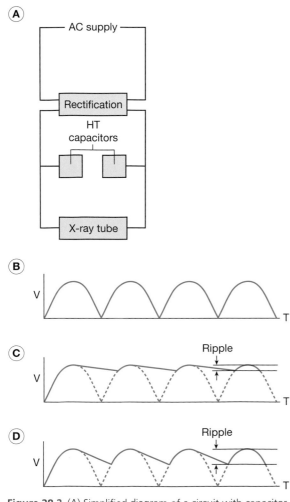

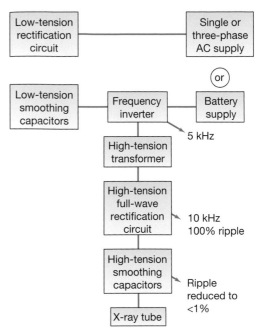

Figure 28.3 Simplified block diagram of a medium-frequency rectification circuit.

Figure 28.2 (A) Simplified diagram of a circuit with capacitor smoothing. (B) Effect of smoothing at different mA values. The shading indicates the effect of smoothing on the voltage ripple.

28.5 MEDIUM-FREQUENCY GENERATORS

The improvement of semiconductor devices in solid-state rectification has led to the development of the medium-frequency generator (see Fig. 28.3). With the exception of intraoral dental units, which use solid-state single-phase full-wave rectification, this technology has superseded the older systems and is now found in almost all X-ray generators, including battery-powered mobile units.

At this point, it is useful to clarify the term 'medium frequency'. Low-frequency systems operate at frequencies of up to 1000 Hz, medium-frequency systems operate in the range of 1000 Hz to 1 MHz while high-frequency systems operate at frequencies of 1 MHz and above.

The rectification system in these generators can be thought of as consisting of a number of subcircuits:

- The initial rectification and smoothing of incoming AC supply (if used).
- A frequency multiplication circuit.
- The high-tension transformer.
- Rectification.
- A smoothing circuit.

Note that the input supply may be from a battery, a single-phase AC or three-phase AC mains supply. If the input is from an AC supply, it is first rectified and smoothed by a large-capacitance low-tension smoothing circuit before passing to the inverter. A DC supply passes directly to the inverter.

The inverter has two functions:

1. It outputs the correct voltage to the fixed ratio high-tension transformer (HTT) to produce the required kVp.
2. It acts as a frequency multiplier, outputting a supply with a frequency of 5 KHz.

This is then rectified by a Gratz bridge rectification circuit producing a supply with a frequency of 10 KHz. This then passes through a capacitor smoothing circuit, which uses high-tension smoothing capacitors, and then passes to the X-ray tube. Because the frequency is so high, the interval while the voltage is dropping and the capacitor is discharging is very short and the ripple present after smoothing is less than 1%. The result can be regarded as an (almost) constant potential output.

These systems have additional advantages. The increased frequency results in improved transformer efficiency. This means that the high-tension transformer can be made less bulky, leading to improvements in the overall design of the unit and the possibility of using a single-tank X-ray tube.

Summary

In this chapter, you should have learnt the following:

- The reasons an AC supply is required for an X-ray generator and why this needs to be rectified before it is applied to the X-ray tube (see Sect. 28.2).
- The rectification used in a single-phase full-wave unit and the voltage waveform produced (see Sect. 28.3).
- How capacitors may be used to smooth a full-wave rectified waveform (see Sect. 28.4).
- How rectification is attained in modern generators using a medium-frequency rectification system (see Sect. 28.5).

FURTHER READING

Ball, J.L., Moore, A.D., Turner, S., 2008. Ball and Moore's Essential Physics for Radiographers, fourth ed. Blackwell Scientific, London (Chapter 13).

Curry III, T.S., Dowdey, J.E., Murry Jr., R.C., 1990. Christensen's Physics of Diagnostic Radiography, fourth ed. Lee & Febiger, London (Chapter 3).

Dowsett, D.J., Kenny, P.A., Johnston, R.E., 1998. The Physics of Diagnostic Imaging. Chapman & Hall Medical, London (Chapter 4).

Thompson, M.A., Hattaway, R.T., Hall, J.D., Dowd, S.B., 1994. Principles of Imaging Science and Protection. W B Saunders, London (Chapter 7).

Chapter | 29 |

Exposure and timing circuits

29.1 AIM

The aim of this chapter is to examine the principles involved in switching the X-ray exposure on and off. It will also consider the physics involved in timing the X-ray exposure.

29.2 PREPARATION FOR EXPOSURE

Before the X-ray tube can deliver an exposure for a predetermined time interval, it must first be prepared for exposure. This is done during the 'prep' stage of the exposure sequence and during this time two major things happen:

1. The appropriate filament of the X-ray tube is raised to its working temperature so that it emits the required number of electrons by thermionic emission (see Sect. 30.7.1) to allow the correct tube current (mA) to flow during the exposure.
2. The anode is made to rotate at the required speed prior to the exposure being made.

If an exposure is made before these processes are completed, there is a risk that the incorrect mA will be delivered or that the target of the anode may be subjected to localized overheating, resulting in damage to the anode. In Sections 13.5 and 13.6, it was shown that selection of a suitable resistance would determine the time taken to charge or discharge a capacitor. This principle is used to provide a delay function prior to the X-ray exposure.

Initiating the prepare sequence causes a switch to open, 'shorting' the capacitor to remove any residual charge present. Current flows in the stator circuits and the anode commences to rotate. The switch then closes, which permits a direct current (DC) supply to charge the capacitor through the resistor. When the capacitor is charged, it operates an electronic switch in the exposure circuits, permitting the exposure to commence.

There are two circuit sections responsible for the actual exposure:

1. The switching section.
2. The timing section.

29.3 THE SWITCHING SECTION

The function of the switching section is to connect the high voltage (kVp) to the X-ray tube during the exposure and to disconnect this supply from the tube at the end of the exposure. Such switching commonly occurs between the autotransformer and the high-tension transformer, where it is known as *primary switching*, or between the high-tension transformer and the X-ray tube, where it is known as *secondary switching*.

29.3.1 Primary switching

All modern X-ray units make use of solid-state switching. This type of switching has the advantage that there are no moving parts, overcoming the problems experienced with earlier mechanical systems. A simple circuit containing a solid-state switching system is shown in Figure 29.1. Silicon-controlled rectifiers (SCRs), a type of thyristor, are used for this purpose. Two thyristors (connected in inverse parallel) are required to switch an alternating current (AC) as each conducts the half-cycle when that SCR is forward biased. At the end of each half-cycle, each SCR will cease to conduct as the potential difference across it drops to zero and so a voltage pulse must be applied to its gate if it is required to conduct during the next half-cycle.

As an alternative to the SCR, a triac may be used. This device acts as two SCRs connected in inverse parallel and, if pulsed with an alternating supply, will conduct in both phases of the AC cycle. Like the SCR, the device will only conduct when the voltage is not at zero volts and the device has been pulsed.

During the exposure, the timer is simply required to apply a sequence of synchronized pulses to the gate of the device at a time slightly later than the mains zero to switch them back on and ensure their continued conduction. At the end of the exposure, these pulses stop and conduction through the device stops at the end of the next half-cycle. The system allows accuracy of one voltage pulse (i.e. an exposure time of 0.01 second in the case of a two-pulse unit, or 0.002 seconds in the case of a medium-frequency unit; see Ch. 28).

29.3.2 Secondary switching

Solid-state devices such as SCRs cannot withstand the very high voltages present in the high-tension circuit, therefore high-tension valves must be used. In the past, special triode valves were used; modern generators make use of a grid-controlled X-ray tube.

As will be seen in Chapter 30, X-rays are produced when electrons flow from the cathode to the anode of the X-ray tube. These electrons are normally focused onto the target of the tube by a focusing cup, which is at a negative potential approximately equal to that of the filament. If a separate additional negative bias is applied to the focusing cup, then it is possible to make it more negative than

the filament. X-ray tubes offering this facility are known as grid-controlled tubes.

If the focusing cup is made about 3 kV more negative than the filament, it will produce a sufficiently large electrostatic field to prevent any electrons from crossing the X-ray tube; this additional negative potential is termed *grid bias*. At the start of the exposure, this bias is removed, electrons may cross from the cathode to the anode and X-radiation is produced. At the end of the exposure, the high negative bias is re-established on the focusing cup, stopping electron flow. The grid-controlled tube acts as an electronic exposure switch as well as a producer of X-rays.

Secondary switching is also used in capacitor discharge units to control the passage of the charge from the capacitor through the X-ray tube during the exposure time. It was also used in cineradiography and pulsed fluoroscopy, where the system is capable of giving up to 500 exposures per second. In such cases, the switch shown in Figure 29.1 does not exist as the X-ray tube will act as the high-tension switch.

Insight

A similar form of grid-controlled switching is used in a number of dental units. In such units, the current through the tube is switched off when the voltage falls below a certain percentage of the peak kV. The principles of the process are shown in Figure 29.2.

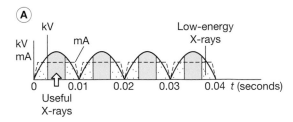

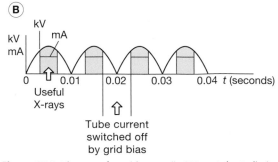

Figure 29.2 The use of a grid-controlled X-ray tube to limit patient dose. (A) Low-energy X-rays are produced which contribute to patient dose but do not contribute to the image. (B) By applying the necessary bias to the cathode, current is prevented from flowing when the tube voltage is below a predetermined limit, preventing production of much of the low-energy radiation.

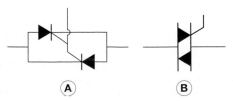

Figure 29.1 Simplified diagram of primary switching using (A) two silicon-controlled rectifiers and (B) a triac.

As we can see from Figure 29.2A, in a conventional X-ray unit, X-rays are produced during each of the voltage pulses but only the X-rays produced at the centre of each voltage pulse (near the peak kV) are of diagnostic value. X-rays produced when the tube voltage is significantly lower than the peak kV have very low photon energies and so will be absorbed by the patient and contribute nothing to the diagnostic image. Preventing production of these low-energy X-rays, we can limit the patient radiation dose and also help to prolong the life of the X-ray tube. This is achieved by applying a strong negative bias to the focusing cup if the tube voltage is below a certain value: no current will flow through the tube and no X-rays are produced. This is shown in Figure 29.2B.

29.4 THE TIMING SECTION

The function of the timing section is to ensure that the appropriate signals are passed to the switching section to allow X-ray production to be switched on and off at the appropriate times. As we can see from Figure 29.3, the resistance is variable; thus, the time taken to charge to a predetermined potential across its plates is determined by the value of the resistance. When this trigger voltage is achieved, a signal is sent to the switching system which terminates the X-ray exposure by stopping current flow through the X-ray tube. If we consider the situation for thyristor switching (see Sect. 29.3.1), then it can be seen

that the exposure can be terminated by simply removing the triggering voltage pulses from the gates of the thyristors. Thus, at the end of the next half-cycle, the thyristors will cease to conduct and the exposure will terminate.

29.4.1 Time-based timers

If the circuit is arranged in such a way that the capacitor receives charge from a fixed single source (e.g. a rectified supply from the autotransformer), then the time it takes to charge the capacitor will be influenced only by the value of resistance selected by the operator. This is the basis of a time-based timer, i.e. a timer where the operator manually selects the exposure time (along with the kVp and the mA). The X-ray output at a given value of kVp is a function of the tube current (mA) and the exposure time (see Ch. 22). As the time-based timer only controls the exposure time, it cannot compensate for any fluctuations in the tube current that would influence the X-ray output from the tube. This problem is overcome by the mAs timer, which will be discussed in the next section.

29.4.2 The mAs timer

A simplified diagram to show the operating principles of an mAs timer is shown in Figure 29.4. Note that on this occasion the capacitor is charged from two sources, V_1 and V_2. V_1 is a stable source of voltage (e.g. a rectified supply from the autotransformer). The amount of charge which the capacitor receives from V_1 is controlled by the variable resistor, R. This supply is connected to the capacitor (C) when the switch moves from position B to position A at the start of the exposure. V_2 is a rectified supply from the midpoint of the high-tension transformer, so that the amount of charge from this source is directly related to the amount of charge passing through the X-ray tube (the mAs). This supply is again switched on with the exposure.

The time taken to charge the capacitor is related to the tube current. A high tube current will result in a short charging time and a low current a longer charging time.

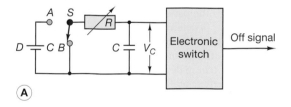

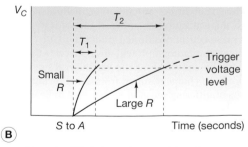

Figure 29.3 Simplified circuit diagram (A) and output graph (B) for a capacitor-controlled timer. Note that when the switch (S) is in position A, the timer is switched off and the capacitor is 'shorted', ensuring it cannot retain any electrical charge. To switch on, the switch should be moved to position B. This will allow the capacitor (C) to receive charge through the variable resistor (R).

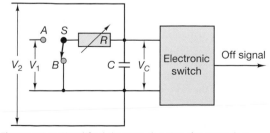

Figure 29.4 Simplified diagram showing the operating principles of an mAs timer. When the timer is switched on, the capacitor (C) receives charge from V_1 and V_2. For further explanation of the operating principles, see text.

217

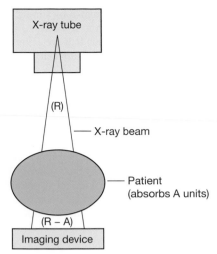

Figure 29.5 Diagram showing the X-ray absorption involved in image production. If R units of radiation leave the X-ray tube and the patient absorbs A units, then $(R - A)$ units of radiation will reach the imaging device.

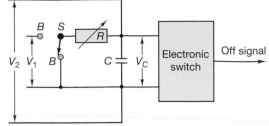

Figure 29.6 Simplified diagram to show the operating principles of an autotimer. When the timer is switched on, the switch (S) is in position B and so the capacitor (C) receives charge from two sources – V_1, a stable voltage supply, and V_2, from an ionization chamber.

When the capacitor is fully charged, an electronic switch terminates the pulses to the exposure switching circuit. The X-ray exposure is then terminated.

These timers can be used on all generators including those where the mAs changes during the exposure such as capacitor discharge and falling load generators.

The mAs timer is manually controlled, with the fundamental problem that the exposure selected depends on the skill and judgement of the operator, who needs to estimate the amount of radiation that will be absorbed by the patient. Ideally the exposure should only deliver sufficient radiation to produce an acceptable image on the image receptor, with the minimum radiation dose to the patient. The principles of this process are shown in Figure 29.5. If R units of radiation leave the X-ray tube and A units are absorbed by the patient, then $(R - A)$ units will strike the imaging device. Thus, ensuring the correct exposure to the film depends on the operator's skill in judging how much radiation the patient will absorb and selecting the duration of the exposure accordingly.

We will now consider automatic timers, which measure the amount of radiation to a small sample of the recording device and terminate the exposure when this radiation has reached a predetermined value. The operator has control of the kV selected, but has no direct control over the *duration* of the exposure.

29.4.3 Automatic timers

There are two basic types of automatic timer. The first, the ionization timer, controls the *duration* of the exposure but permits the operator to select the kV used.

29.4.3.1 Ionization timers

The ionization timer makes use of the fact that X radiation will cause ionization in air. A radiolucent chamber is placed between the patient and the image recording device and as radiation passes though this chamber it ionizes the air within it. The ionized air molecules are attracted to the electrodes in the chamber by a potential difference between them, and as a result, a small electrical current directly proportional to the amount of X radiation flows between the electrodes. This small current is then amplified and used to charge the capacitor (Fig. 29.6). The amount of charge which the capacitor receives from V_1 is controlled by the variable resistor, R. V_2 is an amplified supply from an ionization chamber (or photocell) which can measure the amount of radiation that has passed through the patient. Assuming that the amount of charge from V_1 is determined by the position of the variable resistor, then the remainder of the charge required to raise the potential of the capacitor to the trigger voltage of the switching device must be from the source V_2. As this is directly related to the amount of radiation passing through the patient to the imaging device, this will be constant irrespective of the amount of radiation absorbed by the patient. The timer, in this case, terminates the exposure when the correct amount of radiation has passed through the ionization chamber. If the ionization chamber or photocell is positioned under the correct part of the patient, the radiograph will always receive the correct exposure. The resistance of the variable resistor controls the amount of charge required from V_2, allowing imaging receptors of differing sensitivities (speeds) to be used.

With the ionization timer, although the timer controls the duration of the exposure, the operator has control over the selection of the exposure variables such as the kV, focus used, the image recording medium and, with some units, the mA used.

29.4.3.2 Anatomically programmed timers

With anatomically programmed timers, the operator selects the exposure by body part and projection from

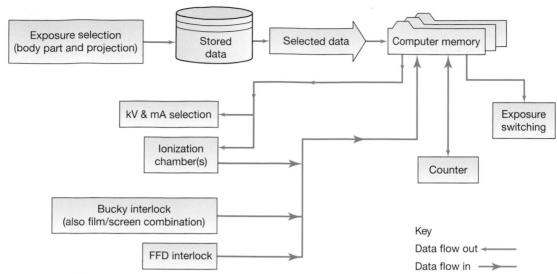

Figure 29.7 Simplified diagram showing the principles of an anatomically programmed timer. FFD, focus to film distance.

a number of preinstalled options. These options will determine the kV, mA, type of image recording medium, focus to film distance and the ionization chamber to be used to detect the radiation that has passed through the patient.

This range of exposures, which is stored in the memory of a microprocessor, is programmed into the X-ray unit by the manufacturer of the X-ray generator. On installation of the unit, a senior operator programs the final selection of exposure factors for each permitted exposure in the range into the computer memory, which is then 'locked' to prevent unauthorized access. A simplified diagram of this type of timer is shown in Figure 29.7. Full details of its operation are beyond the scope of this text.

On exposure, interlocks are used to check that the X-ray tube is at the correct focus to film distance and the recording medium is in place. The radiation detection device is then selected and exposure commences. When sufficient radiation has passed through the detector, the microprocessor terminates the exposure through the exposure switching circuit.

Since the radiation dose received by the patient and the amount of scattered radiation produced are dependent on the quality and amount of radiation delivered during the exposure, this type of timer ensures that the optimum quantity of radiation delivered and kV are used for each exposure, minimizing both the dose to the patient and the amount of scattered radiation produced.

Autotimers are usually used in conjunction with a guard timer. This is a preset time-based timer (see Sect.

29.4.1) which will terminate the X-ray exposure of the autotimer and isolate the generator from the mains supply. The guard timer must be reset by a service engineer before the generator can be reused.

Summary

In this chapter, you should have learnt the following:
- The role of the circuits which prepare the X-ray unit for exposure (see Sect. 29.2).
- The role of the switching section in the X-ray generator (see Sect. 29.3).
- The function and operation of primary exposure switching (see Sect. 29.3.1).
- The function and operation of secondary exposure switching using a grid-controlled X-ray tube (see Sect. 29.3.2).
- The principles of the timing section of the X-ray generator (see Sect. 29.4).
- The principles and mode of operation of time-based timers (see Sect. 29.4.1).
- The principles and mode of operation of the mAs-based timer (see Sect. 29.4.2).
- The principles and mode of operation of autotimers utilizing ionization chambers (see Sect. 29.4.3.1).
- The principles and an outline of the operation of the anatomically programmed timer (see Sect. 29.4.3.2).

FURTHER READING

Carter, P.H., 1994. Chesney's Equipment for Student Operators, fourth ed. Blackwell, London (Chapter 4).

Curry III, T.S., Downey J.E., Murry Jr., R.C., 1990. Christensen's Physics of Diagnostic Radiography, fourth ed. Lee & Febiger, London (Chapter 2).

Webb, S. (Ed.), 2000. The Physics of Medical Imaging, second ed. Institute of Physics, Bristol.

Chapter | 30 |

The diagnostic X-ray tube

30.1 AIM

The aim of this chapter is to discuss the factors involved in the construction of diagnostic X-ray tubes.

30.2 INTRODUCTION

The rotating anode X-ray tube is the most common type of X-ray tube found in diagnostic imaging departments. The reason for this is that it is able to produce higher intensities of X-rays than the stationary anode tube. This is due to two factors:

1. The heat deposited in the anode during an X-ray exposure is spread over a larger area and so there is a smaller temperature rise at the anode surface.
2. The cooling characteristics of the rotating anode are superior to those of the stationary anode and this effective dissipation of heat means that larger loads can be applied without causing thermal damage to the target.

The stationary anode tube has a very low rating (see Ch. 31) and is only found in dental and some portable X-ray units. These units are connected to a 13-amperes mains supply. This limits the amount of electrical power that can be applied to it, preventing overloading of the tube.

30.3 CONSTRUCTION OF X-RAY TUBES

The X-ray tube consists of two main components: the *insert*, which is mounted inside the *tube shield*.

These components and the light-beam diaphragm (we will discuss its role later in this chapter) are shown in Figure 30.1 (see page 222). The components of this tube are discussed individually in Section 30.5. Although the

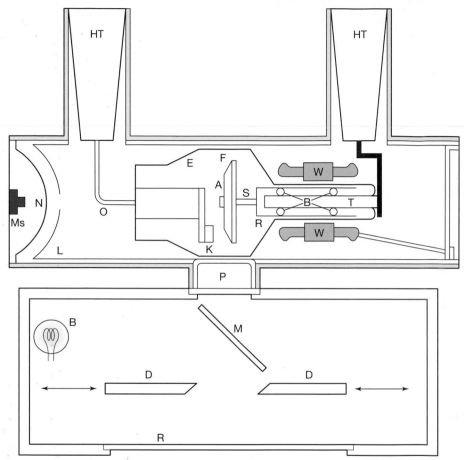

Figure 30.1 Simplified diagram of a rotating anode X-ray tube and diaphragm assembly. A, anode disc; B, light bulb; Br, bearings; D, moveable diaphragms (only one pair shown); E, glass envelope; F, focal track; HT, high-tension socket; K, cathode assembly; L, lead lining; M, mirror; Ms, microswitch; N, bellows; R, rotor assembly; S, anode stem; T, rotor support; O, oil; P, tube port and aluminium filter; R, plastic diaphragm front; W, stator windings.

inserts for the rotating anode tube and the stationary anode tube differ substantially, the shields for both types of tube are very similar in design and function.

30.4 CONSTRUCTION OF THE TUBE SHIELD (HOUSING)

It is necessary to protect the patient and the radiographer from the electrical and radiation hazards posed by the X-ray tube insert while in operation. The insert is incorporated within a suitable container – the shield – which must satisfy the following criteria:

- There must be no danger of electrical shock if the shield is touched during operation of the X-ray tube.
- No significant amounts of radiation should escape from the shield other than the radiation necessary for taking the radiograph.

- The shield must give secure support to the X-ray tube insert, the high-tension cables and the connecting cables within the shield.
- Adequate insulation must be provided between the insert and the tube shield to avoid electrical breakdown.
- There must be adequate cooling of the insert and facilities to allow expansion of the cooling oil.
- There must be facilities at the tube port to allow adequate filtration of the emergent beam so that low-energy radiations may be removed from the beam.

As can be seen from this list, the shield must satisfy many requirements. A schematic diagram of the shield for a rotating anode X-ray tube is shown in Figure 30.1. Note that the insert is held in position by a support at the anode end.

The metal casing surrounding the insert is made of either aluminium or steel and is lined with about 3 mm of lead to provide sufficient radiation protection. This housing is filled with pure oil that acts as an electrical insulator and as a coolant. A neoprene diaphragm at one end of the shield allows for expansion of the oil when the oil is heated. The assembly is usually fitted with a micro-switch, which will prevent further exposures if the oil is very hot. Within the casing there is a radiolucent window – the tube port – which will allow the useful beam of radiation to leave the tube via the light-beam diaphragm.

30.4.1 Electrical safety

Electrical safety is designed around four basic principles:

1. Insulation of live components.
2. Earthling of component housings.
3. Restricted access to live components.
4. Isolation of the circuits from the mains supply when not in use.

All of the above are utilized in the design of the X-ray tube. Insulation exists between the live components and the housing in the form of the oil in the housing. The resistance of an insulator (and so its insulating properties) diminishes as the temperature of the insulator increases and so the role of the oil in heat dissipation is also important from the point of view of electrical safety.

The tube shield is connected to earth via the outer braiding of the high-tension cables (Fig. 30.2) and so the casing will always remain at earth potential. If a live wire within the casing becomes disconnected and touches the shield, then the current will readily flow to earth and the casing will present minimal electrical hazard to someone touching it at the time.

The live components in the X-ray tube are secured inside the tube shield and the ends and the high-tension cable connectors are securely fixed. This means that, under normal circumstances, the operator has no easy access to the live components. In addition, the circuits may be isolated from the mains by switches, fuses or circuit breakers.

30.4.2 Radiation safety

Radiation safety is important for the operators of X-ray equipment and for patients and others who may be in the vicinity at the time of making an X-ray exposure. The lead lining of the tube housing (Fig. 30.1) limits the radiation leakage from the tube and so provides protection to both the operator and the patient. It should be borne in mind that X-rays are emitted *in all directions* from the focus on the anode, but only those which pass through the tube port are allowed to leave the housing. The anode itself has a high absorption and so the lead lining at the anode end of the shield is often absent or thinner than at the cathode end.

The radiation leakage rate from the tube is normally measured at a distance of 1 metre from the housing and should not exceed an air kerma of 1.00 milligray per

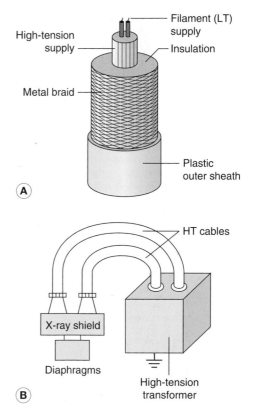

Figure 30.2 (A) Structure of a high-tension cable. Note the thickness of the insulation surrounding the central conductors. LT, low tension. (B) The X-ray tube shield is made electrically safe by connecting the copper braiding of the high-tension (HT) cables to both the shield and the casing of the high-tension transformer tank. The latter is securely earthed.

hour, measured at a distance of 1 metre from the focus (for definitions of the kerma and the gray, see Ch. 27). Any break in the lead lining will result in radiation leakage from the tube, so the leakage levels should be checked at regular intervals as part of the quality checks on the X-ray unit.

Radiation safety means exposing the patient only to the minimum dose necessary to produce a radiograph of acceptable quality. As we saw in Chapter 21, the spectrum of X-rays produced at the target is a continuous spectrum containing a mix of low-, medium- and high-energy photons. Some of the photons have very low energy and will not be able to pass through the patient to reach the image receptor. These photons would contribute to the patient dose but not to the image production. Some of these are removed by the glass envelope of the insert and the oil as the beam passes to the tube port. This is known as the *inherent filtration* of the tube. Further filtration takes place through the aluminium filters placed at the tube port (Fig. 30.1). These are known as *added filtration*. Thus, the *total filtration* of the beam is determined by the *inherent filtration* plus the *added filtration*. Details of this information are frequently marked on the end of the shield.

Scattered radiation contributes to the patient dose and the operator dose and causes degradation in the radiographic image quality. As we have seen in Chapter 23, the amount of scatter produced at a given set of exposure factors is dependent on the volume of tissue irradiated. The volume can be reduced by reducing the area irradiated using a *light-beam diaphragm* (Fig. 30.1). This also means that parts of the body not required on the radiograph can be protected from radiation. In this way, adequate collimation using a light-beam diaphragm (or cones) will reduce the patient dose and the operator dose and produce an improvement in the image quality.

30.5 CONSTRUCTION OF THE ROTATING ANODE TUBE INSERT

30.5.1 Insert envelope

X-ray production is at its most efficient when a vacuum exists between the cathode and the anode of the X-ray tube, so these structures are enclosed within an evacuated metal or heatproof glass envelope, which must be sufficiently strong to preserve this vacuum. Where glass envelope is used, it is joined to the anode spindle at one end and to the nickel cathode support at the other end by *re-entrant seals* – so called because the glass is shaped to point inwards at the area of contact. Slightly different glass seals are used at each end so that the thermal expansion of the glass is similar to that of the metal used in the construction of the anode spindle and cathode. This reduces the stress on the glass when the insert is hot and so limits the chance of cracking. The glass must be a good electrical insulator or a substantial current will flow through it when the high potential difference is applied between the anode and the cathode. However, electrical charges are built up on the inside of the glass during operation and so the glass must have sufficient electrical conductivity to allow these to leak away, usually between exposures, avoiding the build up of high amounts of static charge. The glass is gently rounded so that there are no sharp corners, which would allow the build up of high amounts of static charge (see Ch. 6).

During operation of the X-ray tube, a thin film of tungsten will be deposited on the inside of the envelope as a result of the release of tungsten vapour from the filament and the target. This film acts as a filter to emergent radiation, and where a glass envelope is used, may eventually cause electrical breakdown within the tube as it can act as an electrical conductor around the inside wall of the glass envelope. If this happens, the tube is classed as 'gassy' and is of no further use. The rate of tungsten vaporization can be reduced by not keeping the tube in the 'prep' mode

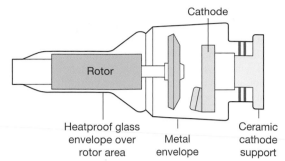

Figure 30.3 Simplified diagram of an X-ray insert with a metal envelope.

(see Sect. 29.2) any longer than is required and by keeping exposures well within the rating of the tube (see Ch. 31).

As shown in Figure 30.3, metal envelopes do not completely surround the insert. The cathode end of the envelope is formed from a ceramic material to provide the necessary electrical insulation between the anode and the cathode. The metal component of the envelope is earthed and, as a result, there is no build up of static charges on the metal envelope. This improves the focusing of the electron beam within the insert and reduces the effect of the build up of vaporized tungsten on the inner walls of the envelope.

30.5.2 The anode assembly

The simplest anode configuration is shown in Figure 30.1 where the anode consists of a disc with an accurately bevelled edge on which is deposited a target track. A number of different materials are used in the design of the anode disc, as shown in Table 30.1 (See page 225). A small amount of rhenium, which has an atomic number and melting point similar to that of tungsten, is alloyed with the tungsten of the target track. This improves the thermal expansion of the target track, making it more resistant to pitting. Tungsten is used as the main component in the target track for the following reasons:

- Tungsten has a high atomic number ($Z = 74$) and so is an efficient producer of X-rays (see Ch. 21).
- Tungsten has a high melting point ($3387\,^\circ$C), so it can withstand the heat generated during the X-ray exposure without melting.
- Tungsten has a low vapour pressure so it does not readily vaporize at its normal working temperature.
- Tungsten can be readily machined to give the smooth surface required for X-ray production.

The bevelled edge permits the use of the *line focus principle*. This results in an effective focus that is smaller than the real focus. The real focus can be longer than the effective focus. Thus, the filament may be relatively long without giving rise to excessive geometric unsharpness. Thermionic emission from the filament is proportional

Table 30.1 Materials used in the design of the modern rotating anode disc

MATERIAL	USE	REASON FOR USE
Molybdenum	Disc	Half the density and twice the specific heat capacity of tungsten
Tungsten	Focal track (90%)	High atomic number. High melting point. Low vapour pressure. Suitable mechanical properties
Rhenium	Focal track (10%)	More elastic than tungsten, therefore less pitting of the focal track
Graphite	Disc backing	Low density. Acts as 'heat sink'. Radiates heat by black-body radiation

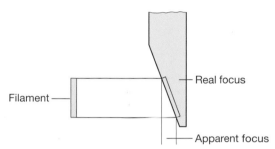

Figure 30.4 The line focus principle. Due to the angulation of the anode, apparent focus is much smaller than the real focus.

to its surface area and so a long filament will provide the high values of mA required by many exposures. The area over which the heat is deposited is the larger area of the real focus as shown in Figure 30.4. This is smaller than the apparent focus. The advantage of the line focus principle is that the temperature rise experienced by a large area for a given amount of heat is less than that experienced by a small area, since more atoms are able to take part in the heat dissipation processes. The line focus principle enables the anode to be designed so that the area of the real focus is about three times the area of the apparent focus. This enables a reasonable compromise between the need to minimize the temperature rise at the target (thus requiring a large focal area) and the need for minimizing the geometric unsharpness (thus requiring a small focal area). The anode face is usually set at an angle between 7° and 15° to the central axis of the X-ray beam. This is called the *target angle.*

The disc has a central hole in it through which it is connected to a molybdenum anode stem and hence to the rotor of the induction motor (see Fig. 30.1). The rotor, stem and anode disc are accurately balanced so that no appreciable wobble occurs when the whole assembly rotates. The rotor is made to spin by the 'rotating' magnetic fields produced by the stator coils situated externally to the insert, using a similar process to the alternating current (AC) induction motor described in Chapter 12. The rotor moves smoothly on steel ball bearings coated in a

soft metal, such as tin or silver, which acts as a lubricant but does not destroy the vacuum inside the envelope; a lubricant such as oil would evaporate and compromise the vacuum. The rotating magnetic field produced by the stator coils causes the rotor (and thus the anode disc) to rotate at the same frequency as the applied voltage.

The rotation of the anode during the exposure has the effect of elongating the area bombarded by the electron beam in a lateral direction, reducing the amount of heat generated per unit area even further. The positive terminal from the high-tension supply is connected to the rotor support, and through this there is a continuous electrical connection to the anode disc.

The conduction of heat from the anode disc to the ball bearings is inhibited by the fact that the anode stem has a small cross-sectional area (see Sect. 5.4.1) and is made of molybdenum (a relatively poor thermal conductor). However, some heat will inevitably reach the ball bearings and could cause sufficient expansion to produce a risk of seizure. This risk is reduced by applying a black coating to the outer surface of the rotor so that it loses heat efficiently by black-body radiation (see Sect. 5.4.4).

Many modern X-ray tubes also have graphite backing on the anode disc. This has a greater thermal capacity than molybdenum and draws heat from the anode and then dissipates it by black-body radiation. This results in the possibility of greater loads being applied to the anode and in reduced heat dissipation to the ball bearings.

30.5.3 The anode heel effect

Consider Figure 30.5 (See page 226). X-rays are produced slightly below the surface of the target material. X-rays passing along path 1 will therefore pass through a smaller section of the target than those passing along path 2. There is absorption of the X-rays as they pass through the target and so the rays that pass through the greatest thickness of target are the more heavily absorbed – there will be a lower intensity of X-rays along path 2 than along path 1. This means that the X-ray intensity at the anode end of the beam will be less than at the central axis, while the intensity at the cathode end will be greater than at the central axis. This is known as the *anode heel effect.* The

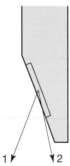

Figure 30.5 The anode heel effect. Ray 2 is more attenuated than ray 1, owing to its longer path through the tungsten target

effect increases as the target angle is reduced and increases with the age of the X-ray tube. This latter increase is caused by the fact that the target becomes pitted with use.

30.5.4 The cathode assembly

The terms *cathode* and *filament* are often interchanged when discussing the X-ray tube. However, the correct usage of the term 'cathode' implies the whole cathode assembly, including the filament, focusing cup, supporting wires and cathode support. The filament is therefore part of the cathode but the cathode is not part of the filament.

The focusing cup, which supports the filaments, is off-set from the central axis of the tube so that the electrons emitted from the filaments are aligned with the bevelled edge of the anode disc. It is made of either nickel or stainless steel, each of which has a high melting point and is a relatively poor thermionic emitter – each has a high thermionic work function. In addition, the thermal expansion of these materials is close to that of certain types of glass, thus reducing the stress on the seals during operation of the tube. When the filaments produce electrons by thermionic emission, these would repel each other by electrostatic repulsion – 'like' charges repel – and so would strike a large area of focal spot. The area of the focal spot is reduced by the negative bias on the focusing cup which 'squeezes' the electrons together.

The filaments are made of a thin tungsten wire for the following reasons:

• Tungsten has a low thermionic work function and so will readily emit electrons by thermionic emission.
• Tungsten has a low vapour pressure and so does not easily evaporate. This helps prolong the life of the filament, as evaporation would cause the wire to become thin. It also prolongs the life of the tube as it prevents the formation of a tungsten film on the inner wall of the glass envelope.
• Tungsten is a strong metal that can be drawn into a thin wire that will not easily distort. This helps to maintain the shape of the filament helix over a period of time.

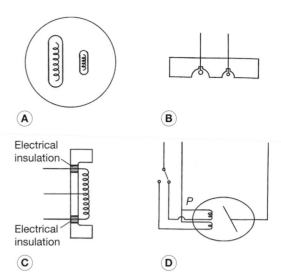

Figure 30.6 Details of cathode filament assemblies. (A) Face-on view of dual filaments; (B) dual filaments viewed from above; (C) in-line filaments viewed from the side; (D) electrical connections.

A rotating anode X-ray tube usually has two filaments. They may be positioned side by side, as shown in Figure 30.6. This is known as a dual-focus tube. Alternatively they may be positioned end to end, which means that the electron beams fall on different parts of the bevelled surface of the anode disc, which can be set at differing angles. This in-line configuration with different anode angles is referred to as a *biangular tube*. In both instances, the differing sizes of filament result in differing sizes of electron foci on the anode. The larger is known as the *broad* focus and would be used in situations where a high radiation output was required from the tube, while the smaller – the *fine* focus – would be used in situations where it is desirable to keep geometric unsharpness to a minimum. One side of each filament is connected to the focusing cup while the other is insulated from it (Fig. 30.6C). This connection between both filaments also forms the common connection between the filament circuit and the high-tension circuit. This is represented by point P in Figure 30.6D. From this diagram, it can be seen that three conductors are required in the high-tension cable coming to the cathode end of the X-ray tube. The secondary side of the filament transformer is also connected to one side of the high-tension circuit and this transformer could be a source of electrical hazard to the operator of the X-ray unit. For this reason and for reasons of ensuring good electrical insulation and heat dissipation, the filament transformer is contained in the same oil-filled tank as the high-tension transformer. All high-tension cables for X-ray units contain at least three conducting wires, even though only one is required at the anode end of the tube. This means that manufacturers only need to make (and X-ray departments only need to stock) one type of cable.

Only one of the three wires at the anode end is used to make an electrical connection to the tube.

30.6 CONSTRUCTION OF THE STATIONARY ANODE TUBE INSERT

30.6.1 The anode

The anode of the stationary anode tube, like the rotating anode, is constructed of two materials, copper and tungsten, and so is known as a *compound anode*. The main part of the anode assembly is made of copper because of its good thermal conductivity. The face of the anode is inclined at an angle of about 15° to the central axis of the insert and has an inset of a thin (about 2–3 mm) tungsten plate known as the *target* on which the electrons are focused.

30.6.2 Cathode and filament

The basic construction of the cathode is the same as that of the cathode of a rotating anode tube. The main differences in construction are that the focusing cup is aligned along the central axis of the insert and there is only a single filament present.

30.7 PRINCIPLES OF OPERATION OF THE X-RAY TUBE

As we have seen in Chapter 21, X-rays are produced by electrons which are accelerated from the cathode to the anode of the X-ray tube. The number of electrons crossing the tube is controlled at the mA selector while the kinetic energy of the electrons – and thus the photon energy of the X-ray beam – is indicated by the kV selector.

30.7.1 Thermionic emission

The electrons are emitted by the heated filament by a process termed thermionic emission. In atoms, the outer shell electrons are more loosely bound than the inner electrons because they are further away from the nucleus (remember $F \propto 1/d^2$). The application of heat to a body increases the kinetic energy of its atoms and so increases the violence of their collisions. Because of these collisions, the outer electrons may be dislodged from the atom. Electrons so released near the centre of a body travel only a relatively short distance, but if they are released near the surface of the material, they may have sufficient kinetic energy to leave the body.

The higher the temperature of a body, the greater the kinetic energy of the atoms, and the greater number of electrons with sufficient energy to break free from the influence of the surface atoms of the body. We have also stated that the electrons, which are released by thermionic emission, are released from the surface atomic layers of the body. It follows that any alteration to these outer layers will alter the ability of a body to perform as a thermionic emitter. This has two practical consequences in radiography:

1. All the surfaces involved in thermionic emission (e.g. the tube filament) must be manufactured to a high degree of purity and must be kept scrupulously clean during assembly.
2. The thermionic emission characteristics of a body may be altered by the deliberate addition of 'impurities' either to the whole body or just to the body surface.

The efficiency of thermionic emitters may be compared by comparing their work function, which is normally expressed in electron volts (eV). The work function is the amount of work that must be performed by an electron in escaping from the body. Alternatively, it can be considered as the amount of work that must be performed on an electron to enable it to escape from the body. Substances which are good thermionic emitters have a lower work function than those that are poor thermionic emitters since, in the former, less work is required to allow the electrons to escape.

From the above discussion, it should be apparent that the amount of thermionic emission from a body is controlled by:

- the temperature of the body
- the material of the body
- the surface area of the body.

The relationship between the temperature of a tungsten filament and the number of electrons liberated in unit time is shown in Figure 30.7.

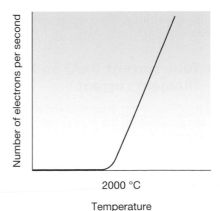

Figure 30.7 Graph of thermionic emission against temperature for a tungsten filament. Note that a small change in temperature produces a large change in emission.

30.7.2 The space charge effect

If we assume that a body is electrically neutral before the application of heat, then each electron which leaves the body by thermionic emission will cause the body to have a net positive charge. After a very short time, a state of equilibrium is set up where electrons leave the body and enter a 'cloud' of electrons near its surface and are then attracted back to the body, i.e. electrons are attracted back to the body as fast as they are emitted. The number of electrons in this cloud remains fairly constant since electrons are entering and leaving the cloud at equal rates. This cloud of electrons is known as the *space charge*. If the temperature of the body is increased, then the number of electrons in the space charge will also increase due to the increased electron emission from the body. If the body is left to cool, it will reduce the space charge to zero by attracting electrons from it back to the body.

Insight
If we take a normal tungsten filament light bulb and switch it on, then the filament of this bulb is producing significant numbers of electrons by thermionic emission. These electrons form a space charge around the filament and return to it in the process described above. If we bring a large positive charge close to this light bulb, we can cause these electrons to 'flash over' to this positively charged body. If we switch off the power supply to the bulb, the filament cools down almost immediately, thermionic emission ceases and no further flash over occurs until the bulb is switched on again.

If a positively charged body is placed close to the space charge, then some of the electrons within the space charge will be attracted towards that body and so an electrical current flows between the heated body and the positive body via the space charge. This property is explored further in Section 30.7.3.

30.7.3 Tube current (mA) and filament current

Figure 30.8 shows a circuit diagram of the X-ray tube and high-tension circuit which has been greatly simplified to illustrate the difference between the tube current (mA) and the filament current (I_f). The relationship between the temperature of the tungsten filament and the number of electrons released by thermionic emission has already been discussed in Section 30.7.2. This section will look at the application of this information to the X-ray tube. In Figure 30.8, B_1 represents the power supply across the X-ray tube and B_2 represents the power supply across the filament. Suppose B_2 causes a current I_f to flow through the

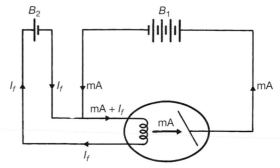

Figure 30.8 Simplified diagram to show the difference between tube current (mA) and filament heating current (I_f).

Table 30.2 Filament heating currents for different tube currents for a typical X-ray tube

FILAMENT HEATING CURRENT (A)	TUBE CURRENT (mA)
5	200
7.5	400
9	800

filament circuit. The passage of this current through the filament causes the filament to heat and the subsequent temperature rise will cause electrons to be emitted by thermionic emission. These electrons are drawn towards the positive anode and constitute the tube current (mA). When all the electrons in the space charge are 'in use', it is said to be operating under saturation conditions. This is the normal operating condition of the X-ray tube. The only method of increasing the tube current is to increase the number of electrons in the space charge by increasing the temperature of the filament, causing more electrons to be released. Thus, the selection of a given mA by the radiographer determines the filament heating current required to produce that mA. A typical set of filament currents for an X-ray tube is shown in Table 30.2.

30.7.4 Electron focusing

During X-ray exposure, the anode of the X-ray tube is positively charged and the cathode is negatively charged. As a result of this, the electron space charge emitted from the filament is repelled from the negative cathode and attracted to the positive anode. The situation, which would arise if both the cathode and the anode were flat plates, is shown in Figure 30.9A (see page 229). The electric force field (see Ch. 6) consists of parallel lines starting at the anode and finishing at the cathode. Electrons are emitted from the filament, *F*, and are attracted to the

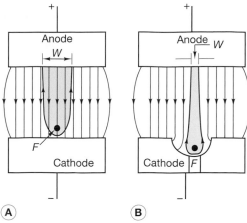

Figure 30.9 Simplified explanation of the focusing of electrons in the X-ray tube. (A) The result of no focusing cup on the cathode; (B) the electrostatic charge around the concave focusing cup directs the electrons from the thermionic emitter, *F*, towards the central axis so they strike a smaller area, *W*, on the anode.

positive anode. However, the electrons repel each other, so the beam of electrons will increase in size as it travels across the X-ray tube. The area, *W*, on the anode represents an unacceptably large focal area as this would produce a large geometric unsharpness on the resultant radiograph. This problem is overcome by the use of a focusing cup (see Sect. 30.5.4), as shown in Figure 30.9B. The thermionic electrons from *F* now experience two forces – one towards the anode and the other towards the central axis of the beam. The force towards the central axis of the beam is greater than the force of electrostatic repulsion between the electrons and so the beam of electrons is focused onto a small area of the anode – *W* in Figure 30.9B. The interactions between the electron beam and the anode are discussed in more detail in Chapter 21.

30.7.5 Tube voltage (kVp)

The kVp selected by the radiographer controls the peak potential difference across the X-ray tube. The higher the kVp, the higher the peak potential difference and so the greater the force of attraction between the anode and the cathode. Because of this, the electrons will strike the anode with greater kinetic energies and so will produce more energetic X-ray photons. This was discussed in more detail in Chapter 21 when we considered X-ray production in detail. In this chapter, we will finish with a brief synopsis of the process so that the construction of various parts of the X-ray tube may be more clearly understood.

30.7.6 X-ray production

In the X-ray tube, electrons are produced at the cathode by thermionic emission. These electrons are then accelerated

towards the anode and are made to give up their energy when they collide with the atoms of the target material. The main mechanism of X-ray production is when the electron is made to lose kinetic energy because of the pull of the positive nucleus of the target atoms. This is known as *Bremsstrahlung radiation*. The intensity (*I*) of the Bremsstrahlung radiation varies with both the energy (*E*) of the electrons striking the target and with the atomic number (*Z*) of the target material, as shown in the equations below:

Equation 30.1

$$I \propto Z \times E^2$$

or

Equation 30.2

$$I \propto Z \times kVp^2$$

The process of X-ray production is very inefficient and up to 99% of the energy of the electrons may be converted into heat, which must rapidly be transferred from the focal area to avoid damage to the target of the tube (see Sect. 5.7.2).

30.8 MODERN TRENDS IN X-RAY TUBE DESIGN

There are a number of modern trends in the design of specialist X-ray tubes that are not within the scope of this text. The reader should consult either more specialist texts on tube design or manufacturers' literature. Specialist designs include:

- the metal/ceramic X-ray tube insert
- grid-biased X-ray tubes
- high-speed anode X-ray tubes
- stress-relieved anodes in rotating anode X-ray tubes
- X-ray tubes which allow automatic measurement of anode temperature
- alteration of the shape of the anode disc to allow improved loading (e.g. discus-shaped discs).

Summary

In this chapter, you should have learnt the following:
- The reasons why the stationary anode X-ray tube is of limited use in the modern X-ray tube and why it has been replaced by the rotating anode X-ray tube (see Sect. 30.2).
- The fact that X-ray tubes consist of two major components – the insert and the shield (see Sect. 30.3).
- The construction of the X-ray tube shield (see Sect. 30.3).

(Continued)

- The methods of ensuring the electrical safety of the X-ray tube shield (see Sect 30.4.1).
- The method of ensuring the radiation safety of the X-ray tube shield (see Sect 30.4.2).
- The construction of the rotating anode (see Sect 30.5).
- The construction of the anode assembly of the rotating anode X-ray tube (see Sect. 30.5.2).
- The reason for and the result of the anode heel effect (see Sect. 30.5.3).
- The construction of the cathode assembly of the rotating X-ray anode tube (see Sect. 30.5.4).
- The construction of the stationary anode X-ray tube (see Sect. 30.6).

- The construction of the cathode and filaments of the stationary X-ray tube (see Sect 30.6.1).
- The principles of operation of the X-ray tube (see Sect 30.7).
- The interrelationships between the X-ray tube current and the filament heating current (see Sect. 30.7.3).
- The requirement for and the method of achieving focusing of the electron beam across the X-ray tube (see Sect. 30.7.4).
- The effect of tube voltage on the emergent X-ray beam (see Sect. 30.7.5).
- A basic description of X-ray production (see Sect. 30.7.6).

FURTHER READING

You will find further information on the rating of X-ray tubes in Chapter 31 of this text and more information on the factors affecting the X-ray spectrum in Chapter 21. In addition, you may find that sections from the following texts provide useful further reading.

Ball, J.L., Moore, A.D., Turner, S., 2008. Ball and Moore's Essential Physics for Radiographers, fourth ed. Blackwell Scientific, London (Chapter 4).

Bushong, S.C., 2004. Radiological Science for Technologists: physics, Biology and Protection, eighth ed.. Mosby, New York (Chapter 10).

Curry III, T.S., Downey Jr, J.E., Murry, R.C., 1990. Christensen's Physics of Diagnostic Radiography, fourth ed.. Lee & Febiger, London (Chapter 2).

Dowsett, D.J., Kenny, P.A., Johnston, R.E., 1998. The Physics of Diagnostic Imaging. Chapman & Hall Medical, London (Chapter 3).

Webb, S. (Ed.), 2000. The Physics of Medical Imaging, second ed. Institute of Physics, Bristol (Chapter 2).

Chapter | **31** |

Monitoring and protection of X-ray tubes

31.1 AIM

The aim of this chapter is to enable the reader to understand the concept of the rating of X-ray tubes and why it is monitored. The chapter will discuss factors which affect tube rating and the effects of single and multiple exposures on rating of the X-ray tube. An example of how a microprocessor is used to monitor these effects and prevent damage to the X-ray tube is illustrated.

31.2 DEFINITION OF RATING

The general term *rating* is used to describe the practical limits that are inherent in any device. An example of this is that a fuse rated at 5 amperes will tolerate currents up to 5 amperes. If a current above 5 amperes passes through the fuse, then the fuse will melt, causing a break in the circuit. A high-tension transformer is a more complicated device than a fuse and so has a more complicated set of rating conditions (see Sect. 14.9). Similarly, the rating of an

X-ray unit – the X-ray tube and the associated equipment – depends both on how it is constructed and how it is being used. The rating may be defined as follows:

> **Definition**
>
> The *rating* of an X-ray unit is the combination of exposure settings which the unit can withstand without incurring unacceptable damage.

All radiographic exposures cause slight wear and tear on the X-ray tube, the anode becomes more slightly pitted and the filament becomes slightly thinner as a result of any exposure. However, in this context, 'unacceptable damage' means damage that would seriously impair the performance of the unit for further exposures or might indeed make it inoperative. In this context, a single short exposure where the mA was above the rating of the tube might damage the anode by melting the focal track. Alternatively, a long exposure at low mA may again damage the anode if the total amount of heat generated in the anode caused a sufficient temperature rise to melt the tungsten. It is also true that multiple exposures, each of which is individually within the tube rating, might damage the tube because of the total heat accumulated in the anode by the exposure series. As the anode takes a finite time to cool after an exposure, the closer the exposures follow each other, the more likely the anode is to suffer thermal damage. For this reason, the rating for single and multiple exposures will be considered separately in this chapter.

31.3 SINGLE EXPOSURES

The rating for a single exposure is affected by a number of different factors; some of these are under the control of the operator while others are not, as shown in Table 31.1 (see page 232).

In any particular unit, the non-selectable factors are fixed, so a rating must be used which is applicable to that set of circumstances, e.g. a rating appropriate to an X-ray tube connected to a two-pulse unit. The rating can be plotted as a graph showing the effect on the rating of varying the quantities in the selectable group. A simplified form of such a graph is shown in Figure 31.1. Here the rating curve corresponds to a 1.2-mm focus selection and a kVp selection of 80 kVp. The curve indicates the upper limit for all combinations of mA and time for this value of kVp. The points below the line are safe, whereas points above the line are unsafe because they would result in unacceptable damage to the X-ray tube. If we consider an exposure of 80 kVp, 100 mA and 0.2 seconds, then we can see that this exposure may be safely made, as the point *P* is below the 80-kVp line. Note that because of the wide range of exposure times possible, it is usual to use a logarithmic scale on the *x*-axis.

It can also be seen from the graph that higher values of mA will be tolerated for short exposure times – 150 mA at a time of 0.1 second is within the rating – whereas, at long exposure times, only lower values of mA are within the rating – for an exposure time of 2 seconds, the maximum mA permissible within the rating is 50 mA. In each case, the limiting factor is the anode temperature. For longer exposure times, there can be significant cooling of the anode during the exposure. This is shown by the flattening-off of the curve at longer exposure times.

In clinical practice, a range of kVp values is applied to the X-ray tube. Rating calculations take this and the focus size into account, producing separate rating graphs for broad and fine focus. Examples of such graphs are shown in Figure 31.2. Figure 31.2A in the chart is for the broad focus and part B is for the fine focus. As can be seen from these graphs, the rating of the tube is lower for the fine focus than for the broad focus. This is because for a fine focus, the electron beam is concentrated onto a smaller area, thus producing a higher temperature rise for the same value of mA.

The figure also shows that larger values of mA are permitted as the kVp is reduced; the difference between the curves is most marked for the shorter exposure times. As was discussed in Chapter 30, electrons are produced at the filament of the X-ray tube and are accelerated towards the anode. The higher the kVp across the tube, the more kinetic energy each electron possesses when it interacts with the anode target. Thus, the same number of electrons per second (mA) will deliver more energy per second to the target and so will increase the possibility of thermal damage. The graph shows this inverse relationship between the kVp and the mA.

Table 31.1 Factors affecting the rating of a particular X-ray tube

SELECTABLE FACTORS	FIXED FACTORS
kVp mA	Rectification type Rating of high-tension transformers
Exposure duration	capacity of anode
Focal spot size	Diameter of anode
Operating mode – fluoroscopy or radiography	Speed of anode rotation Anode angle Thermal capacity of tube shield Efficiency of heat loss from anode and tube shield

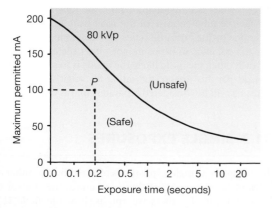

Figure 31.1 Graph of rating at a single kVp.

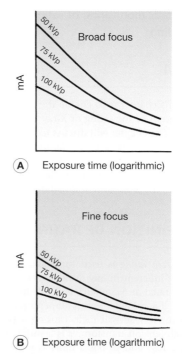

Figure 31.2 Graphs showing the effect of tube focus on rating.

Consider a situation where for a given exposure time (t), the anode may be given a total energy E without causing thermal damage. The energy of a single electron crossing the X-ray tube is proportional to the kVp across the tube. The total number of electrons is related to the current (mA) and the exposure time (t).

$$\therefore E \propto \text{kVp} \times \text{mA} \times t$$

Thus, for a given exposure time, halving the kVp should double the permissible mA.

Finally, the effect of different types of rectification when using the same X-ray tube needs to be considered. (see Figure 31.3) illustrates this effect for four different types of rectification, where the same focal spot and the same kVp have been selected. As can be seen from the graphs, the self-rectified circuit has the poorest rating, while the constant potential (or medium-frequency) circuit has the best rating. Also, note that the differences in rating are most marked at short exposure times. This is because the heating effect of individual pulses is most apparent in this situation. The more constant the heat production, the less the likelihood of thermal damage to the target – hence the best rating for constant potential.

For longer exposure times, the thermal capacity (see Sect. 5.3.2) of the anode disc is the dominating factor. This is independent of the type of rectification and so the curves all tend to come closer together as the exposure time increases. Also, note that for longer exposure times the cooling of the tube shield and the heat dissipation within the high-tension transformer are significant factors in determining the rating of the tube and X-ray unit.

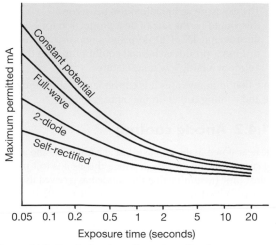

Figure 31.3 Graph showing effect of rectification system on rating.

31.3.1 Rating of stationary anode and rotating anode X-ray tubes

In the stationary anode X-ray tube, the process of conduction loses heat from the target through the copper anode and thence to the oil surrounding the insert in tube shield. The process is limited by the melting point of copper (1083°C) and the rate at which conduction occurs. As a result, the rating of stationary anode X-ray tubes is much lower than that of rotating anode X-ray tubes. Such X-ray tubes have a very limited application. In the rotating anode X-ray tube, heat loss by conduction is discouraged by the design of the anode stem (see Sect. 30.5.2) and the main method of heat loss from the anode is by radiation. Efficient heat loss by radiation is achieved by designing the anode disc so that it can tolerate high temperature rises (remember that the rate of heat loss by radiation is proportional to the fourth power of the kelvin temperature). During large exposures, the anode disc often becomes incandescent and at such temperatures can lose heat effectively by radiation, hence the higher rating of the rotating anode tube.

31.3.2 Effects of anode diameter and speed of rotation on tube rating

When we consider the rating of the rotating anode tube, we must consider not only the material used in its construction and its mass but also the effects of the anode diameter and the rate of anode rotation. In the rotating anode tube, the electrons land on the focal track around the bevelled circumference of the disc. This means that the heat is deposited around the whole disc instead of in the same area, as in the case of the stationary anode tube. Because this heat energy is now deposited over a larger area, there is a smaller temperature rise per unit area and rating is improved.

If we increase the anode diameter, we may increase its mass but this change also increases its circumference. This means that the heat energy is now deposited over a larger area and, as more atoms are involved in cooling, this leads to more efficient cooling, improving the rating. Doubling the diameter of the disc will increase its rating by 40–50%, but this has practical limitations because of the extra mechanical stress this imposes on the bearings. A simplified graph showing the improvement in rating is shown in Figure 31.4A (see page 234). If we double the speed of rotation of the anode, this means that only half the heat energy is deposited onto the anode for each rotation, although it makes twice as many rotations during a given exposure time. If there were no cooling between successive heating of the same point, there would be no advantage of increasing the rotational speed. The effect of increased anode rotation on the tube rating is shown in Figure 31.4B. Doubling the speed of rotation will again increase the rating by about 40–50%.

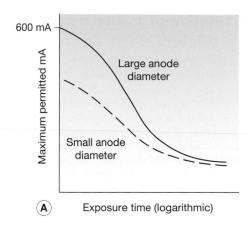

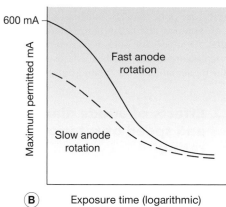

Figure 31.4 Graphs showing effect of (A) anode diameter and (B) speed of anode rotation on rating.

31.4 MULTIPLE EXPOSURES

When single exposures are made, there is a comparatively long interval between exposures. If a series of exposures is made, there may be insufficient time for the anode disc to cool between exposures. While every single exposure in this series may be within the rating of the tube, the heating effect of subsequent exposures could raise the temperature of the anode above the permitted level, resulting in thermal damage to the focal track. In such cases, it is necessary to consider additional factors to be able to predict the safety of any combination of exposures.

31.4.1 Anode heating

The anode disc has a given mass and thermal capacity and so there is a given quantity of heat which will raise the whole anode disc to its maximum desirable operating temperature. This is known as the *heat storage capacity* of the anode and is expressed in kilojoules – in the example shown in Figure 31.5, this is 80 000 kilojoules.

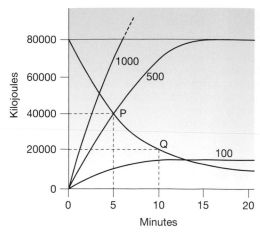

Figure 31.5 Graph showing anode heating and cooling curves.

For long exposures such as during fluoroscopy, the cooling, which occurs during the exposure, becomes important in calculating tube ratings. The anode initially heats up fairly quickly but then tends towards a thermal equilibrium, which occurs when the rate of heat generated in the anode by the electron beam is exactly balanced by the rate of heat loss from the anode. Examples of anode heating curves for a particular tube are shown in Figure 31.5, where the number of kilojoules stored by the anode at any moment is plotted against time. The maximum heat storage capacity of this anode is 80 000 kilojoules. Three different exposure rates are shown:

1. The rate of 1000 kilojoules per second fairly rapidly exceeds the heat storage capacity of the anode and further exposure beyond this time would result in thermal damage.
2. The rate of 500 kilojoules per second establishes thermal equilibrium at the maximum heat storage capacity of the anode.
3. The exposure at 100 kilojoules per second – this would be the rate of heat production for a fluoroscopic kV of 100 kVp and a fluoroscopic current of 1 mA – produces thermal equilibrium with the anode at a fairly low temperature.

Note that in many cases it is convenient to show the heating and cooling curves on the same graphs.

31.4.2 Anode cooling

The heat stored in the anode is lost at a finite rate and a cooling curve showing the rate at which this heat is lost plotted against time (assuming that the anode has received its maximum permitted number of kilojoules at $t = 0$) is shown in Figure 31.5. Suppose an exposure of 40 000 kilojoules is made: the point P shows this in the figure. The anode loses heat, as given by the curve below P, such that 5 minutes later, at point Q, only 20 000 kilojoules remains stored in the anode. An example of the use of such a graph is given below.

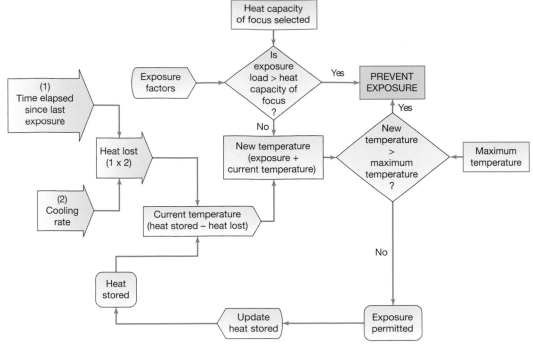

Figure 31.6 Flow chart showing computer monitoring of X-ray tube rating.

Example

An exposure of 60 000 kilojoules is made on the X-ray tube for which Figure 31.5 is the cooling curve. The exposure requires to be repeated as soon as possible. How long must we wait between exposures to ensure that the anode does not exceed its maximum heat storage capacity?

Heat produced by the exposure = 60 000 kilojoules.

The maximum heat storage capacity of the anode is 80 000 kilojoules and so it must cool down till it stores only 20 000 kilojoules before the exposure is repeated. By consulting the graph, it can be seen that this takes approximately 7 minutes.

In the cases discussed so far using cooling curves, it is assumed that no significant cooling of the anode takes place during the exposure. If this is not the case, e.g. during fluoroscopy, then anode heating curves are applied, as described above.

31.5 AUTOMATIC MONITORING OF RATING

With older X-ray generators, it was necessary to use manufacturers' rating charts to ensure that exposures, particularly multiple exposures, were within the rating for the generator. This was a complex, error-prone process. Modern units are fitted with devices such as thermistors (temperature-sensitive resistors) and photo diodes, which can be used to measure the temperature of the oil in the housing and of the anode disc. The electrical output from these is then passed to a microprocessor; this can then calculate whether the proposed exposure is within the rating of the tube. The microprocessor takes into account not only the heat generated by the exposure but also any heat already stored by the anode disc, and includes this in the calculation. This process is shown in flow chart form in Figure 31.6. Using stored data, the first stage checks that the individual exposure is within the permitted loading for the selected focus. The second stage checks that the exposure will not exceed the maximum rating for the X-ray tube. The heat lost between last exposure and current exposure is calculated and subtracted from the current temperature of the X-ray tube. The resultant figure is added to the heat generated by the exposure and this is then compared against the thermal capacity of the X-ray tube. If either of these tests results in an 'overload' condition, the computer activates an interlock, which will prevent the exposure until 'safe' conditions exist.

Summary

In this chapter, you should have learnt the following:
- The definition of rating when applied to the X-ray tube and its associated equipment (see Sect. 31.2).
- The factors affecting single exposures (see Sect. 31.3).
- A comparison of the rating of stationary anode and rotating anode X-ray tubes (see Sect. 31.3.1).
- The effects of the anode diameter and the speed of rotation on the rating of the rotating anode tube (see Sect. 31.3.2).
- Additional factors which affect rating for multiple exposures (see Sect. 31.4).
- Automatic monitoring of rating (see Sect. 31.5).

FURTHER READING

Dowsett, D.J., Kenny, P.A., Johnston, R.E., 1998. The Physics of Diagnostic Imaging. Chapman & Hall Medical, London (Chapter 3).

Johns, H.E., Cunningham, J.R., 1983. The Physics of Radiology. Charles C Thomas, Illinois (Chapter 2).

Chapter | 32 |

Orthovoltage generators and linear accelerators

32.1 AIM

The aim of this chapter is to review the main differences between diagnostic X-ray generators and the orthovolvoltage generator. It will also present an overview of the linear accelerator.

32.2 INTRODUCTION

X-rays at energies of up to 300 kV have been used to treat benign and malignant conditions since the early twentieth century. Historically this has been in two categories:

1. Superficial therapy using energies of up to 150 kV with beam filtration of 1–8-mm aluminium equivalent material at a focus to skin distance (FSD) of 10–30 cm.
2. Orthovoltage or 'deep' therapy with energies of 150–500 kV with 0.5–3-mm copper filtration at a 50-cm FSD.

Superficial units are rarely found in clinical use today, as many of the conditions they were used to treat are no longer common and other more efficient methods of treatment have been developed, many of which do not use ionizing radiation. These units are unable to deliver sufficient dose to areas of significant separation; they produce a high surface dose and a significant amount of scattered radiation is produced outside the beam as a result of Compton scatter. Orthovoltage units, with their increased higher energies and filtration, deliver less surface dose. Although the beam still produces large amounts of Compton scatter, the differential absorption of radiation by tissues of higher atomic number, such as bone, makes orthovoltage treatment suitable for use on patients with metastatic bone deposits and some primary bone lesions.

32.3 THE ORTHOVOLTAGE UNIT

There are a number of similarities and differences between these units and the general diagnostic unit. The orthovoltage unit uses a stationary anode X-ray tube, unlike the rotating anode used in diagnostic radiography. The circuit of a high voltage generator is similar to that of modern microprocessor-controlled medium-frequency diagnostic generators (see Ch. 28). However, the control panel differs in that a number of distinct stages must be followed in sequence before exposure can be initiated; these include the ability to select the additional filtration used – this automatically sets the kV and mA available. The radiographer must then select the dose to be delivered and the exposure time. This determines the setting of the back-up timer, which will terminate the exposure if the elapsed time exceeds the set time by 10%. Other differences are the beam filtration and the way in which the beam is collimated.

32.3.1 The X-ray tube

Unlike the rotating anode design found in diagnostic units, the orthovoltage unit uses a hooded stationary anode (see Fig. 32.1). This is likely to have an insert with a metal–ceramic envelope, which overcomes the common cause of tube failure, which in these units is usually the breakdown of the glass envelope around the insert. As can be seen, the target is surrounded by shielding apart from two ports: the first is in line with the electron beam from the cathode, and the second, covered by a beryllium window, is at 90° to this axis and in line with the tube exit port. This permits the beam of useful radiation to leave the anode and tube. The hood serves two functions: i) it absorbs secondary electrons produced by electron interaction with the target; and ii) it attenuates unwanted radiation, reducing the thickness of the lead required in the tube housing, thus reducing weight of the tube assembly. Note that the anode, which loses heat through conduction to the oil surrounding the insert, has, in addition to a large cross-sectional area, channels in it through which oil is circulated, thus improving the cooling process.

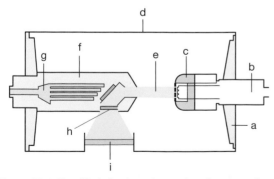

Figure 32.1 Simplified diagram of an orthovoltage metal–ceramic X-ray tube insert. a, ceramic insulate support; b, cathode assembly; c, cathode block and filament; d, metal envelope; e, electron/radiation beam; f, hooded anode; g, oil coolant channels in anode; h, beryllium window; i, insert exit port.

32.3.2 Beam filtration

As with diagnostic X-ray tubes, the orthovoltage tube has both the inherent filtration that attenuates the beam due to the components of the tube and additional filtration produced by filters placed in the beam path after it has left the tube. In diagnostic units, the filtration, which serves to 'harden' the beam by removing low-energy radiation from the beam, is in the form of a thickness of an aluminium-equivalent material. With the orthovoltage tube, this filtration can be changed to suit the energy spectrum used to treat the patient. At lower energies, the filters are usually of a single material – aluminium, copper or tin. At higher energies, a composite filter such as the Thoraeus filter, made of tin, copper and aluminium, is used. With these composite filters, it is important that the material of the higher atomic number is placed near the tube port. The function of the lower atomic number material is to remove the characteristic radiation produced by the filter material of higher atomic number.

32.3.3 Beam collimation

Collimation in the diagnostic unit is provided by the adjustable diaphragms in the form of the light beam diaphragm. The orthovoltage unit uses interchangeable cones or applicators of standard design. These are usually square or circular in shape and produce a beam field of up to $22\,cm^2$. The applicators are attached to the tube housing by a large lead plate with an aperture that determines the field size of the applicator. Specially shaped applicators are often used for specific treatment areas, e.g. the canthus of the eye.

32.4 THE LINEAR ACCELERATOR

32.4.1 Introduction to the linear accelerator

Linear electron accelerators, or LINACs as they are commonly known, accelerate electrons in a straight path and differ from the cyclotron (see Ch. 37), in which electrons follow a circular path. They have been in used in radiotherapy since the 1950s to treat patients with malignant and benign disease. Since their introduction, they have virtually replaced earlier treatment systems such as cobalt units in the UK. The increasing complexity of treatment methods and improvements in technology have seen the LINAC develop from a relatively simple fixed-energy output unit to units with dual and multiple megavoltage output energies of up to 5 MeV, which are capable in some instances of techniques such as conformational therapy treatment methods. Improvements in electronics have resulted in increased unit reliability and stability of output. This is an important factor in radiotherapy treatment.

32.4.2 Construction of a typical linear accelerator and its principal components

The construction of a typical LINAC and its principal components is shown in simplified form in Figure 32.2. As can be seen from the figure, the linear accelerator can be divided into two large structures – a floor-mounted stand and a motor-driven gantry which rotates about the treatment isocentre. These components are discussed individually in the following sections.

32.4.3 The magnetron

As can be seen from Figure 32.3, the is an evacuated cylindrical structure, consisting of a central hollow, indirectly heated, oxide-coated cathode and surrounded by a copper anode containing a number of equidistant cavities that communicate with the space surrounding the cathode. The entire structure is enclosed in a magnetic field running parallel to the long axis of the magnetron. Both anode and cathode are supplied by a pulsed direct current supply from the modulator. The voltage of this supply is selected so that the electron cloud emitted by the cathode forms a rotating field with a number of spoke-like projections. As the 'spokes' pass over the entry to the anode cavities, they lose about 60% of their energy, inducing them to resonate at a radiofrequency, rather in the same way that a musical note is produced by a flute when a musician blows over it.

The resonance, at a frequency of 3000 MHz, corresponds to a wavelength of 10 cm. This results in the production of microwaves that are detected and transmitted into a waveguide. Stability of output is maintained by an automatic frequency control (AFC) which adjusts the size of the resonant cavity to maintain this frequency with an accuracy of ±20 kHz. The pulsed input means that,

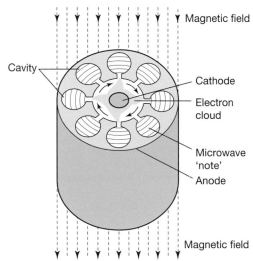

Figure 32.3 Section through a magnetron showing arrangement of anode, cavities, rotating electron field and electron field produced.

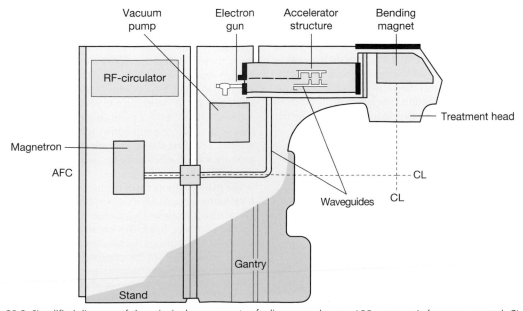

Figure 32.2 Simplified diagram of the principal components of a linear accelerator. AFC, automatic frequency control; CL, centre line; RF, radiofrequency.

although the device operates at an average output of 2 kW, it has a peak output of 2–5 MW.

32.4.4 The waveguides and radiofrequency circulator

Two types of waveguide are found in a linear accelerator: the first are simple hollow tubes that carry the radiofrequency waves from the magnetron to the accelerator section waveguides (at these frequencies, the high impedance of solid conductors would result in significant power losses due to their impedance). The waveguides are sealed at both ends by ceramic discs that are transparent to microwave radiation and the first type of waveguide is filled with sulphur hexafluoride to improve its power-handling capabilities. A radiofrequency circulator is situated between the magnetron and the waveguide; its function is to act as a one-way valve permitting the radiofrequency radiation to pass into the waveguide, but preventing any from passing back into the magnetron, which would be damaged if this occurred. The accelerator waveguide is evacuated and differs in structure and purpose. This will be discussed in more detail in Section 32.4.5.

32.4.5 The accelerating waveguide and accelerator

The accelerating waveguide and accelerator are situated in the gantry of the LINAC. The waveguide uses the radiofrequency wave to accelerate electrons to very high velocities. The principle underlying this process is that an electrical field exerts a force on a charged particle placed in the field. It follows that, for the force to continue to act on the particle, it must move with it. The waveguide is divided into a buncher and a relativistic or accelerating section: the latter forms about two-thirds of the total length of the waveguide. The main difference between the two sections is that the washer-like annular inserts (shown in Fig. 32.4) are closer together in the buncher section. The electrostatic fields in the buncher section slow the passage of the radiofrequency

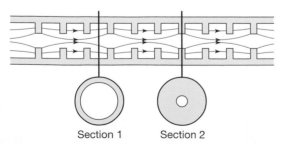

Figure 32.4 Section through the 'buncher' section of an accelerating waveguide showing the annular inserts (sections 1 and 2). The electrostatic fields controlling the electron path are shown by the arrowed lines.

wave to approximately 0.4 C. As already mentioned, this waveguide is evacuated. It is also a resonant structure, which brings the 'injected' electrons into phase with one another. The accelerator is surrounded by a water jacket through which tempered cooling water flows to minimize the thermal contraction and expansion of the guide, which can change its resonance. An electron gun is attached to the buncher section and this injects electrons into the guide in pulses under the control of the modulator, in synchronization with the radiofrequency wave. Typically, only about one-third of the electrons are captured into the optimum part of the radiofrequency wave; however, because of the sinusoidal shape of the wave, the electrons, which are in non-optimal locations, will experience different degrees of acceleration and will decelerate and fall back until they are at the crest of the following wave. On reaching the accelerator section, the electrons gain velocity, reaching speeds of approximately 0.9 C. Because 'like' charges repel one another, the electron beam tends to diverge. This is countered by steering coils positioned externally along the length of the cooling jacket that produce lines of magnetic force running parallel to the long axis of the guide. Focusing coils at the entrance and exit of the waveguide carry out a similar function and ensure that the electron beam is centred to the centre of the guide and target.

32.4.6 The bending magnet and treatment head

The electron beam produced in the accelerator is travelling in a horizontal alignment with the gantry and must be deflected to assume an alignment, which is perpendicular to it. This process is carried out by the bending magnet, which deflects the electron beam through a 270° angle. The magnet is situated externally to the accelerator structure and, like the accelerating waveguide, is an evacuated structure. The radius of the bend depends on the velocity of the electrons; those with higher velocity are deflected in a turn with a larger radius, while lower velocity electrons are deflected in a turn of smaller radius, effectively focusing the beam to a small area at 270° to its original path. The effect is similar to focusing light waves to a point by an achromic lens. For this reason, the magnet is sometimes referred to as an achromic magnet. The effect shown in Figure 32.5 (see page 241) is to produce a small electron beam that yields treatment fields that have well-defined edges.

The main components of the treatment head (which is set for electron therapy) are shown in Figure 32.6 (see page 241). The electron applicator is attached to an external mounting on the treatment head. If X-ray treatment is required, the scattering foil, which is designed to produce a 'flat' electron beam, is rotated out of the electron beam and is replaced by a thin tungsten transmission target and a bell-shaped flattening filter. In both instances, the radiation beam passes through a dual ionization chamber. This monitors beam intensity and is also used to terminate the exposure when the desired amount of radiation has been produced.

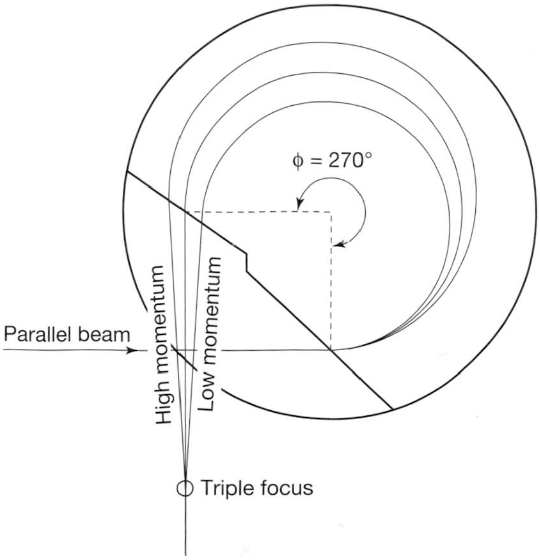

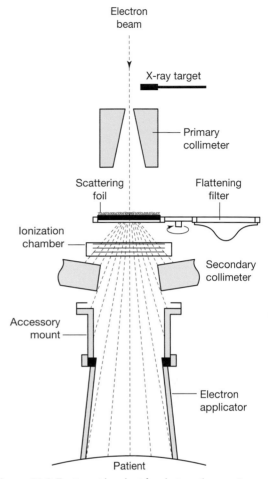

Figure 32.5 Diagram of a 270° bending magnet. Note that electrons of differing speeds are focused to a point on the target (see text for more detail).

Figure 32.6 Treatment head set for electron therapy. For X-ray therapy, the scattering filter is rotated out of the beam and replaced by the transmission target and flattening filter.

Summary

In this chapter, you will have learnt the following:
- Why superficial therapy machines are no longer used for radiotherapy treatment (see Sect. 32.2).
- How the orthovoltage X-ray tube insert differs in design from a diagnostic insert (see Sect. 32.3.1).
- How the tube filtration differs between radiotherapy tubes and diagnostic tubes (see Sect. 32.3.2).
- Why waveguides are used in preference to solid conductors (see Sect. 32.4.4).
- The structures found in the treatment head of a linear accelerator (see Sect. 32.6).

FURTHER READING

Bomford, C.K., Kunkler, I.H., 2003. Walter's and Miller's Textbook of Radiotherapy, second edn. Churchill Livingstone, Edinburgh (Chapters 9 and 10).

Cherry, P., Duxbury, A., 1998. Practical Radiotherapy Physics and Equipment. Greenwich Medical Media, London (Chapters 9 and 10).

Greene, D., Williams, P.C., 1997. Linear Accelerators for Radiation Therapy, second edn. Institute of Physics, Bristol.

Morris, S., 2001. Radiotherapy Physics and Equipment. Churchill Livingstone, London (Chapters 5 and 7).

Chapter | **33** |

Radiotherapy simulators

33.1 AIM

The aim of this chapter is to provide the reader with an overview of the similarities and differences between the radiotherapy simulator and the linear accelerator.

33.2 INTRODUCTION

The radiotherapy simulator is an X-ray generator designed to simulate the treatment beam of a linear accelerator in terms of size and direction, but not the energy. It has the same mobility and accuracy as the linear accelerator, and is capable of producing radiographic images of the treatment area for use in the treatment planning process. The requirement for simulators developed primarily from the development of the linear accelerator, with its ability to deliver X-ray beams with significantly greater percentage depth doses, which resulted in an awareness of the need to avoid radiosensitive areas and the long-term

effects of poorly planned therapy. The need for simulators has been increased by advances in conformational radiotherapy techniques.

33.3 SIMULATOR SPECIFICATIONS

The simulator must comply with the documentation produced by the International Electrotechnical Commission (IEC) as set out in British Standards Institution (BSI) 1993a and 1993b. It must mimic the range of movement (but not energy levels) megavoltage units likely to be found in radiotherapy departments and also be capable of producing radiographic and fluoroscopic images. In addition, it should meet the following general criteria:

- It should be mechanically and geometrically as compatible with as many of the department's treatment units as possible.
- It should be well constructed so that the manufacturer's tolerances are maintained for long periods during routine use.
- The variable focus to film distance (FFD) should match the focus to skin distance (FSD) range of the treatment equipment and techniques available.
- As some treatment techniques use very large treatment fields, the image intensifier should have provision to accept or support cassettes of size that will record these fields.
- It should be Digital Imaging and Communications in Medicine (DICOM) compatible to permit digital communication between it and other imaging equipment in the department.

33.4 GANTRY DESIGN

A conventional standard simulator as described here is found in all radiotherapy departments. (Computed

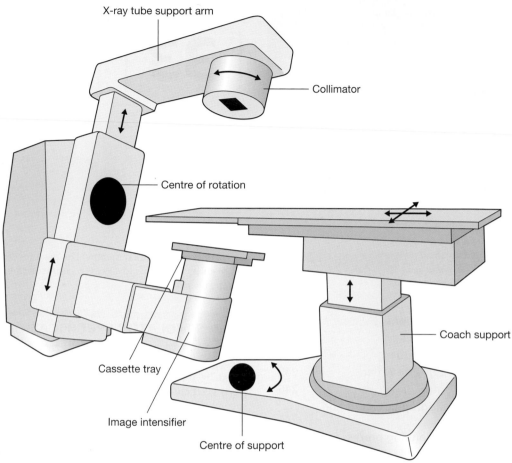

X-ray tube support arm

Collimator

Centre of rotation

Coach support

Cassette tray

Image intensifier

Centre of support

Figure 33.1 Basic gantry configuration and movements (see text for details).

tomography simulators are available, but are not in wide-spread use.)

The basic configuration of a gantry (a U, L arm) is shown in Figure 33.1. The U arm is mounted on a vertical stand and is capable of variable speed ±180° rotation about its central point to reflect the rotation that may be used on the linear accelerator for treatment. The upper part of the arm supports the X-ray tube and collimator, which is always directed to the centre of the input of the image intensifier. The length of this part of the arm is variable to permit the selection of different FSDs that may be used in treatment. The lower part of the arm which supports the image intensifier it is also capable of vertical movement so that it can be moved as close to the support table as possible, reducing image magnification. A scale mounted at the rotation point of the U arm indicates the position of the gantry as it rotates about the patient couch.

The floor-mounted L arm can be rotated horizontally ±90° about its point of rotation. A solid, low-attenuation support table (e.g. fibreglass) which is capable of vertical,

logistical, longitudinal and transverse movement also provides means of attaching the patient-immobilization shells that will be used in treatment. It is important that these attachment points should match (or can be adjusted to match) those on the treatment unit.

33.4.1 The X-ray head

The basic components of the X-ray tube head ares shown in Figure 33.2 (See page 245)(overleaf) are:

- rotating anode X-ray tube
- field-defining wires
- collimation system
- attachments for lead tray and electron applicator
- crash guard (not shown in figure)
- ionization chamber (not shown in figure)
- field-defining light
- collimator rotation scale (not shown in figure).

The X-ray tube is a standard rotating anode tube (see Ch. 31) and is supplied by a medium-frequency rectification

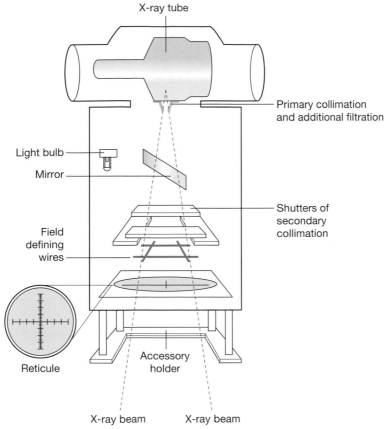

X-ray tube

Primary collimation
and additional filtration

Light bulb

Mirror

Shutters of
secondary
collimation

Field
defining
wires

Reticule

Accessory
holder

X-ray beam   X-ray beam

Figure 33.2 Basic components of the X-ray tube head (see text for details).

circuit (see Ch. 28). The insert has a dual-focus filament with a broad and fine focus. A radiolucent ionization chamber which records the output of the X-ray tube is positioned between the primary collimation and the light bulb, radiolucent mirror and the adjustable shutters of the secondary collimation.

The exact position of the X-ray beam in the radiographic and fluorographic mode is indicted by the light field projected onto the patient. Checking the accuracy of this collimation is a simple, but essential, part of the regular QA checks that should be carried out on the simulator. The radiopaque field-defining wirers are then moved to indicate the planning or clinical target volume depending on the procedure being used. This may be done automatically on newer simulators but has to be done manually on older models.

As the light beam leaves the collimator housing, it passes through a thin interchangeable perspex plate which has a radiopaque reticule engraved on it where the simulator is used at differing FSDs as the reticule represents the geometry of the radiation field at a specific FSD. A 'range-finder' or optical distance indicator (ODI) mounted on the exterior of the collimator housing measures the FSD.

A scale indicating the amount of collimator rotation is also mounted externally to the collimator housing.

33.4.2 The image intensifier

The input face of the image intensifier on the lower part of the U arm is, as already mentioned, always central to the central ray from the X-ray tube and provides a visible real-time image of the structures the X-ray beam is passing through. The actual intensifier may be of the older conventional type or a more modern (and more expensive) flat-panel type. Both are described in more detail in Chapter 35. Flat-panel intensifiers have the advantages of being lighter and occupying less space than the older type. They are also capable of producing 'radiographic images' without the need for a separate recording medium. If radiographic images are required when using a conventional image intensifier, the recording medium must be placed in a cassette holder, mounted above the input face of the intensifier. On exposure, this device automatically centres the cassette to the centre of the input face. The cassette holder carries an ionization chamber which will terminate the exposure when the recoding medium has received sufficient radiation. Both types of intensifier are able to output the data in digital format (DICOM.). The output from a flat-panel intensifier is in digital format while, with the conventional intensifier, the light output from the phosphor can be detected by a charge-coupled device (CCD) array (similar to those in digital cameras) and 'passed on' in digital format for display on a monitor screen or for downloading into the planning computer. The fluoroscopic imaging system should be capable of providing pulsed fluoroscopy, with such features as last image hold or 'frame freeze' facilities.

Over the years, the simulator design shown in Figures 33.1 and 33.2 has become much more compact with the result that modern simulators make greater use of electronic displays and are capable of direct communication of the verified treatment plan to the linear accelerator. An example of such a simulator is shown in Figure 33.3 (below).

33.4.3 The control panel

There are two sets of controls for the simulator. A set of local controls inside the simulator room allow the operator to move the couch, gantry collimator, image intensifier and radiation field, and also carry out operations like adjusting the radiation field, laser and room lighting. A remote set of controls is placed outside the room. This permits the operator to view and communicate with the patient and to make adjustments to the couch, gantry collimator and image intensifier settings. They also have separate controls for fluoroscopic and radiographic procedures,

an emergency stop and mains on and off switches. Finally, they have a control transfer switch or interlock, the function of which is to ensure that only a single set of controls can be in use at any one time.

33.4.4 The radiographic recording medium

The most common recording medium in use today is the photostimulable plate (PSP), which has the advantages of a very wide exposure latitude and the fact that the data on it can be converted into digital format. The plate is exposed in a cassette which is unloaded and processed in an image reader, at which point the stored data are converted into an optical output and then into digital format for display on a monitor or for passage to the planning computer. An alternative recording medium which is becoming more common is the amorphous selenium array. Like the PSP, this is also exposed in a cassette and read by an image reader; the major difference is that the array converts the data directly into digital format.

33.5 THE TREATMENT PLANNING PROCESS

As patient treatment is usually delivered on the linear accelerator in a series of fractionated radiation doses

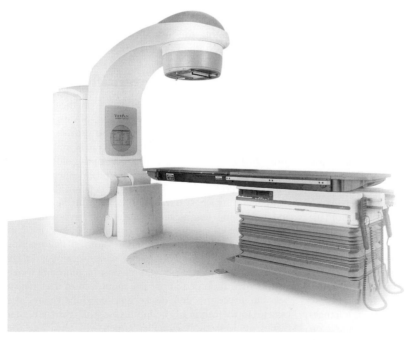

Figure 33.3 A modern radiotherapy simulator.
(Photograph courtesy of Varian Medical Systems.)

spread over an interval of time, it is an obvious requirement that the radiation dose is delivered to the same target volume in the patient. Where this target volume is relatively immobile, such as the head and neck, mediastinal area, spine and pelvic region, immobilization forms one of the most important parts of patient planning and subsequent treatment. This involves the production of tailor-made aids or 'shells' which are used to immobilize the patient during the planning stage on the simulator and subsequent treatment on the linear accelerator. The shell should integrate with the fixation points on the simulator and linear accelerator being used for treatment, as well as with any pre-existing immobilization systems. The shell should be safe and comfortable for the patient, and permit the visualization of any initial fields drawn on the patient as well as allowing any field changes to be drawn on the shell. Finally, the shell should maintain any skin-sparing effect due to the treatment energies used. Once the initial data are obtained, the patient's identity is rechecked and all the data from the simulator passed to a 3D planning computer, together with data from other sources such as computed tomography (CT) or magnetic resonance imaging (MRI) scans.

The planning computer produces a patient cross-section and plots an isodose distribution map (similar to Fig. 1.3 in Ch. 1) of the cross-section, showing the treatment volume, direction of the treatment fields, any wedges to be used and radiosensitive areas in the cross-section. This is passed back to the simulator, where the treatment plan is verified. Verification entails producing radiographs at all the beam entry points specified in outline produced by the planning computer. The resulting data are passed again to the planning computer, where another cross-section is produced; this is compared against the original cross-section to ensure the fields selected are correct and that it complies with the department's treatment protocols.

33.6 CT SIMULATOR

The CT simulator has many advantages over the conventional type of simulator, but is less commonly used in most simulator suites. The CT simulator consists of a CT scanner, laser positioning aids and a 'virtual' treatment planning computer. In common with most of today's generation of CT scanners, it will probably be capable of spiral CT and have 3D imaging software. Once a 3D image of the tumour volume has been produced, this is passed to the virtual planning computer which constructs a cross-section showing the beam entry points, treatment area and isodose curves. The patient data are rechecked by the oncologist and, if approved, the entry points of the treatment beams are transferred to the conventional planning computer where the patient is placed in the treatment position and the treatment plan is verified in the conventional manner.

Summary

In this chapter, you should have learnt the following:
- The basic difference between a simulator and a linear accelerator (see Sect. 33.2).
- The particular requirements of a radiotherapy simulator (see Sect. 33.3).
- The design features and movements of the simulator gantry (see Sect. 33.4).
- The difference between the treatment planning process and the verification process (see Sect. 33.5).
- The advantages offered by CT simulators (see Sect. 33.6).

FURTHER READING

British Standards Institution, 1993a. Part 2: Particular Requirements for Safety, Section 2.129 Specification for Radiotherapy Simulators. BSI, Milton Keynes.

British Standards Institution, 1933b. Part 3, Section 3.1291993,

Characteristics of Radiotherapy Simulators, Supplement 1. Guide to Functional Performance Values. BSI, Milton Keynes.

Farr, R.F., Allisly-Roberts, P.J., 1977. Physics for Medical Imaging. WB Saunders, London.

Morris, S., 2001. Radiotherapy Physics and Equipment. Churchill Livingstone, Edinburgh (Chapter 1).

Part | 7 |

The radiographic image

Chapter | **34** |

Production of the digital radiographic image

34.1 AIM

The aim of this chapter is to introduce the reader to the principles of digital imaging as practised in the radiological department. The assumption is made that the reader has read and understood Chapter 25 which dealt with the basic mechanisms of image production. The consequences of producing a digital image will be discussed in Chapter 36.

34.2 THE DIGITAL IMAGE

The old method of producing a radiograph using film and intensifying screens is an example of an *analogue image*. The information (or data) it contains is represented by a range of continuously varying densities or shades of grey. If such an image is scanned as a series of horizontal lines and the densities plotted on a graph, we would see an appearance similar to that shown in Figure 34.1A (see page 252).

A digital image is divided into a series of small boxes called *pixels*, arranged in a series of rows and columns called a *matrix* (Fig. 34.2, see page 252). The density of each pixel has a numerical integer value. If we consider our initial radiograph, we could allocate the value 0 to the most dense value and 255 to the least dense value giving a digital scale of 256. Thus, any single pixel would have a discrete value between zero and 255 and our line would appear as a series of steps as shown in Figure. 34.1B. The smaller the image size and the larger the number of pixels in the image matrix, the better the spatial resolution of the image. If the pixels are too large, the individual pixels can be seen by the observer and distract from the image information.

Most modern digital imaging systems have a matrix of 1024×1024 pixels; the resultant image has $1\,048\,576$ individual pixels. If such an image was displayed on a 20-cm square section of a monitor, each pixel will be a square of side just under 0.2 mm and so will be below the resolving power of the eye; thus we are aware of the overall image and do not see the individual pixels.

Definition
A *digital image* is any image in which the information is represented in discrete units, with integer values.

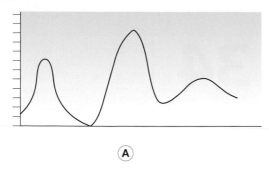

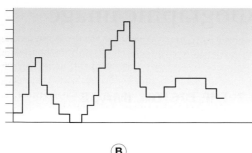

Figure 34.1 A horizontal line drawn across an image. (A) A conventional analogue image; (B) the same line as a digital image.

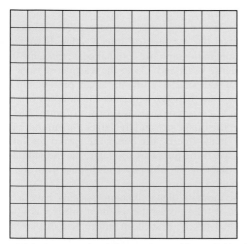

Figure 34.2 An example of the matrix used for a digitized image. Each box of this matrix is a pixel.

Digital imaging is used in all imaging modalities in the modern diagnostic imaging department. The process of converting the analogue radiation image from the patient into a digital image differs with each modality and application. However, the principle of changing this analogue signal into a digital one is common to all modalities and applications.

Digital imaging allows the construction of an image with a high spatial resolution, large dynamic range and good contrast resolution. In addition, the imaged data may also be processed by a computer to enhance the diagnostic value of the 'raw' unprocessed image. The data for these images, as already mentioned, can come from a variety of sources and will be received by some form of image receptor (imaging plate, digital array or transducer, for example). The signal then passes through several basic stages before a visible image is produced.

34.3 DIGITAL IMAGE PRODUCTION

If the image is not already in the form of an electrical signal, the first stage of the conversion process is to convert the image to an electrical signal. (This may not be necessary with all imaging modalities.) The analogue electrical signal is converted into a digital one using a device known as an *analogue-to-digital converter* (ADC). Within the ADC, the signal undergoes three stages: scanning, quantization and coding.

34.3.1 Scanning

The incoming signal is scanned as a series of equally spaced horizontal lines. Each line is divided into a number of equally spaced points producing a series of small 'boxes'; each 'box' forms a single picture cell element or pixel. To eliminate display errors, the scanning frequency must be at least twice the highest frequency present in the analogue image signal. This produces the *image matrix* (as already mentioned, the number of pixels per line), which is important as this controls the horizontal resolution of the image. A high rate of sampling produces a high-resolution image but is more demanding on the computing facilities. The effect of pixel size on resolution can be seen by viewing Figure 34.3 (see page 253). If viewed at close range, the individual pixels are quite noticeable. However, when viewed from a distance of about a metre, the eye cannot resolve the individual pixels.

34.3.2 Quantization

This process allocates a numerical integer to each pixel. On a scale of 1024, for example, each pixel can have an integer value between 0 and 1023. A typical TV camera video signal ranges from zero to 700 mV at peak white intensity. This scale permits the ADC to detect changes in the video signal as low as $0.7\,\text{mV}.10^{-7}$ volts.

34.3.3 Coding

The final stage, coding, converts the numerical value produced by quantization into a binary number as this is the type of number 'understood' by the computer, which

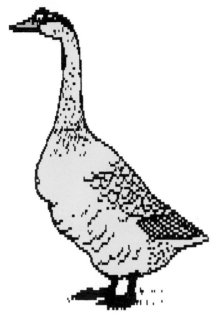

Figure 34.3 An example of a digitized image where the pixels are so large that they can be seen at close range.

cannot understand conventional numbers. The data then pass from the ADC to the computer.

Where the signal is part of a 'moving' image such as produced during fluoroscopy, it is also important that the ADC can sample and process each individual frame of the image before it is replaced by the next frame in the sequence, and therefore it is desirable that the ADC has a high sampling rate.

34.4 SHORT-TERM STORAGE, MANIPULATION AND DISPLAY OF DIGITAL IMAGES

The second stage of the conversion is carried out by the computer. The binary number passes to the central processing unit (CPU) of the computer which directs the data to an area of computer memory termed a frame store. When the data capture for the image is complete, it is recalled by the CPU and, if required, manipulated. This facility allows us, for instance, to alter the contrast and brightness of the image, to window on specific values within the image so that only structures of interest are displayed, to enhance the edges of structures or to subtract one image from another. These facilities are especially useful in studies using a contrast agent. Having manipulated the image as required, the binary values are recalled from the frame store and, if necessary, matched to the display capabilities of the VDU or monitor and passed to an output buffer (a storage area in the computer memory). Finally, once all data are modified

and stored, the CPU monitors the transfer of the data to the appropriate output device. This process is shown diagrammatically in Figure 34.4 (see page 254).

The final stage is the conversion of the digital signals from the computer back into an analogue signal. This process is carried out by a device known as a digital-to-analogue converter (DAC) which operates in a reverse manner to the ADC. As each binary number is received by the DAC it is allocated a discrete absolute numerical value; this current then passes through an output resistor, resulting in an analogue voltage output.

This final stage is only necessary if the monitor is a cathode ray tube (CRT). If the monitor is a liquid crystal display (LCD) (which has a digital input), no conversion is necessary. The digital signal is also sent to a picture archiving and communications system (PACS). The PACS system has many functions: it provides long-term storage facilities for the digital image, and communicates with the departmental and hospital computer networks. This will be further discussed in Chapter 36 which considers the consequences of digital imaging. The digital signal may also be passed to a device such as a laser imager, where it is used to produce hard copy on a film, although this is very rare today.

34.5 DIGITAL IMAGING IN GENERAL RADIOGRAPHY

Digital imaging systems in general radiography tend to be classed under two broad types, computed radiography (CR) or digital radiography (DR) – this latter system is sometimes referred to as direct digital radiography as it does not involve the need to take a digital plate to a plate reader.

34.5.1 Computed radiography

Computed radiography systems use *photostimulable plates* as a temporary store for the radiographic image (see Sect. 24.5). The plates are stored in CR cassettes. After the plate has been exposed to radiation, the operator places the cassette in a *plate reader*. Here the plate is removed from the cassette and scanned in a linear fashion using a laser beam. The information from the plate and patient information are matched and then sent through the computer system to appropriate workstations for viewing and reporting. Finally, the plate is 'cleaned' of any residual image information and inserted into the cassette where it is ready for use in the next imaging situation.

34.5.1.1 Construction and physics of the storage phosphor plates

A cross-section of a typical storage phosphor plate is shown in Figure 34.5 (see page 254). When the atoms in

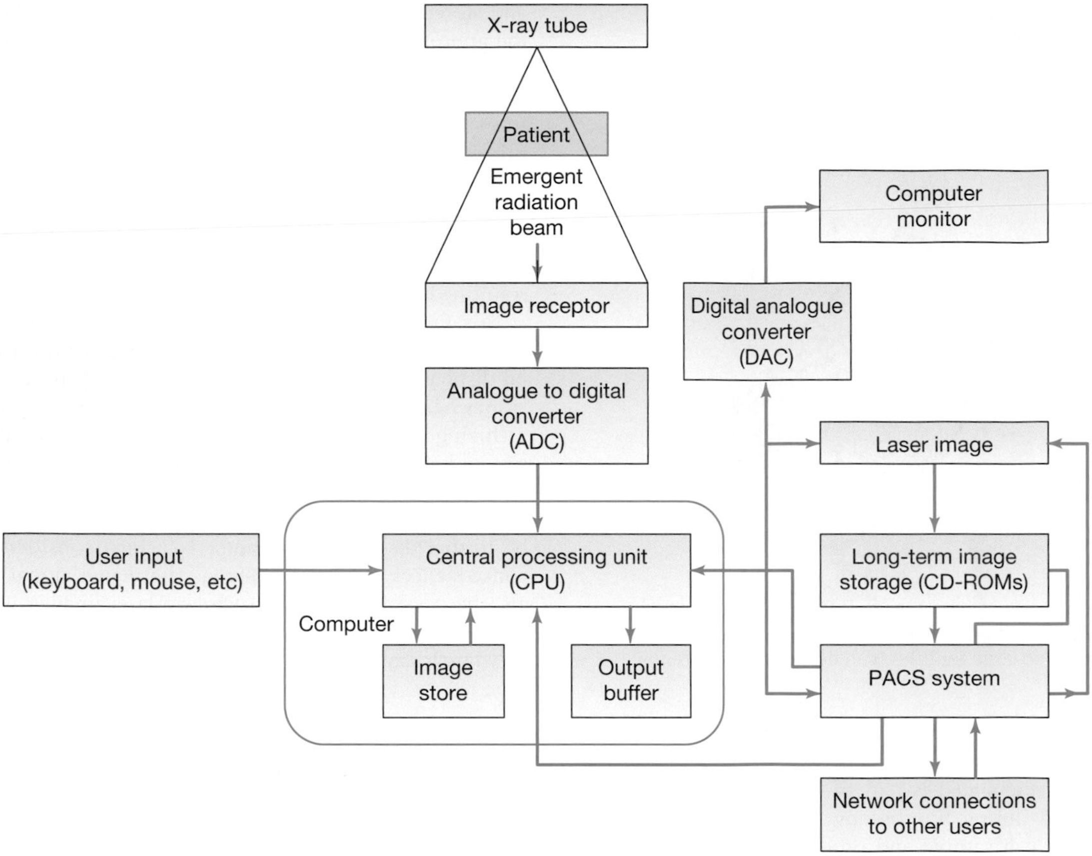

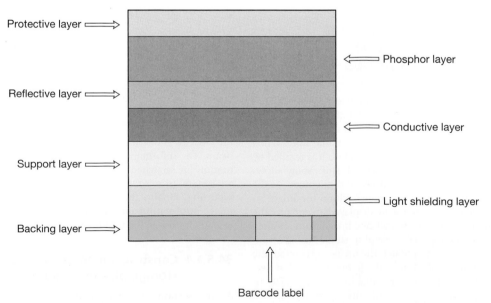

Figure 34.4 Block diagram of the major components of a digital imaging system. Note the picture archiving and communications system (PACS) component functions as an interface between the system and its long-term storage. It also permits communication between the internal departmental network and other hospital and external users.

Figure 34.5 Cross-section through a typical CR imaging plate. The functions of the various layers are discussed in the text.

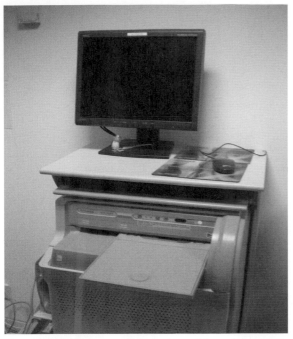

Figure 34.6 This shows a plate reader and the radiographer's workstation. The plates are inserted, after exposure, into the slotted areas shown and the image is displayed on the monitor at the work area.

(Photograph courtesy of The Robert Gordon University.)

the phosphor layer (i.e. europium-activated barium fluoro-halide $(BaF(BrI):Eu^2)$) are stimulated by X-ray photons, then electrons in the valence band are moved to the higher energy of the electron traps in the 'forbidden energy band'. This process has been described in detail in Chapter 24. The greater the number and energy of the X-ray photons inter-acting with the plate, the greater the number of electrons which have their energy raised and so enter the electron traps, and so an 'X-ray image pattern' is created on the plate. The plate is now read in the plate reader by scanning it with a laser beam. The electrons are given sufficient energy to be liberated and eventually drop back to the valence band. This drop in the electron energy causes the liberation of a light photon which is detected by a photomultiplier sys-tem and sent as an electrical signal to the computer system. The amount of light emitted and the strength of the electri-cal signal are proportional to the original intensity of X-rays which interacted with the plate. These samples of electrical signal are used to construct the digital image (see Sect. 24.5).

An example of a plate reader is shown in Figure 34.6.

34.5.2 Digital radiography

Digital radiography does not involve the operator taking an imaging plate to a plate reader. Instead the imaging device (flat-panel detector) is incorporated into the X-ray couch or erect stand and sends the image information to the computer as soon as the exposure is made. The image is then produced on the operator's viewing monitor after a few seconds. Such a set-up is shown in Figure 34.7.

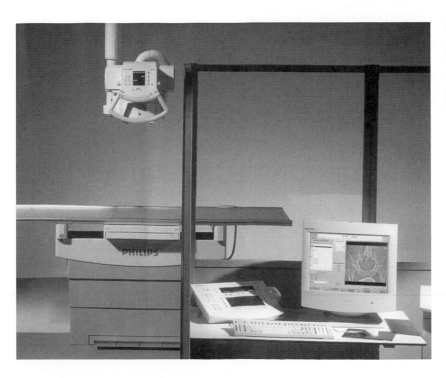

Figure 34.7 This is a typical direct digital technique setup showing the X-ray tube, the table, the operator's console and the monitor with an image displayed on it.
(photograph courtesy of Philips Health care.)

The technology of flat-panel detectors can be divided into two major types – 'direct conversion detectors' and 'indirect conversion detectors'.

34.5.2.1 Direct conversion flat panel detectors

Figure 34.8 shows a section through a typical direct conversion flat-panel detector. The outer layer of the plate is a micro-plated electrode. This allows a charge to be applied via the dielectric layer to the amorphous selenium (a-Se) layer as shown in the diagram. The amorphous selenium layer absorbs X-ray photons and this results in the liberation of electrons. These electrons are directed by the charge pattern towards the silicon thin film transistors (TFTs). The TFTs act as switches which send the signal to the processing system where the software converts it to the appropriate greyscale for that pixel. The image is usually displayed on the display panel in the operator's control area in less than 1 second after exposure.

34.5.2.2 Indirect conversion flat-panel detectors

Indirect conversion flat-panel detectors are similar to the direct conversion detectors except that the conversion is a two-step process. Figure 34.9 shows a section through a typical indirect conversion flat-panel detector. The crystals in the caesium iodide layer are struck by X-ray photons and emit light photons proportional to the energy and intensity of the X-ray photons. Caesium iodide crystals are needle shaped and so limit the spread of light emitted thus improving resolution. The light photons fall onto the amorphous silicon (a-Si) layer and cause the emission of electrons within this layer. These electrons are then directed towards the TFTs and the image is produced in a similar way to the direct conversion method. Because there is the potential for the light to diverge before being captured by the amorphous silicon layer, the resolution of this system may not be as high as the direct conversion system.

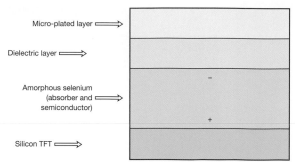

Figure 34.8 This is a diagrammatic representation of the construction of the material which will collect the image information from a single pixel in the matrix of a direct imaging plate.

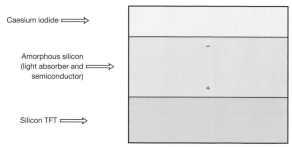

Figure 34.9 This is a diagrammatic representation of the construction of the material which will collect the image information from a single pixel in the matrix of an indirect imaging plate.

Summary

In this chapter, you should have learnt the following:
- What is meant by a 'digital image' in radiography (see Sect. 34.2).
- The main processes in digital image production (see Sect. 34.3).
- The short-term storage, manipulation and display of digital images in radiography (see Sect 34.4).
- The basics of digital imaging as applied to general radiography (see Sect. 34.5).

FURTHER READING

You may find Chapter 36 of this text, which discusses the implications of digital imaging, useful further reading.

Carter, C.E., Veale, B.L., 2008. Digital Radiography and PACS. Mosby Elsevier, Missouri.

Siegel, E.L., Kolodner, R.M. (Eds.), 1999. Filmless Radiology. Springer, New York.

Chapter | 35 |

The fluoroscopic image

35.1 AIM

Fluoroscopy is a technique that is widely used in radiography to produce images of moving structures. These can be used for real-time diagnostic imaging and treatment guidance. The aim of this chapter is to explain how fluoroscopic images are formed, concluding with a consideration of image quality and radiation dose issues. Traditionally the term fluoroscopy has referred to real-time imaging used for guiding procedures, while fluorography produces higher-quality images for organ investigations.

35.2 FLUOROSCOPIC PRINCIPLES

In the process of *fluorescence*, materials called *phosphors* absorb high-energy photons such as X-rays and emit short bursts of visible light photons. The brief nature of the light emissions is useful in radiography, where there is a need to produce sharp images free from 'lag' or blur. It was light from fluorescent crystals of barium platinocyanide that led Roentgen to realise in 1895 that hidden 'X-rays' were being produced from an electrified vacuum tube in a darkened laboratory. The rest, of course, is history.

Phosphor materials are very widely used in radiography and need to have two key characteristics – the ability to strongly absorb X-rays and the ability to convert a percentage of this absorbed energy to visible light. X-ray absorption (by the photoelectric absorption process) is improved by the presence of high atomic number elements like caesium, barium, iodine and the 'rare earths'. These all typically have *K*-shell absorption edges at about 30–35 keV, which are well placed to absorb X-rays produced at about 70–100 kVp (see Ch. 23).

Insight

The greatest intensity of X-rays produced within the continuous X-ray spectrum by Bremsstrahlung is at about one-third to one-half of the peak beam energy (which is determined by the kVp across an X-ray tube). Thus it is useful to match the *K*-edge energies of absorbing materials to this point of greatest intensity, not to the peak beam energy (as very few X-rays are produced at the peak energy).

The overall *luminescent radiant efficiency* (conversion rate of X-ray energy to light energy) is normally only about 10–20% for phosphor materials. This means that considerable intensities of X-rays are needed to produce enough light for a glowing fluoroscopic image to be viewed directly (without any amplification), even in a darkened room. In the first half of the twentieth century, imaging department staff had to do exactly this; view a phosphor screen directly during fluoroscopic procedures, with patient and staff receiving large radiation doses in the process.

35.3 THE IMAGE INTENSIFIER

In radiography, an image intensifier is simply a device which amplifies the visible light resulting from the fluoroscopic process. Such devices were introduced in the 1950s and permitted fluoroscopy to take place in normal room lighting conditions, as well as greatly reducing radiation doses to patients and staff. This section will describe a traditional X-ray image intensifier, which is based around a cylindrical evacuated tube designed to accelerate and focus electrons. These devices have been partly replaced by more modern 'solid-state' devices, but are still widely used in radiography.

The traditional X-ray image intensifier involves various energy changes between the input and output phosphors of the device, as shown in Figure 35.1.

Note: Although X-ray energy is transferred to light energy within the device, it should be noted that light photons are not turned into electrons. At the photocathode, light energy is used to promote the energy of existing electrons within the material so that they are emitted from it.

Table 35.1 indicates the relative numbers of photons or electrons arising at each stage of the process of image intensification.

The *flux gain* of an image intensifier refers to the relative numbers of incident X-ray photons striking the input phosphor to emitted light photons leaving the output phosphor. This is in the general region of $1{:}10^4$ to 10^5. To achieve this, energy is put into the system, largely by accelerating electrons from the photocathode through a vacuum across a potential difference of about 25 kV towards an anode. The speeding electrons have a lot of kinetic energy when they strike the output phosphor, which responds by emitting many light photons.

The conversion of an input of relatively few X-ray photons to an output of many light photons can result in image noise, due to the phenomenon of *quantum mottle*. When individual X-ray photons are very effective at producing an amplified signal and the number of X-ray photons can be reduced as a consequence, random variations in X-ray density can become visible and produce a 'salt and pepper' appearance on the image.

Table 35.1 Approximate relative numbers of photons or electrons arising at each stage of the image intensification process

TRANSFORMATION	NUMBERS OF RESULTANT PHOTONS OR ELECTRONS
1 X-ray photon absorbed in the input phosphor	$\approx 2 \times 10^3$ light photons are emitted by the input phosphor – of these, about half are absorbed in the phosphor material
$\approx 1 \times 10^3$ light photons strike the photocathode	$\approx 2 \times 10^2$ electrons are emitted by the photocathode
$\approx 2 \times 10^2$ electrons are accelerated and strike the output phosphor	$\approx 1 \times 10^5$ light photons are emitted by the output phosphor

The key components of an image intensifier are shown in Figure 35.2 (see page 261). The input phosphor typically contains caesium iodide. Crystals of this material can be needle shaped and transmit emitted light effectively down 'light channels' to the photocathode. Caesium iodide consists of high atomic number elements which encourage X-ray absorption. The photocathode contains caesium–antimony compounds which emit electrons (photoelectrons) from their surface when light is absorbed.

Looking at the diagram, it can be seen that the electrons emitted by a large photocathode are focused down onto a small output phosphor. This size difference contributes to the increase in brightness, or *brightness gain*, which is obtained at the output phosphor relative to the input phosphor. This is in the region of $1{:}10^4$ and is also affected by the previously mentioned flux gain. If the charge on the focusing electrodes (which are sometimes called electrostatic focusing lenses) is adjusted, this will affect the position of the electron beam focal spot F and can produce magnification of the fluoroscopic image. This will take place when the output phosphor occupies only the central part of the full circular area of the focused electron beam. A dual field image intensifier can produce a normal-sized image and a magnified image, while a triple-field intensifier can give two sizes of magnified field. A magnified image is less bright, since it is produced by electron output from only the central part of the photocathode. X-ray tube mA may be increased to compensate for this, but at the expense of giving greater patient dose.

The output phosphor is typically made of zinc–cadmium sulphide with silver as an additive. This phosphor emits light when struck by electrons. The light from

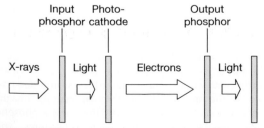

Figure 35.1 The conversion processes that take place within an image intensifier.

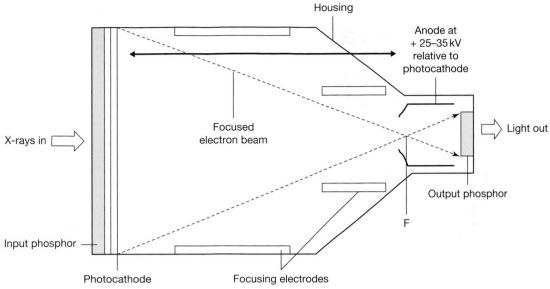

Figure 35.2 A schematic diagram of an image intensifier. *F* is the focal point of the electron beam. In reality, the input phosphor, photocathode and output phosphor are slightly curved and each is circular when seen 'face on'. The housing contains a vacuum.

the output phosphor is fed into components linked to viewing monitors and image recording devices. The latter are now based on digital technology.

35.4 SOLID-STATE IMAGE INTENSIFIERS

Modern image intensification devices are increasingly based on solid-state 'flat-panel' components, rather than on evacuated image intensifier tubes. X-ray energy falling upon a detector array is converted into an electronic output signal. There are two main types of detector:

1. *Indirect systems* include a layer of phosphor material such as caesium iodide, coated on top of an amorphous silicon photodiode. They permit low radiation doses, due to the image amplification of the phosphor layer, but incur possible slight losses in image resolution due to the light spreading that occurs.
2. *Direct systems*, as the name suggests, use an amorphous selenium photoconductor to absorb X-rays directly. Such systems may have a very high image resolution, with a slight radiation dose penalty relative to indirect methods.

A simplified diagram of an indirect X-ray detector is shown in Figure 35.3 (see page 262). Each cell has a top layer of a scintillation crystal made of caesium iodide activated with thallium, which produces light when struck

> **Insight**
>
> In radiographic imaging there is almost always a trade-off between radiation dose and image quality. Intensifying screen phosphors amplify signal and reduce dose but increase image unsharpness. In computed tomography (CT) and digital imaging, a high X-ray tube mA reduces image noise but increases radiation dose. Large-size radiation detectors tend to be more sensitive but provide a reduced resolution. A small pitch value in CT increases both patient dose and image resolution.

by X-rays. The atomic numbers of Cs and I are 55 and 53 respectively and this results in good X-ray absorption. Each absorbed X-ray photon produces $\approx 10^3$ light photons. Below this, an amorphous silicon photodiode converts about 50% of the light into electric charge. This pattern of charge is stored and converted to an electrical signal within a 2D pixel array. Self-scanning of a 2D array of electrodes containing switching elements in a thin film transistor (TFT) reads the stored charge distribution (Fig. 35.4) (see page 262).

In the direct X-ray detector above, there is no intermediate phosphor layer. X-ray absorption in the selenium produces negative charges (electrons) and positive charges (electron 'holes' – essentially absences of electrons) which migrate to the electrodes. Selenium has a relatively low atomic number of 34 and thus its X-ray absorption efficiency decreases at higher X-ray energies.

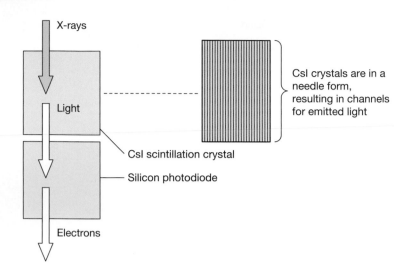

Figure 35.3 Key parts of an indirect detector cell for digital X-ray imaging. A 2D matrix of such cells produces the signal for a pixel display. CsI, caesium iodide.

X-rays

Light

CsI crystals are in a needle form, resulting in channels for emitted light

CsI scintillation crystal

Silicon photodiode

Electrons

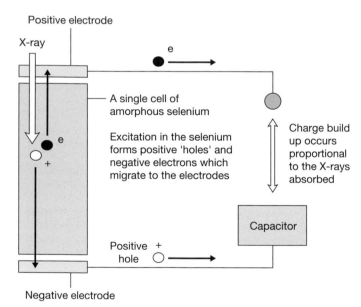

Figure 35.4 Key parts of a direct detector cell for digital X-ray imaging. A 2D matrix of such cells produces the signal for a pixel display.

Positive electrode

X-ray

e

A single cell of amorphous selenium

Excitation in the selenium forms positive 'holes' and negative electrons which migrate to the electrodes

e

+

Charge build up occurs proportional to the X-rays absorbed

Capacitor

Positive +
hole

Negative electrode

35.5 FLUOROSCOPIC IMAGE QUALITY

Traditional image intensifiers suffer from some effects that are a feature of their geometry. Since the photocathode is curved, the image field may appear more magnified towards its edges – this effect is known as *pincushion distortion* and is illustrated in Figure 35.5 (see page 263). Additionally the geometry may result in *vignetting*, in which the centre of the image field appears brighter than the periphery. *Blooming* (excessive brightening) of the image intensifier field, typically when a region of gas or

air is present, occurs due to limitations in the ability of these traditional devices to record a wide dynamic range of image intensity. Solid-state intensifiers are not affected by pincushion distortion, vignetting or blooming, due to their flat geometry and wide dynamic range.

Both traditional and solid-state image intensifiers can be prone to *ghosting* artefact which shows up as a residual image brightness where an object was present in a previous X-ray exposure (but has now left). Previous exposures can alter the performance of detector elements. *Lag* refers to a motion blurring that can occur during fluoroscopy of a moving object, due to time delays in the response of phosphors and amorphous Si or Se. The image resolution of image intensifiers is affected by magnification and by

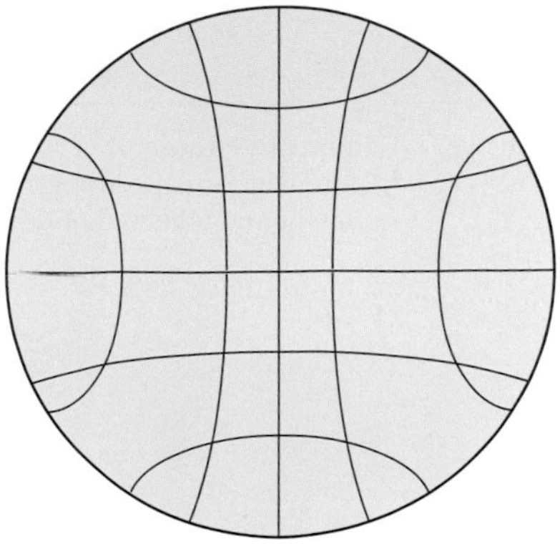

Figure 35.5 Pincushion image distortion (exaggerated here).

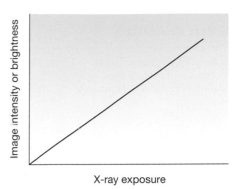

Figure 35.6 The relationship between image intensity and X-ray exposure using solid-state digital X-ray detectors. This relationship is linear (straight line) over a wide range of exposures, resulting in a large dynamic range.

the dimensions of individual digital detector elements or phosphor grains. The performance of a television monitor will also greatly affect image resolution.

Image *noise* can occur in all X-ray detectors and consists of random statistical and electrical fluctuations in the size of a signal across the surface of the image. The *signal to noise ratio* (SNR) is important in imaging as it defines the relative sizes of useful signal (which is based on real features in a patient or test object) to random signal fluctuations. *Detective quantum efficiency* (DQE) is an important measure of imaging performance and is defined as the SNR^2 in the image output divided by the SNR^2 in the X-ray photons at the input of the device. A value of 1 would indicate perfect performance with no loss of SNR but this is never achieved. Typical DQEs for solid-state devices are in the region of 0.5 to 0.7, with direct digital detectors being more prone to electronic noise than indirect digital detectors.

Figure 35.6 shows the relationship between image intensity and X-ray exposure using solid-state digital X-ray detectors.

35.6 DOSE REDUCTION IN FLUOROSCOPY

Fluoroscopic procedures can result in a high radiation dose to patients, especially in long procedures such as interventions (treatments) undertaken with fluoroscopic guidance. Deterministic radiation effects such as radiation erythema (skin reddening) are not normally encountered in diagnostic imaging but can result from prolonged fluoroscopy, especially in a high X-ray tube output mode.

Automatic brightness control (ABC) monitors light output from image intensifiers and increases X-ray output if light levels fall. This feature can increase radiation doses if light output levels fall from any of the following causes:

- Image magnification.
- Ageing and inefficient image intensifiers.

- Large distance between the patient and the image intensifier input.

Solid-state image intensifiers tend to be more efficient than traditional devices and should provide dose reductions. *Pulsed mode* operation provides a periodic 'blipped' X-ray tube output and is a useful means of reducing radiation dose when maximal image quality is not required using traditional image intensifiers. This mode is also standard practice for solid-state image intensifiers. There is a legal requirement for manufacturers to provide dose-reduction measures such as ABC and pulsed fluoroscopy.

Fluoroscopic doses can also be reduced by:

- increasing X-ray tube kVp
- reducing X-ray tube mA
- reducing screening time
- avoiding small X-ray tube to patient distances
- making use of 'undercouch' X-ray tubes and lead-impregnated plastic curtains.

See Chapter 44 for further discussion of dose reduction methods in radiography.

Summary

In this chapter, you should have learnt the following:
- Fluoroscopic imaging converts an X-ray input to a visible light or electrical output (see Sect. 35.2).
- Phosphor materials absorb X-rays and produce visible light emissions (see Sect. 35.2).
- Image intensifiers amplify the output signal and result in large radiation dose reductions to patients and staff (see Sect. 35.3).
- Digital image intensifier devices are replacing traditional evacuated intensifier tubes and these devices are of two types – indirect (involving an intermediary phosphor layer) and direct (see Sect. 35.4).

FURTHER READING

Allisy-Roberts, P.J., Williams, J., 2007. Farr's Physics for Medical Imaging, second ed. WB Saunders, Edinburgh.

Bushong, S.C., 2008. Radiologic Science for Technologists, ninth ed. Mosby, St Louis.

Dendy, P.P., Heaton, B., 1999. Physics for Diagnostic Radiology, second ed. Taylor and Francis, London.

Chapter 36

Consequences of digital imaging in radiography

36.1 AIM

The aim of this chapter is to introduce the reader to the principal consequences of digital imaging in radiography.

36.2 IMAGE PROCESSING

The analogue image produced on a film is not capable of further processing. The digital image, however, is capable of undergoing a number of processes which aid image interpretation. These will now be discussed.

36.2.1 Data clipping

The X-ray pattern which hits the imaging plate covers a wide range of exposures. Processing all this data into an image would produce an image of very low contrast which would make image interpretation difficult. For this reason, an algorithm is applied to the image depending on the area of the body selected by the radiographer when inputting the patient data. This algorithm discards data which are not of clinical interest to the examination and so increases the contrast of the image produced. The effect of this 'data clipping' is shown in Figure 36.1.

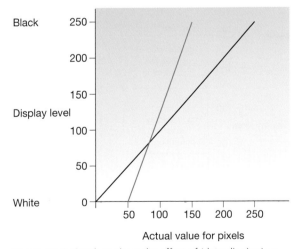

Figure 36.1 Graph to show the effect of 'data clipping' on the contrast. The contrast is represented by the gradient of the coloured line. The black line shows the image as it would be displayed without data clipping. The blue line shows the data as displayed if only pixels with a value between 50 and 150 are used to produce the image. Note the increase in gradient compared to the blue line.

36.2.2 Plate sensitivity

Once the system has clipped the data to data of clinical interest, it then has to correct the image for overall exposure. This is possible because of the linear response of the imaging plates to exposure. This is done by applying a formula which defines the average exposure within the clinically useful range. This is given a different name by different manufacturers – S number (Fuji), Exposure index (Kodak), LogM (Agfa), etc. Thus, if the plate has been overexposed, an image can be produced which has the correct density range displayed on the monitor. The principles behind this are illustrated in Figure 36.2.

36.2.3 Edge enhancement

It is possible to enhance the edges of structures displayed on the digital image. This sometimes makes it easier to see subtle structures like hairline fractures or small catheters in the mediastinum.

36.2.4 Magnification

Because of the digital nature of the image, it is possible to magnify either the whole image or a part of the image.

36.2.5 Image annotation

With the appropriate software, it is possible to annotate the image. This can be a useful tool either to point out structures or to add anatomical data for teaching purposes.

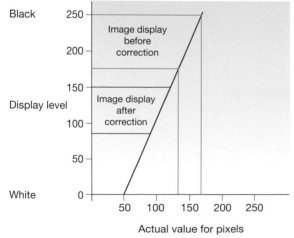

Figure 36.2 Graph to show the effect of altering the plate sensitivity. The original image (shown by the blue lines) has been overexposed and so would produce an image towards the black end of the display range. The corrected image is more in the centre of the display range and so is easier to interpret.

36.2.6 Image stitching

Because of the size limitation of the digital imaging plates (usually about 50 cm × 50 cm), it is impossible to image the whole of the spine as a single image – this may be useful in the imaging of scoliosis. It is, however, possible to take a number of images with the patient in the same position and then to use the software to 'stitch' the images together to produce a composite image. Similar techniques are utilized in lower limb measurement and also for display of the blood supply to the lower limb.

36.3 IMAGE STORAGE AND RETRIEVAL

Because of the digital nature of the image data, there are a number of possibilities for image storage and retrieval. In most cases, the image is stored as part of a picture archival and communication system (PACS) which will be discussed in more detail in the next section of the chapter. This presents a number of possibilities and challenges in terms of the storage and retrieval of this data.

36.3.1 Patient demographics

In order that the correct images are stored and retrieved from the correct files, it is crucially important that the correct patient demographic data are entered into the system. Different systems require different inputs and these can usually be entered from barcode readers or other input devices. In many cases, an important identifier is the patient's NHS number which is a unique identification number given, centrally, to each NHS patient. The same precise data must be entered for the patient each time he/she is examined – e.g. if on one occasion the patient is identified as 'John Smith' and on the next occasion he is identified as 'John S. Smith', then the system will treat these as two separate patients and will allocate separate files.

36.3.2 Sign on and password

The security of data in the store is important both in terms of patient confidentiality and to prevent unauthorized altering of the data. For this reason, most systems require the operator to sign on to the system (usually from a card with a magnetic strip) and to enter an appropriate password. This password may have an expiry date on it. When the person is identified by the signing on signature and password, the system will then give access only to appropriate data.

36.3.3 Bedside image retrieval

There are some situations where it is useful to review images of a patient at that patient's bedside. An example of this may be in the intensive therapy unit (ITU). By having the appropriate monitor and connections systems, it is possible for staff to review images and reports at the bedside. This can be very helpful when images are used to monitor the efficacy of a specific therapy.

36.3.4 Case conferences and teleconferences

When the image is recalled from the image store, it is possible to display this image on a number of monitors simultaneously. This means that a patient may be discussed in a case conference where the staff involved may not be in the same location or even in the same hospital. This facility is especially useful where the possibility of transferring a patient from one hospital to another is being discussed.

36.3.5 Teleradiology

Because the digital image can be transmitted from one site to another by any secure link then it is possible for images produced in one location to be reported by a radiologist or a radiographer in another location. This facility is extremely useful where the geographical spread of hospitals is great or when a second opinion is required outwith normal working hours.

36.4 PICTURE ARCHIVING AND COMMUNICATIONS SYSTEMS (PACS)

Figure 36.3 shows the structure of a typical PACS system. The system is centred around the archive server. Various imaging modalities (or input modules), e.g. digital radiographic (DR), can input data to this server. This image can then be acquired by a radiology workstation where the image appearances are reported. The image and the report are then returned to the archive server. Information from the hospital information system (HIS) can be acquired via the archive server – this could be information required for the image report, e.g. the patient's blood pressure. Similarly, information is available through the archive server from the radiology information system (RIS) – this could be something like a list of any other radiological examinations booked for this patient. Data from the archive server can be sent to remote locations, e.g. peripheral hospitals, via the web server. After an appropriate time, data are transferred from the archive server to the data archive for-long term storage. Because the various components of a PACS must be able to 'speak to each other' then it is important that they comply with Digital Imaging and Communications in Medicine (DICOM)

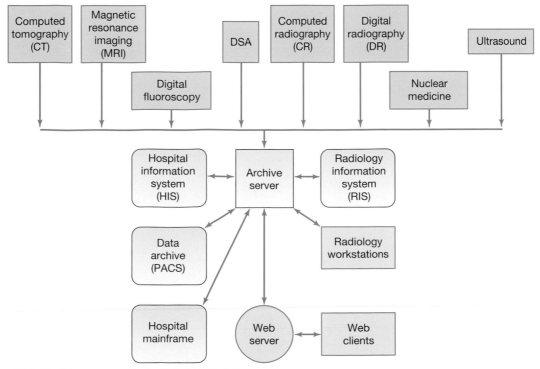

Figure 36.3 Principle components of a typical PACS design.

compatibility. This means that, for example, the RIS may be from a different manufacture to the HIS but both systems are still able to communicate.

36.5 DIGITAL IMAGING AND COMMUNICATION IN MEDICINE (DICOM)

DICOM is a global information technology standard which allows network communication between the various components of a PACS. The DICOM standard covers the handling, storage and transmission of medical information. The DICOM statements were originally written by the National Electrical Manufacturers Association (NEMA) in 1985 and these statements have been modified since then. NEMA still holds the copyright for the DICOM statements. All manufacturers of digital medical imaging equipment boast DICOM compatibility but the statements must be read carefully to determine the extent of the compatibility. If the DICOM standard is properly applied, then scanners, servers, workstations, printers and network hardware from different manufacturers can be incorporated into a PACS.

Summary

In this chapter, you should have learnt the following:
- The possibilities for image processing presented because of digital imaging (see Sect. 36.2).
- Methods of Image Storage and Retrieval (see Sect. 36.3).
- The basis of a PACS and its purpose in Radiology (see Sect. 36.4)
- The importance of DICOM compatibility for components of a PACS (see Sect. 36.5).

FURTHER READING

There are many sites on the Internet where the manufacturers of digital equipment give information on their specific technologies. In addition, you may find the following useful.

Carter, C.E., Veale, B.L., 2008. Digital Radiography and PACS. Mosby Elsevier, Missouri.

Siegel, E.L., Kolodner, R.M. (Eds.), 1999. Filmless Radiology. Springer, New York.

Part | 8 |

Applications of radiographic physics

Chapter | 37 |

Radionuclide imaging

37.1 AIM

The aim of this chapter is to introduce the reader to the basis of the technology used in radionuclide imaging. The information available on a nuclear medicine scan will be compared with the information available on other forms of medical imaging.

37.2 BASIC CONCEPT OF RADIONUCLIDE IMAGING

The basic concept of radionuclide imaging involves a three-stage process:

1. A suitable radionuclide is introduced into the patient – this is usually an artificially produced radionuclide.
2. The radionuclide is allowed to concentrate in a specific organ.
3. The organ is scanned using an appropriate scanner, e.g. a gamma camera.

37.3 PRODUCTION OF ARTIFICIALLY PRODUCED RADIONUCLIDES

There are three common ways of producing artificially produced radionuclides which are then used in radionuclide imaging. These are:

1. irradiating materials in a nuclear reactor
2. using a technetium generator
3. using a medical cyclotron.

37.3.1 The nuclear reactor

The nuclear reactor (or pile) produces heat energy by controlled fission (see Sect. 19.9). The heat generated within the reactor raises the temperature of a coolant which in turn is used to heat water to produce steam. The steam can then drive very powerful electric generators. This is the basis of nuclear power stations.

A simplified diagram of such a reactor is shown in Figure 37.1 (see page 272). The controlled fission is produced by using the neutrons of fissile decay to produce further fission in other atoms. Thus, a sustained reaction can be

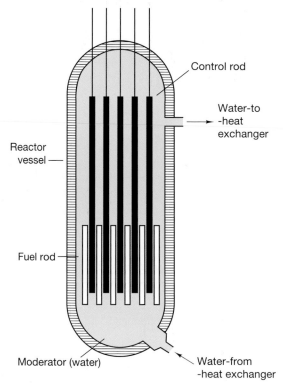

Figure 37.1 Simplified diagram of a pressurised water nuclear reactor.

set up where one neutron released during the fission of a nucleus will interact with another nucleus to produce fission of that nucleus with the release of further neutrons.

Nuclear reactors are important in radionuclide imaging in that they allow us to insert samples into the neutron flux within the reactor. This results in neutrons being inserted into nuclei to allow the manufacture of *artificial radionuclides*. An example of this is that stable molybdenum-98 can be made to absorb a neutron to produce the radionuclide molybdenum-99. The reaction may be shown using the equation below:

Equation 37.1

$$^{98}_{42}\text{Mo} + n \rightarrow ^{99}_{42}\text{Mo} + \gamma$$

37.3.2 The technetium generator

It is not feasible to produce nuclei with very short half-lives at a remote site and then transport these to the hospital. Such radionuclides are produced at the hospital's radiopharmacy either by the use of a technetium generator or by the use of a medical cyclotron.

The *technetium generator* used in nuclear medicine is an important example of the production of artificial radionuclides. As mentioned in Section 37.3.1, if molybdenum-98 is placed in a neutron stream, the nuclei of the molybdenum atoms can be made to absorb the neutrons to produce

molybdenum-99. The capture of a neutron raises the energy of the resulting molybdenum-99 nuclei and each loses this energy by the prompt emission of a gamma-ray.

A molybdenum-99/alumina column is in the centre of the generator, as shown in Figure 37.2 (see page 272). The molybdenum-99 has a half-life of 67 hours and decays to form technetium-99m by β^--particle emission, as shown below:

Equation 37.2

$$^{99}_{42}\text{Mo} \rightarrow ^{99}_{43}\text{Tc}^{\text{m}} + \beta^- + \nu^-$$

The $^{99}_{43}\text{Tc}^{\text{m}}$ is eluted (or flushed) from the generator at regular intervals as sodium pertechnetate. This radionuclide, which is in liquid form, may be used for a number of radionuclide imaging situations. The $^{99}_{43}\text{Tc}^{\text{m}}$ decays to $^{99}_{43}\text{Tc}$ by the emission of a gamma-ray of energy 140 keV. The metastable radionuclide has a half-life of 6 hours. Clearly, after a period of time, the activity of the molybdenum-99, and hence its ability to produce technetium 99m, will be reduced and the technetium generator must have its molybdenum-99/alumina column replaced.

A number of other radionuclides used in nuclear medicine can be produced from stable materials when they are bombarded with particles but further discussion about their production is beyond the scope of this section

37.3.3 Production of radionuclides using a cyclotron

The type of cyclotron used in nuclear medicine to produce artificial radionuclides by the bombardment of stable substances will briefly be described. A simple diagram of such a device is shown (see Fig. 37.3) (see page 272). The cyclotron consists of an evacuated cylinder which has an ion source placed at its centre. Ions from this source are influenced by strong axial and radial magnetic fields. This causes acceleration of the ions in circular paths of increasing radius. This ion beam achieves significant velocity and can be made to interact with materials placed at the exit port of the cyclotron. This interaction causes nuclear changes in these materials and we can produce neutron-deficient nuclei (see Sect. 19.5.1) which are capable of positron emission. Such materials form the basis of the radiopharmaceuticals used in positron emission tomography (PET) scanning. Figure 37.4 (see page 272) shows a photograph of such a medical cyclotron.

37.4 CLINICALLY USEFUL RADIONUCLIDES

Radionuclides are used to diagnose and to treat certain conditions. When they are used for diagnosis, they may be labelled (chemically linked) to a certain *radiopharmaceutical*, thus encouraging their uptake by specific body

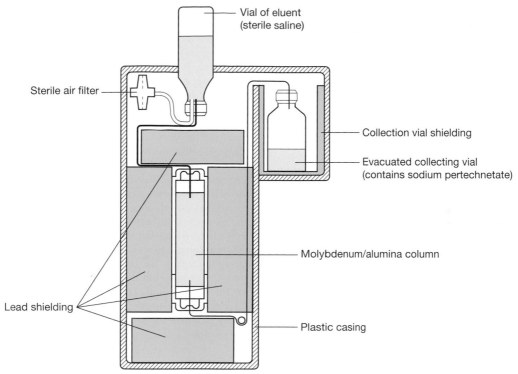

Figure 37.2 Principal features of a technetium-99m generator.

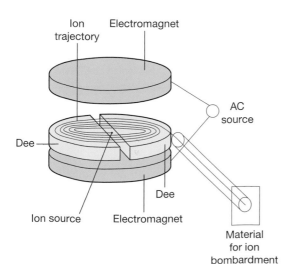

Figure 37.3 The main components of a medical cyclotron.

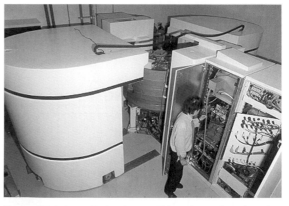

Figure 37.4 A medical cyclotron. This cyclotron is undergoing maintenance. The position of the Dees is clearly visible. *Photograph courtesy of the Department of Nuclear Medicine, Aberdeen Royal Infirmary.*

parts. The labelled radionuclide may then be injected into, or ingested by, the patient. Such diagnostic techniques in nuclear medicine have three main uses:

1. To provide numerical or graphical information on organ physiology, e.g. technetium-labelled diethylene triamine penta-acetic acid (DTPA) will give information on the rate of excretion of this radionuclide by the kidneys, thus giving information on renal function.

2. To produce an image of organ physiology on a gamma camera, e.g. $^{99}_{43}\text{Tc}^{\text{m}}$ as pertechnetate may be injected into the patient to produce images of the skeletal physiology; this is for very useful early detection of metastatic spread into bone.

3. To produce information on organ physiology using PET scanning (see Ch. 40), e.g. brain scans using fluorodeoxyglucose can produce images of cerebral physiology indicating the levels of cerebral activity for specific tasks.

A list of the radioisotopes which are commonly used is given in Table 37.1 (see page 275).

For the diagnostic purposes of imaging or charting organ physiology, only gamma-ray emission or positron emission is useful. This is because particles (α or β) emitted are absorbed very efficiently by the patient's tissues. If the particles are absorbed by the patient and do not reach the imaging or counting device, they contribute a radiation dose to the patient but give no diagnostic information. In the case of positron emission, the positron itself is rapidly annihilated by collision with an electron (see Sect. 27.5.3) but the annihilation radiation is detected by suitable detectors in a PET scanner (see Ch. 40).

The ideal radionuclide for imaging should:

- have a short half-life – approximately twice the length of time from injection into the patient to completion of the scan
- emit gamma-rays of relatively low energy, so that these are easily detected and do not pose a major hazard to others because of their penetrating power
- emit no particles as part of its decay pattern as these add significantly to the patient dose
- be readily labelled to allow its uptake by specific organs
- be readily excreted by the patient
- be easily generated in the radiopharmacy.

In many ways $^{99}_{43}\text{Tc}^m$ is the almost ideal radionuclide for scanning purposes.

37.5 ORGAN SCANNING

37.5.1 NaI crystals and photomultipliers

A crystal of sodium iodide with a thallium activator is one of the most efficient scintillators developed. The thallium impurities act as luminescent centres (see Ch. 24) and about 10–15% of the energy deposited in the crystal is converted to light energy. The maximum light emission is in the blue part of the spectrum with a wavelength of 420 nm. The sodium iodide crystals are mounted in containers called cans to prevent them absorbing moisture from the atmosphere and becoming cloudy. One face of the crystal is attached to a transparent glass window and all other surfaces are in contact with a white reflective powder (magnesium oxide) so that as much light as possible is directed at the back of the crystal.

The back of the crystal is in optical contact with a photomultiplier tube, as shown in Figure 37.5 (see page 276). If a gamma-ray is absorbed by the crystal (at point P on the diagram), this results in the emission of light in all directions. A fairly high percentage of this light reaches the photocathode of the *photomultiplier tube*. The photocathode consists of a thin coating of a mixture of alkaline salts deposited on the inner wall of the face of the photomultiplier tube. About 10–25% of the light photons reaching the photocathode cause it to emit electrons by the photoelectric effect (see Sect. 23.5) and these electrons are accelerated through the tube to a series of positively charged plates called dynodes. The surface of these dynodes is coated with a layer of a secondary electron emitter so that each dynode produces approximately six times as many electrons as fall on it. As a result of this process, one electron released at the photocathode may result in one million electrons being collected by the anode of the photomultiplier. The collection of this charge occurs at a very short time interval after the initial electron is released by the photocathode (normally $<10^{-6}$ s) and so a pulse of electricity is produced, the magnitude of the pulse being proportional to the energy of the absorbed gamma-ray photon.

Insight

If the photomultiplier tube contains n dynodes, each of which releases six electrons for one incident electron, then the electron gain in the photomultiplier tube is 6^n. Thus, for a 10-dynode tube, the gain would be 6^{10} which is just over 60 000 000 electrons and represents a charge at the anode of about 10 picocoulombs.

A spectrum of these pulses will not produce the discrete gamma energies emitted by the radioactive source because of the statistical nature of the light production in the crystal and the electron multiplication in the photomultiplier. This is shown in Figure 37.6 (see page 276), where the numbers of pulses of a given height are plotted. The true spectrum would be a line at the centre of the photopeak, as this corresponds to the energy of the gamma-rays absorbed by photoelectric absorption. In addition to the gamma-rays absorbed by photoelectric absorption, some of the gamma-rays undergo Compton scattering (see Sect. 23.6) within the crystal and then escape from the crystal with no further interactions. Such scattering interactions result in energy being deposited in the crystal which is

Table 37.1 Radionuclides commonly used in medicine

APPLICATION	NUCLIDE	$t_{1/2}$	DECAY MODE	GAMMA ENERGY (MeV)	MAXIMUM BETA ENERGY (MeV)	USES
Diagnostic						
Organ physiology	$^{131}_{53}I$	8.04 days	β^-, γ	0.364	0.61	Thyroid uptakes (NaI)
	$^{132}_{53}I$	2.3 h	β^-, γ	0.67, 0.78	2.12	Renal function studies (iodohippurate)
	$^{99}_{43}Tc^m$	6 h	IT	0.140	–	Renal function studies (DTPA)
	$^{99}_{43}Tc^m$	6 h	IT	0.140	–	Imaging of brain, kidney, liver, lung, spleen, skeleton
	$^{113}_{49}In^m$	90 min	IT	0.390	–	Imaging of brain, kidney, liver
	$^{75}_{34}Se$	121 days	EC	0.14, 0.27	–	Imaging of pancreas
	$^{68}_{31}Ga$	68 min	β^+, EC	0.51	1.89	Imaging of tumours and inflammatory lesions
	$^{81}_{36}Kr$	13 s	IT	0.19	–	Pulmonary function (ventilation) studies
	$^{133}_{54}Xe$	5.3 days	β^-, γ	0.081	0.34	Cerebral blood flow, pulmonary function (ventilation) studies
Tracers	$^{3}_{1}H$	12.3 years	β^-	–	0.018	Used for a large variety of studies
	$^{14}_{6}C$	5760 years	β^-	–	0.115	Used in the estimation of cellular volumes
	$^{35}_{16}S$	87.2 days	β^-	–	0.167	
	$^{43}_{19}K$	22 h	β^-, γ	0.37, 0.61	0.83	Used for a variety of blood studies
	$^{51}_{24}Cr$	27.8 days	EC	0.32	–	
	$^{59}_{27}Fe$	445 days	β^-, γ	1.10, 1.29	0.46	
	$^{57}_{27}Co$	270 days	EC	0.112	–	Used for the investigation of pernicious anaemia
	$^{58}_{27}Co$	71 days	β^+, EC	0.51, 0.81	0.485	
Therapy						
By injection	$^{32}_{15}P$	14.3 days	β^-	–	1.71	Phosphate used for the treatment of polycythaemia vera
	$^{90}_{39}Y$	62.2 h	β^-	–	2.27	Used as a colloid for the treatment of some lymphatic cancers
By ingestion	$^{131}_{53}I$	8.04 days	β^-, γ	0.364	0.61	Treatment of hyperthyroidism or thyroid cancer
Interstitial	$^{182}_{73}Ta$	115 days	βs, γs	Wide range	Wide range	Localized treatment of cancer by insertion of needles, tubes or wires of the radionuclide
	$^{192}_{77}Ir$	74 days	βs, γs	Wide range	Wide range	
	$^{137}_{55}Cs$	30 years	β^-, γ	0.662	0.51	
Teletherapy	$^{137}_{55}Cs$	30 years	β^-, γ	0.662	0.51	External beams of gamma radiation from the nuclides are used to treat cancers
	$^{60}_{27}Co$	5.3 years	β^-, γ	1.17, 1.33	0.31	
Radioimmunoassay						
	$^{125}_{53}I$	60 days	EC	0.027, 0.035	–	Used to detect small quantities of hormones

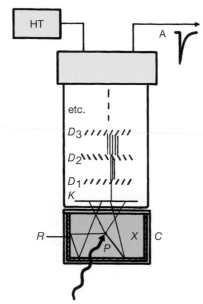

Figure 37.5 A scintillation detector using sodium iodide. D_1, D_2, etc., dynodes; *C*, crystal can; *K*, photocathode; *R*, powdered reflector; *X*, NaI(Tl) crystal.

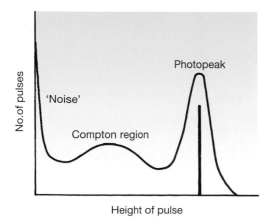

Figure 37.6 A typical gamma-ray spectrum using sodium iodide.

at the dynodes which may strike the photocathode and cause it to release electrons. The electrons produced by both of the above mechanisms produce no useful signal and are referred to as 'noise pulses' (see Fig. 37.6).

37.5.2 The use of solid scintillation counters in medicine

It is usual practice to count only the pulses which occur in the photopeak of the spectrum, particularly when investigating the activity and distribution of a radionuclide within a patient's body. This is achieved by the use of a *pulse height analyser* (PHA) which will only produce an electrical output signal if the input pulse lies within a certain range – this range is adjusted to cover the photopeak for the particular radionuclide. Pulses from the PHA are counted on a scalar for a time determined by the timer (see Fig. 37.7). The number of counts obtained is directly related to the activity being measured and may be compared to a normal range of values for that structure.

An example of such a study will now be considered. The patient is given iodine-131 in the form of sodium iodide. The iodine component of this is taken up by the thyroid gland. The thyroid uptake may then be counted using equipment similar to that illustrated in Figure 37.7. The gamma-rays emitted from the thyroid are detected by the lead-shielded sodium iodide crystal and those which lie within the photopeak are counted as described above.

The possibility of gamma-rays emitted outside the thyroid (see rays 3 and 4) being counted is reduced by the lead collimator – this is the shaded area in Figure 37.7. The selection of a specific photopeak by the PHA allows the counter to reject radiations which impinge on the crystals as a result of Compton scattering of the gamma-rays (see ray 2). The uptake count is obtained by expressing the thyroid uptake as a percentage of the total radiation ingested by the patient. Typical figures for a '24-hour uptake' lie between 10% and 25%. An overactive thyroid will give a higher figure and an underactive thyroid has a lower figure.

37.5.3 The gamma camera

The gamma camera was first developed by HO Anger in 1958 and the camera and its associated technology have shown considerable progress since then. Many modern gamma cameras are dual headed so that scanning information in two plains can be collected simultaneously (see Fig. 37.8). The structure of the gamma camera and its associated circuitry is shown in Figure 37.9 (see page 278). The gamma camera is a specialized type of scintillation counter where the position as well as the count of the scintillations within a thin NaI(Tl) crystal (or multiple

less than the energy of the gamma-rays and so smaller pulses are produced in the photomultiplier. These pulses produce a 'Compton peak', as shown in Figure 37.6.

Some very-low-energy pulses are produced by the release of electrons from the photocathode by thermionic emission. There are also some positively charged ions produced

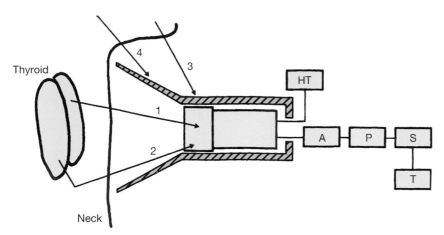

Figure 37.7 A scintillation detector used to measure activity within the thyroid gland. *A*, amplifier; *P*, pulse height analyser (PHA); *S*, scalar; *T*, timer.

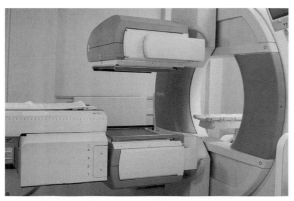

Figure 37.8 Photograph of a modern gamma camera. Note that the camera is double headed so that information from two surfaces of the body (e.g. anterior and posterior) can be collected simultaneously. *Photograph courtesy of the Department of Nuclear Medicine, Aberdeen Royal Infirmary.*

crystals) are obtained using a number of photomultipliers. A multichannel parallel collimator similar to that shown in Figure 37.7 ensures that only gamma-rays which are at right angles to the crystal face can enter the camera. A geometrical arrangement of photomultiplier tubes – of which there are typically around 120 – allows the position and the intensity of the scintillation produced in the crystal to

be measured. This allows us to display a picture of certain physiological processes within the body. This ability to image a dynamic physiological process makes the gamma camera a very powerful tool in the detection of pathologies where the physiology of the structure is disrupted.

37.5.4 SPECT imaging

The acronym SPECT stands for *single photon emission computed tomography* and is now a useful tool in many nuclear medicine departments. Here a gamma camera is mounted on a suitable gantry so that it can either rotate round the patient or can move along the long axis of the patient. If the camera rotates around the patient, it produces a series of axial scans whereas the camera moving over the body produces a longitudinal scan (not unlike the scans produced by the old rectilinear scanners). If we consider the production of an axial scan, the camera is made to rotate around the patient as a series of stepped rotations. Each step is an equal arc e.g. 1° and information is collected at each step of the rotation. In the stepped rotation described, 360 different images would be collected in a complete rotation and these are then reconstructed to produce an axial image. The reconstruction techniques are similar to those used in CT scanning. This technique has a number of uses in nuclear medicine, mainly in cardiac profusion imaging and in oncology.

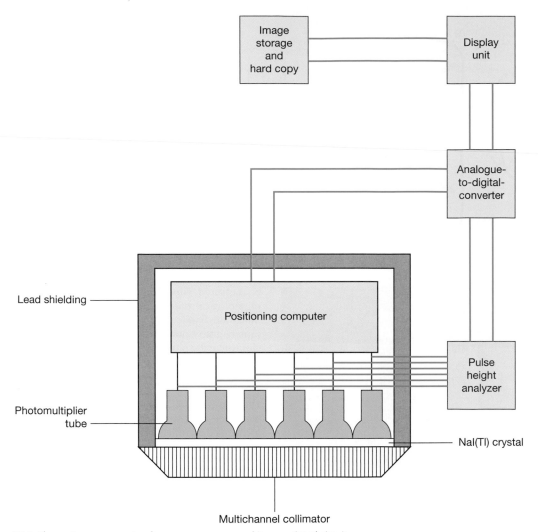

Figure 37.9 The main components of a gamma camera and its associated circuitry.

Summary

In this chapter, you should have learnt the following:
- The basic concept of radionuclide imaging (see Sect. 37.2).
- The production of artificially produced radionuclides (see Sect. 37.3).
- An overview of clinically useful radionuclides (see Sect. 37.4).
- The basis of radionuclide organ scanning (see Sect. 37.5).

FURTHER READING

Early, P.J., Sodee, D.B., 1995. Principles and Practice of Nuclear Medicine, second ed. Mosby, St Louis.

Chapter | 38 |

CT scanning

38.1 AIM

The aim of this chapter is to provide its readers with an overview that will enable them to understand the basics of the complex computed tomography (CT) scanning process.

38.2 INTRODUCTION

It is difficult for today's radiographers and radiologists to imagine working in an imaging department without a CT scanner, which was first demonstrated in 1973 by its inventor, Sir Godfrey Hounsfield. It revolutionized many imaging procedures, making dangerous interventional techniques unnecessary. It also gave improved demonstration of other body parts, especially soft tissue and overlying structures, which are difficult to demonstrate using conventional techniques. The physics and mathematics of CT imaging is a complex topic. This chapter provides the reader with an overview that will enable them to understand the basics of the process.

38.3 THE DEVELOPMENT OF THE CT SCANNER

The first generation of CT scanners was of the translate–rotate type. A single source consisting of a finely collimated pencil beam was focused on a single detector that moved on a frame in a transverse direction across the body, the gantry on which the source and detector was mounted then rotated through 1° and another transverse movement was made. As can be imagined, this was a very slow process requiring approximately 5 minutes to produce a single slice. This restricted scanning to the demonstration of skeletal structures and soft tissues in which movement did not take place.

The second-generation scanners were still of the translate–rotate type. These used a fan-shaped beam and an arc of about 30 detectors. To compensate for the reduced beam attenuation at the periphery of the body, a 'bow tie' filter was placed between the source and the patient. The increased area covered in each translation and by the arc of detectors permitted rotation of 10° on each rotation producing a substantial reduction in the time per slice. However, because of the complexities of the translation–rotation movement, and due to the mass to be moved in the gantry, imaging times were still in the order of 2 seconds per slice.

The third-generation scanners were known as the rotate–rotate design. The width of the radiation beam and the arc of the detectors was increased to 60°. The geometry of the detector arc produced a constant source to detector distance, an advantage in image reconstruction, and also permitted better beam collimation reducing scatter formation. The increased detector arc had the effect of reducing time per slice to the order approximately 1 second, substantially reducing the risk of motion artifacts. The one major disadvantage with this system was that the failure of a single detector would result in the production of a 'ring' artefact. This could often be corrected by the image processing software.

The current (fourth-generation) scanners (see Figure 38.1) have what is sometimes termed a stationary–rotate

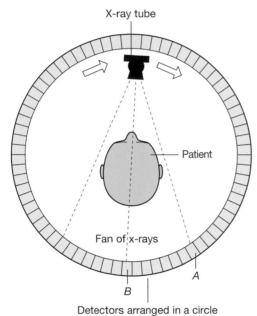

X-ray tube

Patient

Fan of x-rays

A

B

Detectors arranged in a circle

Figure 38.1 Section through the gantry showing the geometry of the X-ray tube and detectors.

geometry, in which the X-ray tube rotates within a stationary circle of detectors. The earlier sodium iodide scintillation detector linked to a photomultiplier tube has been replaced by ceramic scintillation detectors. These detectors have a better response to radiation of the energy range used in CT. The photomultipliers have been replaced by solid-state photodiodes. The photodiode is far smaller than the photomultiplier tube and requires considerably less power to operate.

The reduction in size has permitted the detectors to be arranged in a continuous circular array containing as many as 40 000 individual detectors while the X-ray tube rotates around the patient within the circle of detectors. Fourth-generation systems are free from the ring artefact problem associated with third-generation scanners and are capable of subsecond slice production times.

The medium-frequency generator has permitted the development of 'slip ring' technology. The low-tension supply is supplied to a stationary ring of contacts, while the high-tension (HT) transformer, rectification system and X-ray tube are mounted on a second ring which rotates about the stationary ring. This innovation has eliminated the need for the X-ray tube to return to its starting position to commence another rotation.

38.4 SCANNER SUBSYSTEMS

38.4.1 The patient support couch

This is about 1.5 metres long: the end nearest the gantry is often narrowed to pass through the aperture of the gantry. Prior to the scan, couch position height and longitudinal movement can be adjusted by the user; during the scan, couch movement is computer controlled.

38.4.2 The gantry

The gantry (see Fig. 38.1) consists of a large box-like structure with a central aperture through which the patient is passed during the scan. Within the gantry are the X-ray tube, HT transformer, rectification system, collimators, detectors and the motor drive and control system to move the X-ray tube during the scan.

38.4.3 The X-ray generator

This uses a three-phase mains supply collected from the slip ring and has a medium-frequency output. Radiation output is often pulsed, with each pulse lasting for about 3 milliseconds. Pulsing permits the cooling of the X-ray tube between pulses and permits a higher generator rating. Generator output is monitored and controlled by an on-board microprocessor.

38.4.4 The X-ray tube

The X-ray tube is very different in design from the tube used for conventional radiography. It has a much larger and thicker anode and a higher heat capacity in the order of 6000 kilojoules with a cooling rate of 1000 kilojoule per minute. The heat load on the focal spot is calculated by a computer algorithm which automatically adjusts the mA to prevent overloading.

38.4.5 The computer subsystem

The computer subsystem is possibly the most important part of the scanner and has many different functions (Fig. 38.2 see page 281). The monitoring part of the system accepts input from input devices on the operator console and controls

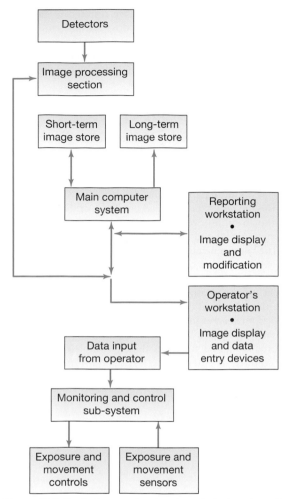

Figure 38.2 Block diagram showing the principal sections of the CT computer system.

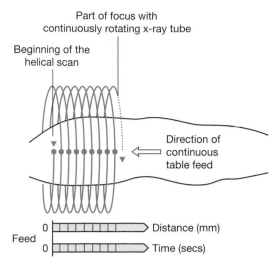

Figure 38.3 The principle of helical CT scanning (see text for details).

exposure and movement of the scanner during the scan. The main part of the system is concerned with data collection and manipulation. It collects the incoming data from the detector system and processes it. This requires the capacity to solve 25 000 simultaneous equations per second. It then passes the data to short-term storage and also displays the data as an image on the operator and reporting workstations. These data can be passed back to the image manipulation section to be reformatted to produce a different image on the workstations before the image is passed to long-term image storage.

38.5 ADVANCES IN CT TECHNOLOGY

The forth-generation configuration has made the development of helical and multislice techniques possible. These will now be examined in more detail.

38.5.1 Helical or spiral CT

Helical or spiral CT was first introduced in the early 1990s following the development of slip ring technology. This meant there was no longer a need for tube rotation to stop and return to its starting point and advance the patient table into the gantry before commencing another rotation, effectively ending the necessity for the 'shoot-move' sequence followed with conventional CT. In conventional CT, slice width was determined by the collimation of the beam. This is not possible with helical CT in which the data are produced as a continuous spiral of information (see Fig. 38.3).

With helical CT, the slice width is determined by two factors: beam collimation and pitch – the rate of longitudinal movement of the table through the gantry per revolution of the X-ray tube. The effect of varying pitch is shown in Figure 38.4 (see page 281). As with conventional CT, collimation and pitch are fixed for a given examination.

The *apparent* slice width is determined by a factor termed *index* used in the image reconstruction process. As index is a software function then it is variable and an image can be reconstructed using different index values, producing separate, contiguous or even overlapping 'slices'.

The major advantage of spiral CT is speed. A large patient volume can be scanned in a short period of time, typically 6–20 seconds. The patient can hold their breath for the entire exposure and artefacts due to motion blur are eliminated. With contrast studies, it is possible to demonstrate contrast flow through a complete system.

The major disadvantage of spiral scanning is loss of image resolution on the z-axis due to the continual couch movement. Higher resolution can be obtained by slowing down the rate of couch movement, but this prolongs scanning time and increases patient dose.

38.5.2 Multislice CT

The first multislice CT scanner, called the C TWIN, was developed in 1993 and, as the name implies, it employed a double ring of solid-state detectors, separated by an annular ring of tungsten to prevent cross-scatter between each ring of detectors.

This was rapidly followed by scanners using 4, 8, 18 and up to 64 rings of detectors. Instead of acquiring data from all the rings in multisclice array, improved technology makes it possible to select the rings that are activated, effectively producing different 'slice' widths as well as using all the elements in the detector array, producing separate, contiguous or even overlapping 'slices'. Multislice CT has been of particular benefit in CT angiography which relies on precise timing to ensure good demonstration of the arteries.

Other improvements in CT technology have resulted in reduction in component weight with faster rotation times of up to three rotations a second. Software improvements mean that it is now possible to resolve 0.35-mm voxels at a transverse speed of 19 cm per second on the z-axis.

The most recent innovations (2009) are multislice scanners with 320 detector rings. Detector arrays of this size enable cardiac CT angiograms and whole-brain perfusion studies to be carried out in a single exposure. One manufacturer has even produced a mobile CT scanner with 266 detector rings for use on hospital wards.

All of these improvements have resulted in the benefits of reduction in radiation dose to the patient and improved image resolution.

Improved software technology has resulted in the introduction of 3D imaging and the use of colour in the resultant image.

38.5.3 Dual-output CT

The pulsing of the X-ray tube output has meant that is has been possible to develop dual-output CT scanners using the output of the X-ray tube in which one exposure is made at 150 kVp followed by an exposure at 90 kVp. The resulting data from the detectors are merged. This technique results in increased emphasis of the differences in the absorption edges (see Ch. 23) between tissue and contrast agents and differing tissues.

The latest generation of dual-energy scanners makes use of two X-ray tubes operating at different energies and two banks of detectors resulting in a better balanced arrangement on the rotating ring. This has permitted increased rotation speeds of 0.28 seconds per rotation. As a result, couch movement in the z-axis can be increased by up to 43 cm per second. The combined result of this is much shorter scanning times so that a complete thorax can be scanned in 0.6 seconds (less than a heartbeat) and a whole body scanned in less than 5 seconds.

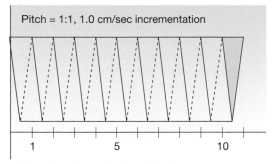

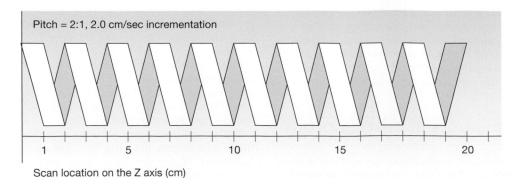

Figure 38.4 Effect of pitch (speed of couch movement) slice spacing for a given examination.

38.6 FORMATION OF THE CT IMAGE

The CT image differs from the image produced by other imaging modalities, in that the image is reconstructed from the data received by the image detectors in the image processing section of the computer system. The image processing section receives the data from the detectors as a continuous data stream. The first task it carries out is to convert thess data into picture elements or *pixels*; this is done using a complex mathematical function called *convoluted back projection*. The value of each pixel is in turn the summation of the attenuation of the X-ray beam by the tissues in the volume element or *voxel* to which the pixel relates (see Fig. 38.5). Each pixel is then allotted a CT number based on

the attenuation of the X-ray beam of the voxel. CT numbers range from −1000, which corresponds to air, to +4000, which corresponds to dense compact bone. Water has a CT number of zero. Table 38.1 indicates the approximate relationship between tissues and CT number (Hounsfield unit). The exact CT number for a given substance or tissue can be calculated using the formula:

Equation 38.1

$$CT\ number = \frac{k(\mu_t - \mu_w)}{\mu_w}$$

where μ_t is the attenuation coefficient of the substance or tissue, μ_w the attenuation coefficient of water and k a constant that determines the scaling factor of the range of CT number. The linear attenuation of a substance or tissue is, in turn, dependent on the kVp used for the examination.

The result of this process, which requires considerable computer processing power, is a 'slice' of data in which the bit depth of the image is approximately 2^{12}. This is beyond the range of shades of grey that can be displayed on the monitor screen and also the range of grey that can be perceived by the human eye.

Once this task is completed, the data pass out of the image processing section into a short-term image store where they are stored as a 'stack' of individual 'slices' and the bit depth is reduced to one within the display limitations of the monitor. The data are then copied to the operator's and radiologist's consoles where they are displayed according to the window selected.

Two factors are used in windowing: the window level which selects the CT number that will occupy the midpoint of the window, and window width which determines the total range of CT numbers displayed on the monitor. A wide window produces a low-contrast image with little difference between adjacent CT values, while a narrow

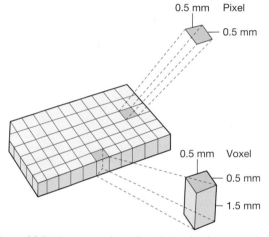

Figure 38.5 Diagram to show the relationship between pixels and voxels.

Labels in figure:
0.5 mm Pixel
0.5 mm
0.5 mm Voxel
0.5 mm
1.5 mm

Table 38.1 Approximate relationship between tissues and CT numbers	
Tissue	CT Number
Cortical bone	1,000
Fresh Blood (associated with acute trauma)	200
Muscle	50
White matter	45
Grey matter	40
Cerebrospinal fluid (CSF)	15
Water	0
Fat	−100
Lung tissue	−200
Air	−1,000

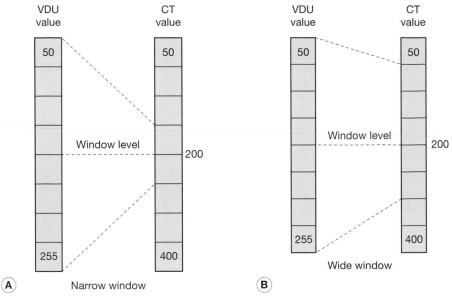

Figure 38.6 Diagram showing the effect of window width on the contrast range displayed on the monitor screen.

window produces a high-contrast image. CT numbers above and below the selected window depth are displayed as black or white respectively (see Fig. 38.6).

Because the data are only copied to the operator's and radiologist's consoles, they can be modified by either the operator or the radiologist to emphasize different tissues leaving the original data in the short-term image store. However, in addition to independent windowing operations, the radiologist console can carry out further operations. Additional software options permit the viewing of the images in the 'stack' as a series of projections in a longitudinal or even a transverse plane. This includes the selective masking of CT values to produce virtual 3D images.

For these operations to take place, the data in the short-term image store is copied back into the image processing system where the required algorithms are applied and the modified data are copied back to the radiologist's console. Once the radiologist has completed their part of the examination, the modified data are transferred in the final format to the long-term image store and the data in the short term image store are erased.

38.7 CT AND RADIATION DOSE

CT offers many advantages over conventional projection radiography. It eliminates the superimposition of structures in the area of interest and, because of its high-contrast resolution, differences between tissues with a difference of less than 1% in physical density can easily be distinguished. Finally, multiplanar reformatting permits the data from a single contiguous multislice scan or spiral

scan to be viewed as images in the axial, coronal or sagital planes, or even to perform 3D reconstructions from the data acquired. This has made examinations such as virtual colonoscopy possible, which is of particular value as it delivers a lower radiation dose than a conventional barium enema. Virtual bronchography (using argon gas as a contrast medium) is also possible, making this examination far less invasive and reducing the contrast medium risks associated with bronchography.

Angiography, both cardiac and abdominal, are also procedures which have become far less invasive through the use of CT. Pulmonary angiography in particular has proved very useful in ruling out pulmonary embolism because of its high sensitivity (greater than 90%). These factors have resulted in CT becoming the modality of choice for these procedures. CT is also a sensitive method for diagnosis of abdominal disease. It is used frequently in the staging of cancer and the follow up of its progress.

It is also a useful test to investigate acute abdominal pain (especially of the investigation of suspected aortic aneurysm and bowel obstruction). Other non-ionizing modalities such as magnetic resonance imaging (MRI) and ultrasound are used for investigations of the liver and renal stones. Unfortunately, despite improvements, CT remains a relatively high-dose modality, and although the latest dose-reduction software can result in significantly lower doses so that the dose from a CT of the chest can be reduced to below 1 mSv, this software is not yet available on all scanners.

Unfortunately, the greatly increased availability of CT, together with its value for an increasing number of conditions, has been responsible for a large rise in its popularity. So large has this rise been that the comprehensive

2000/2005 survey of medical radiation dose in the UK revealed that, although CT scans only constituted 7% of all radiological examinations, they contributed 47% of the total collective dose from medical X-ray examinations. Thus, increased CT usage has led to an overall rise in the total amount of medical radiation used, despite reductions in other areas.

This trend is not just restricted to the UK. In the United States, for example, in 1996 there were 64 CT scanners per 1 million population. In 1980 there were about 3 million CT scans performed compared to an estimated 62 million scans in 2006.

Table 38.2 shows typical radiation doses linked to different examinations.

As with all examinations involving the use of ionizing radiation, a major problem is the reduction of radiation dose. This can be achieved by the following:

- Where practicable, new software technologies should be used to reduce random noise and enhance

structures. These can reduce dose by as much as 70% while still producing high-quality images.
- All CT examinations should observe the diagnostic reference levels (DRLs) recommended by the Department of Health.
- The clinical benefit to the patient should be evaluated carefully against modalities such as ultrasound and MRI that do not use ionizing radiation.

Summary

In this chapter, you should have learnt the following:
- The differences between the first-, second- and third-generation CT scanners (see Sect. 38.3).
- The contents of the scanner gantry (see Sect. 38.4.2).
- The functions of the computer system (see Sect. 38.4.3).
- What is meant by 'slip ring technology' (see Sect. 38.5.1).
- How helical CT differs from conventional CT (see Sect. 38.5.1).
- The advantages of dual-energy CT scanning (see Sect. 38.5.3).
- The process of the formation of the CT image (see Sect. 38.5.6).
- The link between attenuation of the X-ray beam and CT number (see Sect. 38.6).
- Comparison between typical radiation doses from different CT and conventional radiographic examinations and means of reducing radiation dose from CT (see Sect. 38.7).

Table 38.2 Link between examination and radiation dose

EXAMINATION	TYPICAL DOSE (MSV)
Chest radiograph	0.1
Abdominal CT	5.3
Cardiac CT angiography	7 (although lower with the latest dose-reduction software)
Barium enema	15
Virtual CT colonoscopy	3.6

FURTHER READING

Bushong, S.C., 2008. Radiologic Science for Technologists: Physics, Radiobiology and Protection. Mosby, St Louis (Chapter 23).

Chapter | 39 |

Magnetic resonance imaging

39.1 AIM

The aim of this chapter is to describe the technique of magnetic resonance imaging (MRI), which is a powerful imaging tool capable of providing both anatomical and functional information on living tissues. Some key adjustable MR imaging parameters, such as TR (time to repetition) and TE (time to echo), are introduced and the appearances of standard MR image sequences are presented in order to allow their recognition in clinical practice. Available scanner technologies and MRI safety issues are summarized.

39.2 KEY PRINCIPLES OF MRI

From the middle of the twentieth century, the technique of *nuclear magnetic resonance* (NMR) was widely used in laboratories to study the signatures and concentrations of chemicals. Bloch and Purcell, working independently, had noted in 1946 that chemical samples placed in a strong magnetic field, when subjected to radiofrequency (RF) radiations at specific *resonant* frequencies, returned detectable and characteristic radiofrequency signals. At this point it would be useful to explain why this occurs. Atomic nuclei (hence the term *nuclear* in NMR) have an angular

momentum or *spin*, which means that they rotate on their axes, rather like tiny planets. They also have *magnetic dipole moments*. Note that a 'moment' in this context means a vector quantity with magnitude and direction, not a brief moment of time! In MRI, the term 'spin' is commonly used to refer to the rotating magnetic field orientation of an individual atomic nucleus, although strictly the term magnetic dipole moment is more correct.

> **Insight**
>
> Moving charges such as electrons produce a magnetic field and similarly a spinning positively charged proton can possess a magnetic field. It may seem surprising that spinning neutrons also possess magnetic fields. This is because they, like protons, are composed of smaller subatomic particles, some of which are charged. So we can think of both protons and neutrons contributing to the overall magnetic properties of atomic nuclei.

Normally the magnetic dipole moments of individual atomic nuclei, whether in a chemical sample or in a human body, are aligned randomly in all directions. There is no overall net magnetization. But if a powerful and uniform magnetic field is applied, the individual magnetic dipole moments tend to align:

- *either* with the external magnetic field (which is referred to in MRI as parallel or 'spin-up'). This is a low-energy state.
- *or* against the external magnetic field (which is referred to in MRI as antiparallel or 'spin-down'). This is a high-energy state.

There is normally a slight excess of magnetic dipole moments in the low-energy 'spin down' state, an excess which increases as the external magnetic field strength increases. These states are illustrated in Figure 39.1 (see page 288). The rotational or *precessional frequency* of the magnetic dipole moments is directly proportional to the external magnetic field strength. The Larmor equation describes this relationship:

Equation 39.1

$$\omega = \gamma B_0$$

where ω is the precessional frequency in Hertz, B_0 is the magnetic flux density of the external magnetic field in tesla and γ is a constant known as the *gyromagnetic ratio*. This dependence of precessional frequency on local magnetic field strength (since γ is constant) is a very important principle in MRI and has a host of applications.

The gyromagnetic ratio is set according to which chemical element is being used in NMR or MRI. The gyromagnetic ratio of hydrogen-1 is 42.6 MHz (million cycles per second) per tesla. Thus, hydrogen-1 nuclei precess at 42.6 MHz at a magnetic flux density of 1 tesla. Hydrogen is very abundant in water and biological molecules like fats, proteins and carbohydrates. This, coupled with the fact that its most common (H-1) nucleus has a strong magnetic signal, enables us to visualize many body tissues effectively.

Table 39.1 lists the gyromagnetic ratios of some nuclei used in MRI and magnetic resonance spectroscopy (MRS). MRI provides images of human anatomy, while MRS is an adaptation of NMR used to measure the strength of chemical signatures in living tissues, by providing spectra. Only hydrogen-1 has sufficient abundance and signal in the body to provide images.

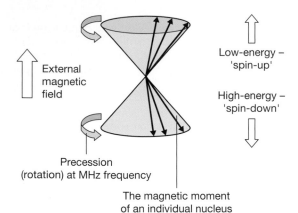

Figure 39.1 The precession of individual magnetic dipole moments placed in a strong external magnetic field.

Insight

It can be seen in Table 39.1 that nuclei which return a useful signal in MRI and MRS all have an odd number of nucleons (odd mass numbers). This is not a coincidence. The magnetic moments of individual nucleons tend to 'pair up' and cancel each other out in nuclei with even mass numbers, leaving no net magnetization. This is rather analogous to a situation that occurs among electrons orbiting atomic nuclei – these electrons tend to pair up in 'spin-up' and 'spin-down' states in chemical bonds, while unpaired electrons are chemically reactive.

The frequency of the returning radio wave signals received from nuclei in chemical samples or living tissues is influenced by the local chemical environment. This is largely due to the presence of electrons in chemical

Table 39.1 Some atomic nuclei used in MRI and MRS			
NUCLEUS (MASS NUMBER)	**GYROMAGNETIC RATIO (MHz PER TESLA)**	**RELATIVE SIGNAL STRENGTH**	**NOTES**
Hydrogen-1	42.6	100	The main nucleus used in MRI and MRS, since it is very common in the human body and has a good magnetic signal Consists of just a single proton
Carbon-13	10.7	1.45	Only 1% of carbon occurs as the magnetically useful C-13 isotope Used in MRS only C-12 has no useful magnetic properties
Fluorine-19	40.1	83	Not naturally present in the human body but can be used to label drugs and other molecules Used in MRS only
Phosphorus-31	17.2	6.6	Very useful for studying metabolic processes in molecules like ATP and ADP Used in MRS only

bonds, which slightly 'shield' nuclei to varying extents from the external magnetic field. Thus hydrogen nuclei (for example) in different chemical molecules (such as water, lactate, fat) precess at very slightly different speeds, according to the Larmor equation. This creates frequency shifts, known as *chemical shifts* in the radio wave signals received within a spectrum. This effect is the basis of nuclear magnetic resonance and magnetic resonance spectroscopy. In MRI, the chemical shift effect can result in artefacts. Figure 39.2 shows a hydrogen-1 spectrum obtained in an MRS procedure.

Magnetic resonance spectroscopy is a powerful tool for providing chemical information on lesions such as tumours, but requires large voxels, high magnetic field strength, a very homogeneous magnetic field and cannot provide 2D or 3D images of human anatomy.

Insight

A high magnetic field strength in the order of 1.5 tesla or greater is needed in MRS in order to increase the frequency shift (chemical shift) between chemicals so that they show up more clearly as distinct spectral peaks. For example, although the shift between water and fat is always 3.5 parts per million, the actual frequency difference is three times greater at a field strength of 3 tesla (where hydrogen-1 precessional frequency is $42.6 \times 3 = 127.8\,MHz$) than at 1 tesla (where hydrogen-1 precessional frequency is $42.6\,MHz$).

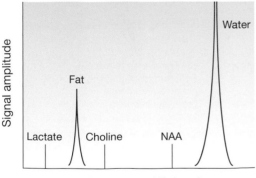

Figure 39.2 A hydrogen-1 (proton) spectrum obtained from MR spectroscopy. Note that, to avoid confusion, frequency is plotted from low (left) to high (right) on the *x*-axis, although in practice this would be plotted in reverse order. Units of frequency are typically parts per million (ppm) frequency shift. The shift between fat and water is 3.5 ppm. The peaks for water and fat are very large (larger than shown) relative to other chemicals. Lactate levels increase in anaerobic conditions, for example in tumours. Choline is a substrate for cell synthesis and reflects cell proliferation. NAA (N-acetyl aspartate) is a marker for neurons.

In 1971, Raymond Damadian provided an impetus to the development of actual clinical imaging using strong magnetic fields (magnetic resonance imaging or MRI) by suggesting that the radio wave signal *relaxation times* of different tissues might be indicative of the degree of tumour malignancy. Paul Lauterbur provided the first 2D MR image of a chemical sample in 1973 and suggested the term *zeugmatography* for the technique. Developments in clinical MRI continued in the United States and in the United Kingdom, led by Peter Mansfield and colleagues in the latter, with the first clinical scanners appearing in about 1980.

Clinical MRI almost always uses hydrogen-1 nuclei as the 'MR-active' signal source in the human body. When radiofrequency (RF) radiations are applied to a patient's body, placed in a powerful magnetic field, *at precisely the Larmor or precessional frequency of the hydrogen nuclei*, then *resonance* occurs and energy is transferred to the nuclei. Subsequently two types of tissue 'relaxations' or releases of radio energy from the patient (resulting in signals) occur *simultaneously*.

- The *longitudinal relaxation* process occurs relatively slowly over a time period typically up to several hundred milliseconds. In this process the overall tissue magnetization, which has been briefly 'flipped' by a *flip angle* α towards 90° from the external magnetic field direction by the RF energy input, subsequently returns to a position of 0°, parallel to the magnetic field. This is the basis of the T1 signal component in MRI.

- The *transverse relaxation* process occurs relatively quickly over a time period typically up to several tens of milliseconds. In this process the rotating magnetic moments of individual nuclei, which have been brought briefly into line (or *in phase*) by the RF energy input, subsequently fan out (or *dephase*). This is the basis of the T2 signal component in MRI.

These relaxation processes are illustrated in Figures 39.3 and 39.4 (see page 290).

Insight

The two processes of i) 'flipping' the overall magnetization towards 90° relative to the external magnetic field, and ii) putting the magnetic moments in phase, induces a strong electrical signal in a receiver coil placed at 90° to the main magnetic field. The frequency of this signal matches the precessional frequency of the magnetic moments of the nuclei. When they are all in phase, a powerful alternating current is induced in the receiver coil. For an analogy, we could think of the way a bright rotating lighthouse beam sweeps periodically towards an observer. Imagine if the light fanned out and went diffuse – the beam would be less effective. As the magnetic moments of the nuclei dephase in MRI, the signal in the receiver coil similarly fades out. This is called a *free induction decay* (FID).

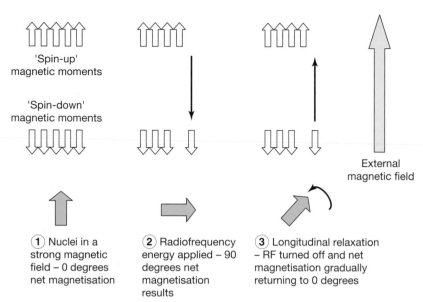

Figure 39.3 The *longitudinal relaxation process* for the magnetic moments of hydrogen nuclei in a strong magnetic field. Before RF energy is applied, there is a small excess of low-energy 'spin-up' magnetic moments, giving an overall magnetization of 0° (up in the diagram) parallel to the magnetic field. On the application of RF at the resonance frequency, some spins are promoted to the higher-energy 'spin-down' state and net magnetization is towards 90°. Removal of the RF energy causes gradual 'recovery' of overall net magnetization to 0°, with some spins returning to the low-energy state.

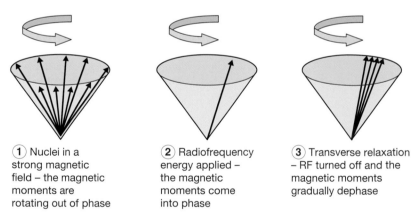

Figure 39.4 The *transverse relaxation process* for the magnetic moments of hydrogen nuclei in a strong magnetic field. Before RF energy is applied, the magnetic moments of individual nuclei are all precessing at the Larmor frequency and 'out of step' (out of phase) with each other. Think of them rotating at points occupying every minute of a clock face. When RF energy is applied, the magnetic moments all come briefly 'into step' (in phase), as if they were all rotating together in the 12 o'clock position on a clock face. When the RF energy is turned off, the magnetic moments all dephase.

The longitudinal relaxation process is also termed longitudinal recovery, or spin–lattice relaxation. It occurs relative to the longitudinal plane (0°) and involves transfer of energy to the atomic lattice of the material. Note that although RF energy causes heating of human tissues, this is via electromagnetic induction and not flipping of the magnetic moments of nuclei.

The transverse relaxation process is also called spin–spin relaxation, because the process of dephasing occurs within the transverse plane and occurs between magnetic moments (spins).

Some important practical features of the longitudinal and transverse recovery processes are summarized in Table 39.2 (see page 291).

Table 39.2 Relaxation of the radiofrequency signal in MRI

LONGITUDINAL RELAXATION	TRANSVERSE RELAXATION
Occurs slowly overall	Occurs quickly overall
Fat relaxes relatively quickly and water slowly	Fat relaxes relatively quickly and water slowly
Is the basis of T1 weighted imaging	Is the basis of T2 weighted imaging
Using T1 image weighting, fat appears bright and water appears dark	Using T2 image weighting, fat appears grey and water appears bright
Good for depicting anatomy	Good for depicting pathology (fluid filled)
Tissues which enhance with gadolinium contrast agent appear bright with T1 weighting	Tissues which enhance with iron oxide contrast agent appear dark with T2 weighting

39.3 IMAGE WEIGHTINGS, SEQUENCES AND APPEARANCES

Leaving the physics aside for a moment, it is very important to be able to interpret the appearance of MRI images. In this section, we will first consider the appearances of T1, T2, proton density and fat or fluid 'saturated' images.

Remember that on a T1 weighted image, in terms of the longitudinal recovery process, fat relaxes quickly and appears bright. Fluid relaxes slowly and appears dark.

Look at Figure 39.5, a *T1 weighted image*. The subcutaneous fat appears bright. Cerebrospinal fluid in the lateral ventricle appears dark. White matter in the corpus callosum of the brain appears relatively bright, because it contains axons with fatty myelin sheaths. Cortical bone appears dark, because its hydrogen-1 atoms are tightly bound within a crystalline lattice and transverse relaxation between spins occurs so quickly that no signal can be sampled. But bone marrow appears bright, because it contains fat. Flowing blood in the sagittal venous sinus appears dark, because in spin echo imaging the flowing hydrogen atoms pass through an imaging slice before they can return a signal. This is known as the *time of flight effect*.

On an MRI image, you may see the terms TR (time to repetition) and TE (time to echo) stated. The TR is the time in milliseconds between one radio wave excitation of the atomic nuclei and the next. The TE is the time in milliseconds between a radio wave excitation and the received signal (which is called an *echo*). This is not to be confused with echoes in ultrasound! T1 weighted images use a short TR and short TE and this contributes to making a T1 image relatively quick to acquire. It is often relatively free from motion blur. Figure 39.6 (see page 292) illustrates the terms TR and TE.

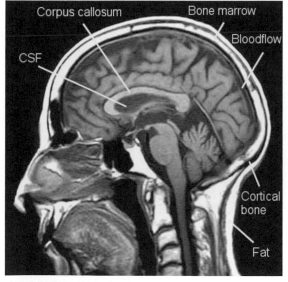

Figure 39.5 A T1 weighted sagittal spin echo image of the head and neck.

Now let's look at Figure 39.7 (see page 292), a *T2 weighted image*. On a T2 weighted image, fluid appears bright. Fluid relaxes more slowly than fat in terms of the transverse recovery process. The bright signal from CSF in the lateral ventricles and oedema surrounding a brain tumour can be seen. Notice that fat and cortical bone appear grey or dark (the latter for the reason considered above) and are not well seen here. Grey matter, which contains many fluid-containing cell bodies, appears relatively bright, while the fatty myelinated axons of white matter appear grey. Once again flowing blood, seen here in two end-on blood vessels, does not give a signal as this

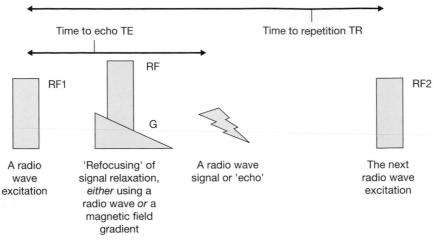

Figure 39.6 The TR is the time between two RF excitation pulses. The TE is the time between an RF excitation pulse and a signal. Adjustment of the TR and TE affects the image weighting in MRI.

Insight

In MRI, a *gradient* is a linear and regular variation in magnetic flux density, from low to high. There are many uses of gradients in MRI. In *gradient echo* imaging, a magnetic field gradient is used to refocus a signal, giving a *gradient echo*. Gradient echo MRI sequences are fast and have the characteristic that flowing blood appears bright. (Spin echo sequences, which use an RF pulse to refocus the signal and give a *spin echo* are relatively slow, high contrast and give no signal from flowing blood.) Gradients are also used in MRI to obtain slices in the sagittal, coronal and axial planes. Changing a gradient in a regular way across a patient alters the local precessional frequencies and phases of the rotating magnetic moments of hydrogen-1 nuclei. This enables a unique 'address' of the nuclei to be obtained. Direct multiplanar imaging is a major strength of MRI.

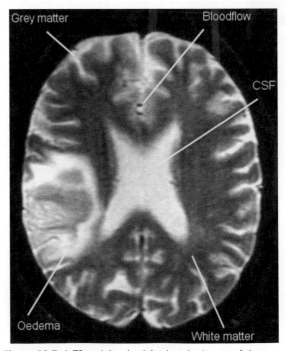

Figure 39.7 A T2 weighted axial spin echo image of the brain.

is a spin echo image. T2 weighted images use a long TR and long TE and this contributes to making a T2 image relatively slow to acquire. It is more often affected by motion blur than a T1 image.

You may also encounter *proton density weighted* images in MRI. Such images tend to appear rather low in contrast compared with T1 or T2 images and are simply based on the number of 'protons' (in fact the numbers of hydrogen-1 nuclei) present within the image. Tissues with a high 'proton density' such as fluid and fat appear relatively bright. To achieve a proton density image, the contribution of T1 and T2 weighting must be minimized and so a long TR (to reduce T1 weighting) and a short TE (to minimise T2 weighting) are used.

There are a number of imaging techniques commonly used in MRI, as summarized in Table 39.3.

Table 39.3 Common imaging techniques used in MRI

TECHNIQUE	EXPLANATION
Spin echo (SE)	A standard MRI technique which uses a signal refocusing RF pulse to generate a spin echo
STIR (short time inversion recovery)	A spin echo sequence based on RF pulses which reduces fat signal and increases the conspicuity of fluid-containing pathologies
FLAIR (fluid attenuated inversion recovery)	A spin echo sequence based on RF pulses which reduces fluid signal and increases the conspicuity of pathologies which could otherwise be masked by fluid
Fat saturation or 'fat sat'	An alternative means of reducing fat signal which works by targeting RF pulses at the precessional frequency of fat
Inversion recovery (IR)	A spin echo sequence which enables contrast between different tissues to be amplified and finely controlled
Dual echo	A spin echo sequence which contains two refocusing RF pulses and simultaneously provides proton density and T2 image information
FSE (fast spin echo), also called TSE (turbo spin echo)	A rapid spin echo sequence which includes several signal-refocusing RF pulses rather than just one
RARE (rapid acquisition with relaxation enhancement) or single-shot FSE	A very fast spin echo sequence which uses a very long train of refocusing RF pulses and obtains all information from an imaging slice in a 'single shot'
Gradient echo (GE)	A standard and fast MRI technique which uses a signal refocusing gradient to generate a gradient echo. Results in T2 weighting in which magnetic susceptibility effects are strong Flowing blood appears bright
Echo planar imaging (EPI)	A very fast gradient echo sequence which uses a very long train of refocusing gradients and obtains all information from an imaging slice in a 'single shot' or 'multi-shot'
Magnetic resonance angiography (MRA)	A gradient echo technique in which flowing blood signal is amplified and stationary tissue signal is suppressed Includes time of flight (TOF) and phase contrast (PC) techniques which do not use gadolinium contrast media and contrast enhanced (CE) techniques which do

39.4 MRI EQUIPMENT – SCANNERS AND COILS

There are three main types of MRI magnet systems in clinical use, with most systems being *superconducting*, since these offer the greatest field strength and image quality. High-field magnets, which typically operate at magnetic flux densities of 1.5 to 3 tesla, offer the advantages of high signal-to-noise ratios (which permit good image resolution and image scanning) and suitability for a range of applications including MR spectroscopy, diffusion imaging and functional imaging.

- Superconducting magnets typically operate at magnetic flux densities up to 3 tesla for clinical use.

They are powerful electromagnets whose coils of wire (typically niobium–tin or niobium–titanium alloy) show the phenomenon of zero electrical resistance at temperatures of around 4 Kelvin ($-269\,^{\circ}$C) when cooled by liquid helium. The magnetic field is typically parallel to the floor, along the long axis of a patient, and is homogeneous over a wide volume. Signal-to-noise ratio is excellent. Drawbacks include large purchase and running costs, a large *fringe magnetic field* (which increases hazards and interference) and claustrophobia. Once 'ramped-up', such magnets cannot be switched off, except via a costly boil-off or 'quench' of liquid helium.

- Resistive magnets are powerful electromagnets which rely on a large current density to create a strong magnetic field and operate at room temperature.

Combination with permanent magnet materials can permit magnetic flux densities up to about 1 tesla. Such magnets often have a magnetic field vertical to the floor and provide the advantages of reduced claustrophobia (being 'open' designs) and reduced fringe field (which reduces hazards). They can also be switched off. However they tend to suffer from poor field homogeneity and low signal-to-noise ratio.

- Permanent magnet designs are based around large ferromagnetic iron or alloy cores and may be quite bulky if even a moderate field strength is to be achieved. Relatively little used in clinical practice, they provide advantages of low fringe field and running costs but suffer from poor signal-to-noise ratio and field homogeneity.

Coils found in MRI are tuned to radio wave frequencies in the megahertz range employed. *Transmit coils*, as the name indicates, transmit RF waves into the patient at a finely controlled range of frequencies which affect slice thickness and image quality. They tend to be of 'volume coil' or bird cage designs which surround an area of patient anatomy. They may also have transmit–receive qualities. *Receiver coils* are designed to permit a good signal-to-noise ratio and should be positioned parallel to the external magnetic field and as close as possible to the anatomy of interest. Like transmit coils, they utilize Faraday's laws of electromagnetic induction. Small coils tend to provide good signal-to-noise ratios but poor volume coverage. This can be addressed by *phased arrays* of individual coils. Whole-body imaging can be provided by extended arrays of coils.

objects, tending to align them with the field and draw them towards greater magnetic flux densities. An exclusion zone of 5 gauss surrounds an MRI scanner, designed to prevent objects like scissors and oxygen cylinders from becoming projectiles and also to prevent damage to magnetically sensitive devices like pacemakers. The static field also affects the T-wave amplitude in the cardiac cycle.

Time-varying (gradient) fields can induce electrical currents and cause resistive heating effects in patients, particularly if 'loops' are created in wires or even by a patient clasping their hands or legs together. Current and heating are greatest in conductors. Induced currents can cause tingling or spasm but are not sufficient to cause fibrillation of the heart. Flexing of the gradient coils due to changing current flow creates the loud banging sounds which may reach 120 decibels and require patients to use ear protection (recommended above 85 decibels).

Radiofrequency waves can cause heating of body tissues, especially shallow tissues, by electromagnetic induction. The *specific absorption rate* (SAR) is controlled in MRI to prevent temperature rises above 1 degree centigrade. The power, repetition rate and wavelength of the RF pulses, as well as the size of the patient, are factors which influence heating.

Finally, it should be noted that MRI is not recommended for use in the first trimester of pregnancy. Although no studies of pregnant radiographers or patients have indicated increased adverse effects, some animal studies have suggested caution, albeit at exposure durations greater than those likely to be encountered in MRI practice.

39.5 MRI BIOEFFECTS AND SAFETY

Although MRI does not generate ionizing radiation and is not thought to induce cancers, there are a large number of biological effects of MRI scanning, some of which can be fatal. This is a surprise to many people. Thus MRI must be operated within strict guidelines, although most effects are transient and reversible. Sources of hazard in MRI arise from:

- the static (time-invarying) external magnetic field which operates at magnetic flux densities of several tesla
- varying magnetic fields applied by magnetic field gradients
- radiofrequency electromagnetic fields used to excite nuclear spins.

The *projectile effect* is the most dramatic demonstration of the influence of the static magnetic field. This exerts a rotational torque and translational force on ferromagnetic

Summary

In this chapter, you should have learnt the following:
- Magnetic resonance imaging grew from an earlier non-imaging technique called nuclear magnetic resonance which is still used today in magnetic resonance spectroscopy (see Sect. 39.2).
- MRI makes use of the relaxation properties of hydrogen nuclei placed in a powerful magnetic field and subjected to RF energies. These relaxation properties provide characteristic signals from different body tissues (see Sect. 39.2).
- T1 and T2 weighted images are the standard visualization method in MRI (see Sect. 39.3).
- There are many available techniques in MRI, which enable visualization of stationary tissues and flowing blood (see Sect. 39.3).
- Most magnets utilize superconductivity (see Sect. 39.4).
- MRI has many biohazards (see Sect. 39.5).

FURTHER READING

Hashemi, R.H., Bradley, W.G., Lisanti, C.J., 2003. MRI – The Basics., second ed. Lippincott, Williams and Wilkins, Baltimore.

McRobbie, D.W., Moore, E.A., Graves, M.J., Prince, M.R., 2007. MRI from Picture to Proton, second ed. Cambridge University Press, Cambridge.

Westbrook, C., Roth, C.K., Talbot, J., 2005. MRI in Practice, third ed. Wiley–Blackwell, Oxford.

Chapter | **40** |

Positron emission tomography (PET) scanning

40.1 AIM

The aim of this chapter is to introduce the reader to the principle of positron emission tomography (PET) scanning as practised in diagnostic imaging. The assumption is made that the reader is familiar with the mechanisms of positron production from a radionuclide as described in Chapter 19 (Section 19.5.2.).

40.2 REVISION OF POSITRON PHYSICS

As was discussed in Chapter 19, if a nucleus has too few neutrons for stability, it is possible for the nucleus to achieve a more stable configuration by the emission of a positron. Positrons are the antiparticles of electrons and the positron and the electron will interact (within a very

short distance in tissue), annihilating each other and producing two photons of annihilation radiation. These photons each have an energy of 0.51 MeV (511 keV) and detection of these photons forms the basis of positron emission tomography. Each photon is produced at an angle close to 90° to the direction of travel of the positron (see Fig. 19.7).

40.3 DETECTION OF POSITRONS

If a positron-emitting radionuclide is introduced into the patient, it can be labelled in such a way that it concentrates in specific structures. The number of positrons emitted by these structures can be related to the activity of the cells within the structure. If we surround the patient with a ring of positron detectors (see Fig. 40.1) then each annihilation radiation from the positron–electron interaction can be registered and the intersections of these points can be 'back-projected' to indicate the positron-emitting tissue in the patient.

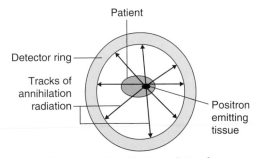

Figure 40.1 Detection of annihilation radiation from a positron-emitting source within the patient.

40.3.1 Types of coincidence

For the annihilation radiation from the positron–electron interactions to give useful information, the two photons must travel in straight lines from the source of the radiation to the detectors. The photons in (A) of Figure 40.2 are of this type.

Because the photons all travel with the velocity of electromagnetic radiation, they will each be detected by a detector almost at the same time – within $<10 \times 10^{-9}$ sec of each other. These photons are said to be coincident. It is possible for one of the photons to be scattered (see Fig. 40.2B). If the position of these two photons were back-projected, it would be an incorrect position for the origin of the annihilation radiation. Because the scattered photon travels along a slightly longer route, the two photons will not be detected within 10×10^{-9} sec of each other and so they are not said to be coincident and the imaging computer can be programmed to ignore them. Similarly, in Figure 40.2C, one of the photons has been absorbed. Because there is no matching coincident photon, the imaging computer will again ignore this event.

40.3.2 Detector materials

In the gamma camera (see Ch. 37), the radiation is detected using a sodium iodide crystal. The radiation from technetium-99m has an energy of 140 keV. The energy of the annihilation radiation from the positron–electron interaction is 511 keV. The greater energy of this radiation requires a material of higher density and/or higher atomic number. Bismuth germinate (BGO) is the material of choice for the detector crystals.

40.3.3 Detector mechanisms

The basic components of the detector mechanism are BGO crystals over which photomultiplier tubes or photodiodes are positioned as shown in Figure 40.3. These arrangements are known as blocks. Each photomultiplier tube detects the light emission as the result of the radiation photons interacting with the crystal. Groups of blocks (see Fig. 40.4) arranged with shared electronics form detector cassettes and a number of these detector cassettes form a detector ring around the patient.

Normally there is more than one ring so that we can detect information from a number of slices simultaneously. To avoid oblique rays from one slice interfering with the image on another ring, the rings are separated by septa made of lead or tungsten (see Fig. 40.5).

40.4 RADIONUCLIDES USED IN PET SCANNING

Three of the common radionuclides used in PET imaging are the following:

- 18-Flurodeoxyglucose (FDG) is a useful nuclide for cerebral metabolism and can also be used to demonstrate tumour activity.

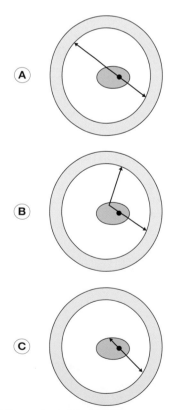

Figure 40.2 Types of coincidence. (A) is a true coincidence. In (B), one of the photons is scattered and in (C), one of the photons is absorbed. This makes (B) and (C) false coincidences.

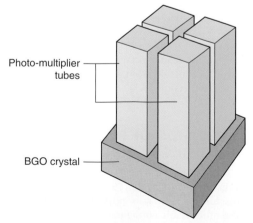

Figure 40.3 Arrangement of BGO crystal and photomultiplier tubes to make an imaging block.

Photo-multiplier tubes

BGO crystal

- $^{13}NH_3$ is useful for myocardial perfusion.
- $H_2^{15}O$ is useful for imaging of cerebral blood flow patterns.

40.5 MODERN TRENDS IN PET SCANNING

There are two modern trends in PET scanning which will be discussed.

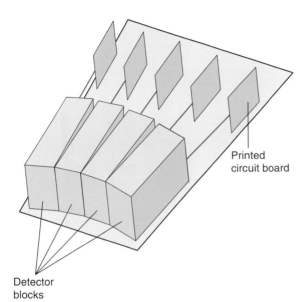

Figure 40.4 Arrangement of imaging blocks to make an imaging 'cassette'.

40.5.1 Time of flight (TOF) profiles

If we consider the method of producing images of the positron annihilation discussed so far, the radiation is detected by two detectors thus establishing the line in which the positron emission has taken place. The image of this event is then produced by 'back projection' of the information along the whole of this line. In TOF scanners, the precise time taken for each of the photons to reach its detector is measured. As can be seen in Figure 40.6 (see page 300), the distance D_1 is greater than the distance D_2 so this first photon will take slightly longer to reach the detector than the second photon. If we know the velocity of electromagnetic radiation $(3 \times 10^8\,m.s^{-1})$ then we can get a more accurate calculation of the distance travelled by each photon. Thus, in the back projection of the image, instead of simply saying the photons were emitted somewhere along this line, we can say more precisely the position of the emitted radiation on the line. This is illustrated in Figure 40.7 (see page 300).

No timer is 100% accurate so there is always some degree of positional uncertainty. The fact that we are able to more accurately calculate the positions of the emitted radiation photons means that we get improved resolution in the image.

40.5.2 Hybrid scanners

PET scanning gives us information regarding the position of high physiological activity. It, however, gives little or no information about related normal anatomy. This makes the interpretation of the images and the management of the patient a more difficult task. For this reason, scanners have been constructed which give anatomical information (e.g. from a computed tomography or magnetic resonance imaging scan) and physiological information (e.g. from

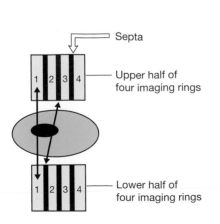

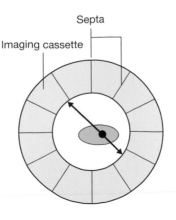

Figure 40.5 Arrangement of detection rings separated by septa which avoid detection of oblique rays.

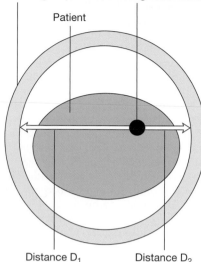

Figure 40.6 Line diagram to explain TOF technology. The distances D_1 and D_2 from the source of activity to the detectors is shown by the open arrows.

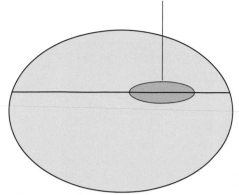

Figure 40.7 Back-projected image showing the probable position of the area of increased activity from the TOF calculations.

a PET or single photon emission computed tomography (SPECT) scan. The images from each modality may be superimposed to give a composite image of the anatomy and physiology of a region. These scanners are known as *hybrid scanners* and will form the topic for Chapter 41.

Summary

In this chapter, you should have learnt the following:
- A basic revision of positron physics (see Sect. 40.2).
- Methods of detecting positrons in PET scanning (see Sect. 40.3).
- Some of the more common radionuclides used for PET scanning (see Sect. 40.4).
- Some of the modern trends in PET scanning (see Sect. 40.5).

FURTHER READING

Chapter 41 of this text will discuss hybrid scanners. Addition information on PET scanning may be found in:

Bailey, D.L., Townsend, D.W., Valk, P.E., 2005. Positron Emission Tomography. Springer, London.

Wahl, R.L., Buchan, J.W., 2002. Principles and Practice of Positron Emission Tomography. Lippincott, Williams and Wilkins, Baltimore.

Chapter | **41** |

Hybrid scanners

41.1 AIM

The aim of this chapter is to introduce the reader to the basic principles and development of hybrid scanners.

41.2 BACKGROUND

In medical imaging, we wish to produce images which will enable us to diagnose, treat (if possible) and monitor a disease process. Some images will produce good anatomical images (e.g. computed tomography (CT) and magnetic resonance imaging (MRI)) of pathology but will give little information about the physiological process occurring around the pathology. Other imaging devices will produce good images of the physiological processes involved in pathology (e.g. radionuclide imaging (RNI) and positron emission tomography (PET)) but give little information about associated changes in the anatomy around the pathology. Hybrid scanners attempt to collect both anatomical and physiological data and to merge this information to give a composite image, and for this reason they are sometimes referred to as *multimodal imaging* (MMI). Such has been the success of hybrid scanners that no manufacturer now produces a 'stand-alone' PET scanner.

41.3 HISTORICAL DEVELOPMENT

Historically there have been two approaches to producing the composite images. These will now be discussed.

41.3.1 The software approach

The software approach took images produced by two different scanners and then merged these images using appropriate software. To achieve effective fusion of the images, accurate spatial and temporal alignment is crucial. This is difficult to achieve when the images have been produced on two separate scanners and so this approach is susceptible to differences in patient position and noise artefacts because of the patient being in different phases of the respiratory cycle. In recent years, this has been superseded by the hardware approach.

41.3.2 The hardware approach

The hardware approach utilizes a hybrid system where two (or more) scanners are housed in a single device. The principal advantage of this system is that the imaging modalities collect data sequentially while the patient is in the same position on the couch thus limiting noise artefacts caused by inaccurate alignment. These systems will now be discussed in more detail.

41.4 THE SPECT/CT HYBRID SCANNER

This system consists of a patient couch and two gamma cameras ring mounted in front of an adapted CT scanner. The system has been around in various forms since 1999 but has seen significant improvement over the years. Figure 41.1 shows the layout of such a scanner.

The gamma cameras can rotate around the patient and so can collect single photon emission computed tomography (SPECT) scan data. This produces an axial SPECT scan. The CT scanner part will produce an axial CT image of the same area. The two images can be displayed separately and a merged image can also be displayed. The ability to collect anatomical and physiological information simultaneously has great merit in oncology and also has potential in cardiac studies.

41.5 THE PET/CT HYBRID SCANNER

This is again an example of a hybrid scanner which will collect functional data (from the PET scan) and anatomical data (from the CT scan). The first of these entered clinical use in 2001 and at least 2000 have been installed worldwide. Figure 41.2 shows such a scanner.

There is a patient couch and a gantry which contains the PET scanner (normally at the front) and a CT scanner. Data from both scanners can be displayed separately or merged to produce a composite image of the anatomy and physiological detail of a lesion. The main use of this type of scanner is in cardiac studies and in oncology where it gives useful data on the anatomy and activity of tumours.

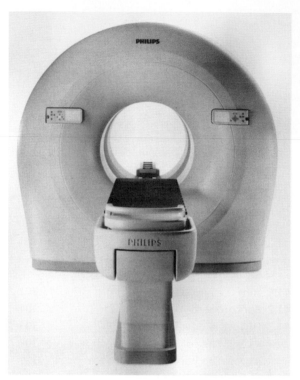

Figure 41.2 An example of a PET/CT hybrid scanner.
(Image courtesy of Philips Healthcare.)

41.6 THE PET/MRI HYBRID SCANNER

Images from a PET/MRI hybrid scanner were first published in 2007. The logic of moving from a PET/CT hybrid to a PET/MRI hybrid is that MRI can often provide better anatomical detail of soft tissue structures than CT. MRI can also deliver specific information about molecular cell structure. One of the problems in designing such a hybrid scanner is that the photomultiplier tubes used in conventional PET scanners are very sensitive to magnetic fields. These photomultipliers are replaced in the hybrid scanner by silicon avalanche photodiode detectors. Again the unit consists of a PET scanner and a CT scanner in the same housing. The images from this type of scanner are still being evaluated but are producing encouraging results in neurological studies, where tumours are revealed earlier and in more detail than with other scanners, and in oncology.

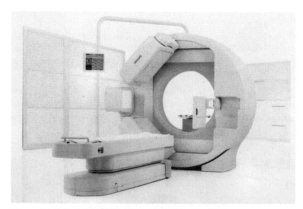

Figure 41.1 An example of a SPECT/CT hybrid scanner.
(Image courtesy of Philips Healthcare.)

41.7 OTHER HYBRID SCANNER COMBINATIONS AND CURRENT RESEARCH

Efforts to develop an ultrasound/MRI hybrid are currently ongoing although no results have been published at the time of writing.

Another area of current research in hybrid imaging is the development of a multimodal contrast agent. These could be used to enhance specific areas in both scans and could also be used as markers to produce better control points for image alignment. At present only very limited clinical studies have been published.

Summary

In this chapter, you should have learnt the following:
- The historical development of hybrid scanners (see Sect. 41.3).
- The general operation of the SPECT/CT hybrid scanner (see Sect. 41.4).
- The general operation of the PET/CT hybrid scanner (see Sect. 41.5).
- The general operation of the PET/MRI scanner (see Sect. 41.6).
- Areas of current research in the area of hybrid scanners (see Sect. 41.7).

FURTHER READING

Most of the up-to-date material regarding hybrid scanners can be found on the Internet by searching for that particular mode of hybrid scanner.

Ultrasound imaging

42.1 AIM

The aim of this chapter is to discuss the key properties of sound and explain how sound can be used to produce a diagnostic image. The Doppler principle, by which the velocity of moving tissues can be determined, is introduced. The clinical applications and advantages of ultrasound are described.

42.2 SOUND PROPERTIES

We tend to be more familiar with sound than with the other radiations used in radiography. From our own experience, we may have noticed that the light from a lightning bolt arrives more quickly than the following loud clap of thunder. This tells us something important about sound – it travels at about 340 metres per second in air, while light, like other electromagnetic radiations (including X-rays), travels at a staggering 300 000 kilometres per second in a vacuum. Sound, unlike electromagnetic radiations, needs a physical medium to travel through, since it consists of a travelling series of vibrations passing through atoms and molecules. It cannot pass through the vacuum of space and hence (perhaps fortunately!) we cannot hear the sun's activity, although we are bathed in its light and

heat radiations. Sound, unlike light and X-rays, cannot be considered as discrete packets or quanta of energy.

The speed and amplitude of sound is greatly affected by the medium through which it passes, much more so than in the case of electromagnetic radiations such as light. You may have noticed the very different pitches of sound that you hear when your head is under water, compared with when your head breaks back above the surface. Sound travels at slightly different speeds in different body tissues. The speed of sound is affected by the compressibility of the medium. It travels faster in more rigid materials which resist being compressed, and more slowly in materials such as fluids and gases which can be compressed easily. As an analogy, think of how much easier you can push an object using a firm rod made of wood, compared with using a bendy rod made of rubber. Table 42.1 lists

Table 42.1 Approximate speeds of sound in different materials and tissues

MATERIAL OR TISSUE	SPEED IN METRES PER SECOND
Air at 20°C and normal atmospheric pressure	340
Lung	650
Fat	1460
Pure water	1500
Salt water	1530
Kidney	1560
Blood	1570
Muscle	1580
Bone	3000

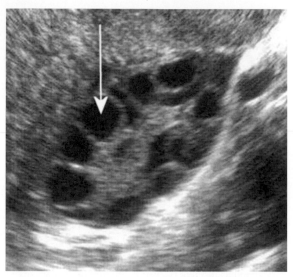

Figure 42.1 The cysts within this polycystic ovary contain watery fluid and appear anechoic (echo free).

Table 42.2 Acoustic impedance (*Z*) values for air and body tissues

MATERIAL OR TISSUE	ACOUSTIC IMPEDANCE (KG.M^{-2}.S^{-1})
Air	0.004×10^6
Fat	1.34×10^6
Water	1.48×10^6
Liver	1.65×10^6
Blood	1.65×10^6
Muscle	1.71×10^6
Bone	7.8×10^6

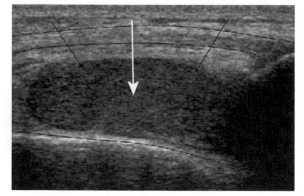

Figure 42.2 This haemorrhage into a joint returns many small bright echoes from the substances within it, such as blood cells and proteins. It is echogenic (echo producing).

the speed of sound in air and biological tissues and it can be seen that the more rigid substances allow sound to travel faster. Reflection and refraction of sound can occur at boundaries between materials or tissues.

Reflection is a very important property of sound waves, as it provides echoes at tissue boundaries, and these are used to depict structures in diagnostic ultrasound. It also gives some information about the nature of tissues. A cyst, which mostly contains fluid, will return few or no echoes (the signal is termed *hypoechoic* or *anechoic*) from within itself, as shown in Figure 42.1, while a haemorrhage will return echoes from within itself (the signal is *echoic* or *hyperechoic*), as shown in Figure 42.2. This is because a haemorrhage also contains blood cells and proteins (which return echoes) in addition to just fluid. The walls

of a cyst may return strong echoes at the capsule–fluid boundary.

Whenever an ultrasound beam reaches a boundary between two materials with different *acoustic impedances*, some of the beam will be reflected, and the remainder transmitted. The acoustic impedance, symbol *Z*, refers to the amount of opposition that a medium presents to sound waves trying to pass through it and is affected by the compressibility and density of the medium. *The greater the acoustic impedance between two tissues, the greater is the amount of sound reflection at the boundary between them.*

- Soft tissue/air interface – large *Z* difference = large reflection.
- Soft tissue/bone interface – large *Z* difference = large reflection (about 100%).

The acoustic impedances of body tissues can be seen in Table 42.2.

Large *Z* differences return good strong echoes *but* will prevent sound waves from penetrating beyond the boundary to show deeper structures. For this reason it is almost (but not quite) technically impossible to see deep structures through the skull using diagnostic ultrasound in adults. The air-filled lungs and ribs also present barriers to ultrasound. Muscle/liver, muscle/fat and muscle/air boundaries reflect back about 2%, 10% and 99% of sound respectively. Good ultrasound images of deep structures result when there are moderate but not huge *Z* differences between tissues.

The process of reflection of sound at a boundary is illustrated in Figure 42.3. Dense objects such as gallstones reflect back large amounts of sound, due to the large acoustic impedance difference between themselves and surrounding substances. This may lead to the appearance

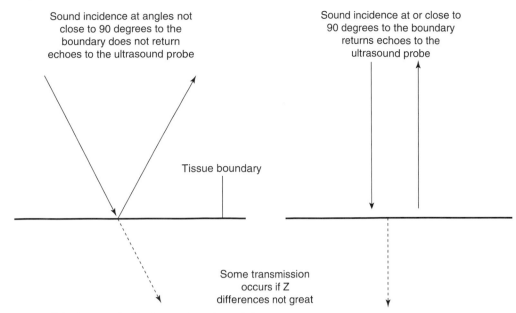

Sound incidence at angles not close to 90 degrees to the boundary does not return echoes to the ultrasound probe

Sound incidence at or close to 90 degrees to the boundary returns echoes to the ultrasound probe

Tissue boundary

Some transmission occurs if Z differences not great

Figure 42.3 Possible ultrasound reflections at tissue boundaries.

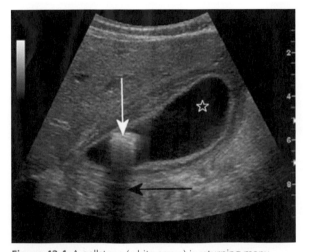

Figure 42.4 A gallstone (white arrow) is returning many echoes and has a bright hyperechoic appearance on its leading face. Behind this there is an acoustic shadow (black arrow) where no sound has been transmitted. There are also bright echoes at the boundary between the wall of the gall bladder and its contained fluid, which appears dark and anechoic (star).

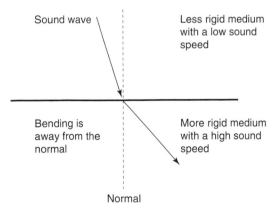

Sound wave

Less rigid medium with a low sound speed

Bending is away from the normal

More rigid medium with a high sound speed

Normal

Figure 42.5 The process of refraction at a boundary between two media. In this case the sound is refracted away from the normal (the normal is at 90° to the boundary).

of an *acoustic shadow* on an ultrasound scan. This takes the form of a dark echo-free band radiating out behind the stone, in a region where no sound has penetrated. An acoustic shadow can be seen in Figure 42.4.

An alternative effect, refraction, although important for visible light, is not a major process in diagnostic ultrasound

and so sound reflections are much stronger than sound refractions at tissue boundaries. In the process of refraction, a wave carries on from one material to another – it isn't reflected back. Refraction is an alteration in propagation direction (direction of travel) which occurs at a boundary between two materials in which the speed of the wave differs. The wave is bent 'towards the normal' if the new speed is slower than the original, and 'away from the normal' if the new speed is faster. The process of refraction at a boundary is shown in Figure 42.5.

Compression waves passing through molecules

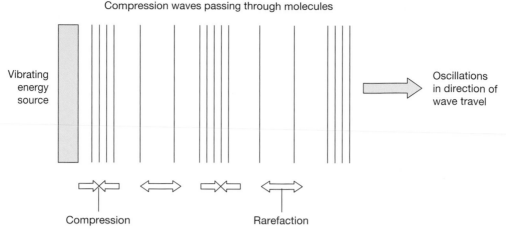

Figure 42.6 Passage of a longitudinal wave through a medium. The waves radiate out from the source, like ripples moving away from where a pebble has splashed in a pool.

Insight

Although all electromagnetic radiations *in a vacuum* travel at the speed of light, c, which is about 299 792 000 metres per second (2.998×10^8 m.s^{-1}), visible light travels at slightly different speeds in different media. In water and glass, visible light travels at speeds of about 2.25×10^8 m.s^{-1} and 1.98×10^8 ms^{-1} respectively. The alteration in speed of light (and sound) at boundaries is part of the process of refraction and, in the case of light, explains the production of a rainbow spectrum in a glass prism, with different light wavelengths being refracted to different extents. X-rays have a much higher frequency and energy than visible light. As a result, although they do experience changes in speed in different media; this is to an infinitesimal degree of no practical significance. X-rays experience absorption and scattering in matter, rather than refraction and reflection, although diffraction effects can be seen in very low-energy X-rays whose wavelength is similar to the spacing between atoms in crystal structures.

Table 42.3 Similarities and differences between sound, light and X-rays

SOUND	VISIBLE LIGHT	X-RAYS
Velocity = $f\gamma$	Velocity = $f\gamma$	Velocity = $f\gamma$
Slow velocity	Velocity is light speed, c, in vacuum	Velocity is light speed, c, in vacuum
Velocity much affected by medium	Velocity slightly affected by medium	Velocity not affected by medium
Longitudinal waves	Transverse waves	Transverse waves
Vibrations in atoms and molecules	Photons (quanta)	Photons (quanta)
Mainly absorbed, reflected	Mainly absorbed, reflected, refracted	Mainly absorbed, scattered
Non-ionizing	Non-ionizing	Ionizing

Sound shares some properties with electromagnetic radiations, in that all of them can be considered as waves with a frequency, wavelength and amplitude. In all of these cases, the velocity of the wave (in metres per second) is equal to the frequency (in Hertz) multiplied by the wavelength (in metres).

$$\text{velocity} = \text{frequency} \times \text{wavelength}$$

A key difference between sound and electromagnetic waves is that sound is regarded as a *longitudinal wave*. This means that the oscillations of the wave (in this case, compressions and rarefactions in a medium) are in the direction of travel rather than at right angles to it. Figure 42.6 shows the process of sound transmission through a medium.

Other examples of longitudinal waves include waves in slinky springs, ripples in a water tank, trucks shunting into each other on a rail track, a trick shot with a row of snooker balls!

The frequency of medical ultrasound is in the range of 2–20 MHz (megahertz). In medical ultrasound, low frequencies in this range penetrate deeper into the body but have a low resolution, while high sound frequencies can only penetrate a shallow depth in the body but have a high resolution. The term *ultrasound* means sound that is above the audible range of hearing for humans (the human range is roughly 20 Hz to 20 kHz).

Table 42.3 summarizes some key properties of sound, light and X-rays.

42.3 THE DOPPLER EFFECT

When an object which is emitting sound approaches an observer at speed, the waves become 'bunched-up' and the frequency (or pitch) of the sound increases. Similarly if an object which is emitting sound moves away from an observer at speed, the waves become 'drawn out' and the frequency (or pitch) of the sound decreases. This effect is shown in Figure 42.7.

This principle has important clinical applications in diagnostic ultrasound, since the altered sound frequency of moving tissues, such as heart valves and flowing blood, can be used to determine their speed of movement relative to the ultrasound probe. In colour-coded Doppler imaging, motion towards the probe is traditionally depicted as red, while motion away from the probe is depicted as blue.

Insight

The Doppler effect can be observed when the speed of wave-emitting objects is significant relative to the speed of the waves. Doppler shift of light occurs in space when galaxies are moving away from us at tremendous speeds. At these high speeds, visible light becomes shifted towards the red end of the spectrum and this effect can be used to measure the expansion of the universe.

42.4 PRODUCTION AND APPLICATION OF ULTRASOUND

An ultrasound transducer (probe) typically consists of an array of individual elements. Each element contains a piezoelectric crystal, typically made of ceramic material combinations of lead titanate ($PbTiO_3$) and lead zirconate ($PbZrO_3$). An alternating voltage applied across the crystal will cause it to flex and emit sound vibrations at an adjustable frequency. Also the crystal will generate an alternating voltage across itself in response to a returning sound wave, resulting in a signal. The crystal can be thought of as acting both as a sound speaker and a sound

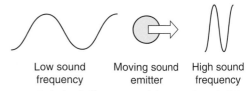

Low sound frequency   Moving sound emitter   High sound frequency

Figure 42.7 A simple illustration of the Doppler principle.

recorder. The elements of the transducer array can be focused to receive signal from shallow or deeper structures in the body.

The various modes of ultrasound scanning available include the following:

- *A mode* – amplitude modulated. Produces a graph plot whose height on the *y*-axis shows the strength of the echoes received from the reflective boundary and whose position on the *x*-axis shows the depth of the boundary. Can be used to show motion in structures such as heart valves, if the data are converted to an *m mode* (motion) trace where the position of a reflective boundary is plotted against time.

- *B mode* – brightness modulated. Produces a 2D anatomical slice through the body with a greyscale brightness based on the amplitude and frequency of reflected sound. This is the most common type of ultrasound scan and the most easy to interpret visually. The depth of the reflective structure (as with A mode scanning) is determined from the time it takes for the echo to return to the transducer.

- *Doppler ultrasound* – change in sound frequency indicates speed of tissue motion and may be plotted as a colour display plot. A spectral plot may be included, to indicate motion on the *y*-axis over time on the *x*-axis. *Pulsed wave Doppler* enables the operator to adjust the depth of tissue being visualized, by only accepting returning echoes with time lags in a particular range.

- *Duplex scanning* combines a Doppler scan with a B mode display which is used for localization purposes.

- Endoscopic ultrasound uses small intracavity transducers which can show the insides of structures like the oesophagus and blood vessels.

- 3D transducer arrays provide a 3D depiction of structures and are most popularly used to depict the fetus in utero.

Ultrasound imaging of tissue structures produces harmonic frequencies, which are multiples of the fundamental (or basic) returning sound frequency. For example, the 2nd harmonic is twice the frequency of the fundamental. Harmonics are of great importance to the tones of sound we hear in music. In ultrasound, filters can be used to separate out the 2nd harmonic, which, being of higher frequency, also provides greater resolution. Microbubble contrast agents in ultrasound include bubbles of gas just a few microns in size and are more compressible than surrounding substances. Thus, they return echoes and can

Table 42.4 Features of clinical ultrasound

STRENGTHS	WEAKNESSES
Inexpensive	Operator dependent
Quick	Images may be hard to interpret
Mobile	Suffers from image artefacts
Non-invasive	May be prone to giving 'false positives'
Can depict free fluid and aneurysms, e.g. in acute emergencies	Not good for deep structures
Can differentiate between solid and fluid structures	Cannot penetrate through bone or air
Can depict flow and motion	
Good for shallow structures	

The biological effects of ultrasound are mainly heat and cavitation. Cavitation occurs in oscillating gas bubbles that can be produced and then collapse in tissues. To reduce these effects on the developing fetus in utero, there are recommended restrictions on the power output, scan time and duty cycle (pulse length and repetition frequency) in pregnancy. Although some researchers have proposed that dyslexia, left-handedness and reduced birth weight can result from ultrasound use in pregnancy, these studies have not been verified and there is no proven long-term harm resulting from ultrasound.

be used to improve the visualization of blood vessels and tissues such as the liver. The microbubbles resonate and produce harmonic frequencies in response to ultrasound waves and this further improves depiction.

Some of the clinical strengths and weaknesses of ultrasound are summarised in Table 42.4.

Summary

In this chapter, you should have learnt the following:
- Medical ultrasound employs high-frequency sound waves which show boundaries between tissues by being reflected at them (see Sect. 42.2).
- Sound waves are unlike the other radiations used in radiography and require a medium for transmission (see Sect. 42.2).
- Reflections are strongest when there are sound transmission differences between tissues, but large differences may be unhelpful by preventing sound transmission to deeper structures (see Sect. 42.2).
- Doppler ultrasound provides information on the speed of moving tissues (see Sect. 42.3).

FURTHER READING

Allisy-Roberts, P.J., Williams, J., 2007. Farr's Physics for Medical Imaging, second ed. WB Saunders, Edinburgh.

Hoskins, P.R., Thrush, A., Martin, K., Whittingham, T.A., 2003. Diagnostic Ultrasound Physics and Equipment. Greenwich Medical Media, London.

Chapter | **43** |

Mammography

43.1 AIM

The aim of this chapter is to explore the modifications of standard X-ray tubes which are specifically designed to image breast tissues. The physics of X-ray beams consisting of a narrow range of low-energy photons is described, since these beams emphasize photoelectric absorption differences between soft tissues.

43.2 INTRODUCTION

X-ray mammography depends upon the ability to display small-density and atomic number differences between soft tissues. This particularly applies to the microcalcifications which can be an early sign of breast carcinoma. So thousands of symptomatic women and those participating within breast screening programmes rely upon X-ray physics to provide an accurate diagnosis. Conventional radiography, which uses X-ray tubes with tungsten targets (see Ch. 30) and tube kilovoltages of 40 and upwards, has difficulty in showing small soft tissue differences. This situation has been somewhat improved with the advent of high-resolution digital imaging methods which provide a wide 'dynamic range' of signal intensities, but despite this advancement, alternative techniques must be employed to demonstrate breast pathologies. These consist of microcalcifications and altered soft tissue densities in glandular, lactiferous and fatty structures. Mammography X-ray units must be compact and maneuverable in order to image all parts of the breast, including the axillary tail.

43.3 TISSUE X-RAY ATTENUATION CHALLENGES FOR BREAST IMAGING

Atomic number differences (calcification ≈ 14, water ≈ 7, fat ≈ 6) can be accentuated using photoelectric attenuation of X-rays (see Ch. 23) which predominates at low X-ray photon energies, and is *directly proportional* to atomic number cubed ($\propto Z^3$). It is also known that photoelectric absorption is *inversely proportional* to X-ray energy cubed ($\propto 1/E^3$). Thus the keV values (energy values) of X-ray photons must be very small if they are to experience much photoelectric attenuation in the low atomic number soft tissues of the breast. A good source of low keV X-ray photons is required, without producing rays which are of such very low energy that they will be absorbed in the skin and increase radiation dose. Although it will never be possible to produce a purely monoenergetic (single energy) X-ray beam, since the Bremsstrahlung process of X-ray production provides a continuous X-ray spectrum (see Ch. 21), it would be ideal of we could produce a 'narrow band' X-ray spectrum, with the bulk of X-rays being found across a small range of energies. This would reduce radiation dose to the breast and also enhance X-ray absorption differences between tissues, increasing image contrast.

43.4 X-RAY BEAM ADAPTATIONS FOR BREAST IMAGING

The requirements for a narrow and low beam energy range for mammography can be met in part by using molybdenum rather than tungsten as an X-ray tube target material. Some of the key properties of tungsten and molybdenum are summarized in Table 43.1.

The intensity of the 'continuous X-ray spectrum' (see Ch. 21) which results from Bremsstrahlung in the X-ray tube target is proportional to the target atomic number Z. Thus there will be less continuous spectrum X-rays from a molybdenum target than from one made of tungsten.

Insight

Bremsstrahlung is a more effective process in high atomic number X-ray tube targets since the electrostatic attraction between unlike charges is proportional to their magnitude. An electron passing through the X-ray tube target has a charge of -1 and will experience a greater attraction to a tungsten nucleus of charge $+74$ than to a molybdenum nucleus of charge $+42$. The nuclear charge, of course, is determined by the number of protons. The greater attraction will result in more 'braking' of the electron and thus more loss of energy in the form of X-ray photons.

X-ray spectra that could be expected from tungsten and molybdenum targets operating at a tube voltage of 30 kVp are shown in Figure 43.1.

It can be seen that molybdenum provides a spectrum in which the characteristic K-lines of 17.5–19.5 keV are important relative to a minor continuous component. The tungsten spectrum mostly consists of continuous X-rays and the characteristic K-lines are absent at a tube kVp of only 30 (since tungsten K-lines only occur at 59 keV and up). However, there is a small characteristic L-line from tungsten at about 11 keV. For mammography, we want a narrow spectrum of useful X-rays of about 17–25 keV and thus the molybdenum output is best.

The X-ray spectrum from a molybdenum target can be further improved by inserting a molybdenum filter into the X-ray beam exiting the tube. This is because a filter made of an element is relatively transparent to the characteristic X radiation emitted from an X-ray tube target made of that same element. This principle is illustrated by Figure 43.2.

In Figure 43.2, it can be seen that the use of a molybdenum filter further suppresses the continuous spectrum, but preserves the characteristic K-line X-ray emissions. Note that the energies of the K-lines in keV correspond to a 'low point' in the absorption curve for molybdenum. Little

Table 43.1 Features of tungsten and molybdenum targets for X-ray production

TUNGSTEN	MOLYBDENUM
Atomic number $Z = 74$	Atomic number $Z = 42$
Characteristic K-lines at ≈59 and 69 keV	Characteristic K-lines at ≈17.5 and 19.5 keV
K-shell absorption edge at 69.5 keV	K-shell absorption edge at 20 keV

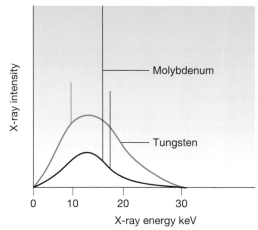

Figure 43.1 X-ray spectra from tungsten and molybdenum targets operating at 30 kVp.

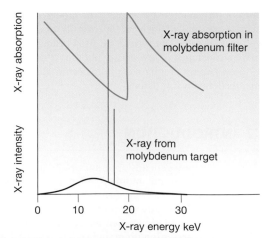

Figure 43.2 An X-ray spectrum (in black) from a molybdenum target, after passing through a molybdenum filter. The blue line shows the relative absorption of Mo at different energies and is NOT a spectrum – it is superimposed on the spectrum to show absorption effects.

X-ray absorption takes place in molybdenum at these energies and thus the characteristic X-rays from a molybdenum target can pass through easily. But just above the energy of these characteristic lines there is a sudden jump in X-ray absorption at 20 keV, which is the K-shell 'absorption edge' for molybdenum.

Insight

An 'absorption edge' occurs when the energy of X-ray photons is just equal to the binding energy of an electron in a shell orbiting the nucleus of an atom. At this energy, the X-rays can ionize an electron from the shell (for example, from the K-shell) and a lot of X-ray absorption takes place. At just below this energy level, relatively little absorption takes place, since the X-rays don't have enough energy to ionize the electron. The binding energy is that energy which must be put in to overcome the attractive force from the atomic nucleus which holds an electron in place in a shell. It is always greatest for inner (K) shell electrons and increases with the atomic number of the atom. The characteristic K-line X-ray energy is equal to the *energy difference* between an electron in the iK-shell and an electron in an outer (usually L or M) shell. Remember that in characteristic X-ray production an electron transfers between shells. The energy difference between the K- and L-shells is slightly less than the K-shell binding energy.

Rhodium, with an atomic number of 45 and K-line emissions of about 20 keV, has sometimes been used as an alternative X-ray tube target material for mammography, with a rhodium filter. Tungsten targets can be used in conjunction with a rhodium or palladium filter which effectively removes X-ray photons of about 24 keV and upwards.

43.5 IMAGE QUALITY CONSIDERATIONS

In mammography, a very small X-ray tube focal spot is necessary in order to reduce geometric unsharpness and maximize resolution. The use of relatively low tube kVp values helps to permit focal spots of small physical size, since heating stresses on the target material are small at low tube voltages. An additional tactic is to tilt the anode angle in order to obtain a small effective focal spot, using the 'line focus' principle (see Ch. 30). Use of a large source to image distance (SID) further reduces geometric unsharpness. Positioning of the anode end of the X-ray tube towards the nipple permits a slightly larger X-ray intensity towards the chest wall, using the 'anode heel effect'.

Compression of the breast tissue is very valuable in mammography as it permits immobilization, reduces tissue thickness and reduces X-ray scattering.

Improvements in digital imaging technology have allowed high-resolution images with an extended greyscale to be obtained. Digital imaging provides a wide dynamic range, thereby enabling a range of image densities to be recorded on a single image. This, when coupled with post-processing capabilities such as subtraction and edge enhancement, increases the visibility of breast lesions.

Although digital mammography promises radiation dose reductions, it must be remembered that too low an X-ray tube mA value might increase image noise and reduce breast lesion detection capabilities. Breast screening programmes provide an interesting example of the 'risk–benefit' relationship that must be considered when delivering ionizing radiations. Screening of asymptomatic younger women is undesirable as it would detect relatively few cancers and carry a relatively high risk of cancer induction from ionizing radiation.

Summary

In this chapter, you should have learnt the following:
- Breast pathology is best imaged making use of photoelectric absorption at low X-ray tube kVp (see Sect. 43.2).
- X-ray mammography employs a number of adaptations of conventional X-ray tubes, especially the use of molybdenum targets and low beam energies (see Sect. 43.3).
- These are designed to increase image contrast between breast lesions and normal tissues, by emphasizing the X-ray attenuation differences that occur due to photoelectric absorption.

FURTHER READING

Bushong, S.C., 2008. Radiologic Science for Technologists, nineth ed. Mosby, New York.

Dendy, P.P., Heaton, B., 1999. Physics for Diagnostic Radiology, second ed. Taylor and Francis, London.

Karellas, A., Vedantham, S., 2008. Breast cancer imaging: a perspective for the next decade. Med. Phys. 35 (11), 4878–4897.

Part | 9 |

Radiation protection

Chapter | 44 |

Practical radiation protection

44.1 AIM

The aim of this chapter is to introduce the reader to the basic legal requirements for the safe use of ionizing radiation. This will cover the main documents involved in the UK and the basic organization of radiation safety in a hospital trust, and will then examine the practical ways in which these are implemented in radiology or radiotherapy departments.

44.2 PURPOSE AND SCOPE OF RADIATION PROTECTION

Radiation dose rises from two sources: natural sources, which constitute the dose received by the whole population, and artificial sources. Radiation protection procedures can do little or nothing to reduce the dose from natural sources.

The principal component of radiation from artificial sources is received from exposure to radiation from *medical sources*. It follows from this that one of the basic tasks of radiation protection is to establish levels of risk to the population due from this source and then to take steps to keep these levels of risk from this source as low as possible.

The purpose of radiation protection in medicine is to produce and maintain an environment, both at work and in the outside world, where the levels of ionizing radiation from this source pose a minimal acceptable risk for human beings. Before beginning any discussion on radiation protection, it is important to realise that our environment can only be described as *relatively safe* from the effects of radiation from artificial sources.

Once the levels of risk from such radiation have been determined, appropriate dose-equivalent limits (see Sect. 44.6) may be set so that the risk associated with such radiations is no greater (and frequently is much less) than other aspects of life, e.g. the risk of injury as a result of a traffic accident. Establishing such dose-equivalent limits, and ensuring that staff work within these limits, helps to prevent suffering.

A full study of radiation protection would need to cover:

- radiobiology
- genetics

317

- statistical analysis of risk
- the fate and decay patterns of radioactivity released into the environment
- the absorbing power of different materials to different radiations.

Such a vast scope of study cannot be covered in a single chapter, or even in one book. Only a simplified review of practical methods of reducing radiation doses to radiation workers and their patients from the medical use of ionizing radiation will be considered here. These points are covered in the core of knowledge which all radiographic staff are expected to learn as part of their education. This consists of 11 key items as summarized in Table 44.1. Items 1–9 are of particular importance to the operator, while items 10 and 11 have particular reference to the role of the practitioner.

44.3 LEGAL ASPECTS

The legislation governing radiation is often confusing to the student. The International Commission for Radiation Protection (ICRP) has produced *recommendations* on radiation protection. These recommendations do not have the force of law. Laws based on these recommendations are then produced by the nations of the world.

In the European Union (EU), this is attained through directives, and all member states in the EU are required to implement these directives. In the UK, the following acts and regulations are concerned with radiation safety:

- Health and Safety at Work Act [HSW 1974].
- Ionizing Radiation Regulations [IRR 1999] Statuary Instrument 1999/3232.

- Radioactive Substances Act 1993 [RSA 1993].
- Ionizing Radiation (Medical Exposure) Regulations 2000 [IR (ME) R 2000] Statuary Instrument 2000/1059.
- Radioactive Substances (Hospitals) Exemption (Amendment) Order [RS (H) EO 1995].
- Ionizing Radiation (Medical Exposure) Regulations 2006 [IR (ME) R 2006] Statuary Instrument 2006/2523.

The inspectorate of the Health and Safety Executive (HSE) is responsible for ensuring that employers and employees comply with the above regulations. IRR 1999 applies to all radiation work and radiation workers in both the private and public sectors of the nuclear industry and those who may be affected by such work activities. In contrast, IR (ME) R 2000 applies whenever humans are irradiated for diagnostic, therapeutic, research or other medical or dental purposes, and where in-vitro medical tests are conducted. These regulations apply to staff, students, patients and their friends and relatives who are acting as comforters or carers, and to volunteers in research projects and members of the public. The above are all legal documents, and are often difficult for the layman to understand. 'User friendly' methods of meeting the requirements of these laws have been published as the *Approved Codes of Practice* and *Guidance Notes*. These do not have the force of law, but in a prosecution the defendant must be able to prove that their method of work is as good as, or better than, that recommended in the code or guidance notes.

44.3.1 Organization of radiation safety

The employer (e.g. the hospital trust) is ultimately responsible for maintaining radiation safety for staff,

Table **44.1** Core of knowledge	
1	Nature of ionizing radiation and its interaction with tissue
2	Genetic and somatic effects of ionizing radiation and how to assess these risks
3	The ranges of radiation dose given to a patient during the course of a particular procedure, the main factors affecting dose and methods of measuring dose
4	Principles of dose limitation and optimization
5	Principles of quality assurance applied to equipment and techniques
6	Specific requirements of children and of women who are or may be pregnant
7	Precautions necessary when handling sealed and unsealed radioactive sources
8	Organizational aspects of radiation protection and the procedure for suspected overexposure
9	Statutory responsibilities
10	Knowledge of the clinical value of the procedure requested, in relation to other available techniques
11	Importance of using radiological information, e.g. reports and images from a previous investigation

patients and others who may be affected by their work active activities. They have specific obligations under the regulations and meet these through a number of radiation safety experts:

- The Radiation Protection Adviser (RPA): an accredited, medically qualified physicist who is appointed by the employer to advise the employer on radiation safety and compliance with the regulations. This includes the production of local rules and written systems of work, the designation of work areas, the supervision of quality assurance programmes and acceptance testing of new equipment.
- The Radiation Protection Supervisor (RPS): every area of the trust in which ionizing radiation is used must have an RPS appointed by the employer. Each RPS must understand the specific requirements of radiation safety as applied to their area of work. Since the RPS is responsible to the employer for ensuring the safety measures are implemented and maintained, such individuals are usually departmental superintendants as they have the authority necessary to do this.
- The Radiation Safety Committee (RSC): this committee oversees all radiation safety issues, including research, and ensures that the reports of the RPA are implemented and radiation safety standards are maintained.

44.3.2 Responsibilities of the manufacturer

The manufacturers have obligations that are designed to improve the radiation protection offered by their equipment. These include such features as limiting radiation leakage from the X-ray tube so that it does not exceed $1\,\text{mSv.h}^{-1}$ at a distance of 1 metre in any direction from the focus of the tube, the provision of suitable antiscatter protection, the use of low-absorption interspacing material in secondary radiation grids, the use of a high-output rectification system, provision of an automatic (preferably anatomically programmable) timer and 'dead-man operation' of exposure switching so that releasing the exposure switch during an exposure automatically terminates the exposure. If the equipment is capable of fluoroscopy, a pulsed fluoroscopy system must be used.

44.4 DOSE-EQUIVALENT LIMITS

Table 44.2 summarizes the dose-equivalent limits specified by the Ionizing Radiation Regulations 1999.

Note: These limits exclude any dose received from natural radiation sources or medical treatment of the individual concerned.

44.4.1 Designated radiation workers

If an employee is likely to receive a whole-body dose equivalent of ionizing radiation which exceeds 6 mSv per annum then that person must be designated as a *classified radiation worker* by the employer. A person who is a classified radiation worker must be subject to *medical surveillance*, with periodic reviews of health at least every 12 months.

It is not sufficient to rely on an individual's history of doses received if they are less than the three-tenths limit. The *potential doses* which may be received in a set of circumstances must be assessed. The reason for designation may be that the individual works in *controlled areas* (see Sect. 44.5.1) but this is not, on its own, sufficient reason for designation. Even if the local rules (see Sect. 44.5), when strictly obeyed, indicate that doses in excess of the three-tenths limit will not occur, persons who work with radiation sources that are capable of producing an overdose in a few minutes will need to be classified.

Table 44.2 Dose-equivalent limits (in mSv) per calendar year specified by Ionizing Radiation Regulations 1999

CATEGORY OF PERSON	DOSE TO WHOLE BODY	DOSE TO LENS OF THE EYE	DOSE TO SKIN AVERAGED OVER AN AREA OF 1 CM²	DOSE TO HANDS, FOREARMS, FEET AND ANKLES
Employee aged 18 or over	20	50	500	500
Trainees aged under 18	6	50	150	150
General public	1	15	50	50

Comforter or carer: no dose limit, however the Health Protection Agency (HPA) (formerly the National Radiological Protection Board) recommends the dose should not exceed 25 mSv over a 5-year period or 5 mSv in a single exposure.
Women of reproductive capacity who are at work: dose equivalent to the abdomen is 13 mSv in any 3-month period. The dose must not exceed 1 mSv from the date the conception is declared.

The radiation dose which the classified person receives should be measured using a suitable *personal dosimeter* (see below) – the doses must be assessed by an approved *dosimetry service* on the basis of accepted national standards.

The above discussion does not mean that radiation workers who are not classified should not be monitored, but monitoring is a precaution and one which may be used to justify non-classified status, although there is no legal requirement for this.

44.4.2 Personnel dosimetry

The monitoring of radiation dose to staff is carried out by the use of thermoluminescent dosimeters (TLDs). The basic principles of thermoluminescence have already been discussed in Chapter 27. An example of a TLD badge and holder used for monitoring purposes is shown in Figure 44.1.

Figure 44.1A shows the plastic Harshaw card, without its Melinex wrapping (which has a number stamped on it in normal numbers). This wrapping protects the lithium fluoride/polytetrafluoroethylene (PTFE) TLD inserts on the card from light and alpha radiations, as well as providing chemical protection and a measure of physical protection. The card contains two discs of thermoluminescent material. One disc is positioned behind the open window of the badge while the other disc is behind the

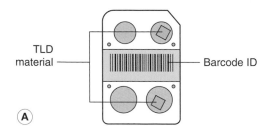

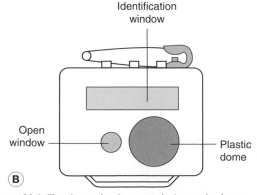

Figure 44.1 The thermoluminescent dosimeter badge as supplied by the Health Protection Agency (HPA; formerly the National Radiological Protection Board).

plastic dome. *Note:* the card is designed so that it can only be inserted into the holder in the correct way. Each card is identified by a unique barcode strip used in the automated dose-reading process.

The cardholder has two windows (Fig. 44.1B) – a long rectangular window along the top edge to display the wearer's identity number and a circular open window that lies directly over one of the TLDs on the card. This TLD records all weak and strongly penetrating radiations, including beta radiation. This dose reading produces the Hp0.7 or whole-body dose. The other TLD lies under the dome, which is made of thick ($90 \, \text{mg.cm}^{-2}$) plastic. This TLD is used to record the more penetrating and gamma radiations producing the Hp10 dose or depth received by the wearer.

Thermoluminescent materials may also be used to measure doses to specific organs, e.g. they can be wrapped round a finger to measure the dose to that finger.

The major disadvantage of TLDs is that they are retrospective monitors and are processed and read after exposure.

'Real-time' dosimeters (often called pocket dosimeters, because they can be worn in pockets of laboratory coats) can give an instant readout on a digital display. Some can provide additional data, such as a breakdown of the rate at which the dose was received, or even sound an audible alarm to indicate that radiation is being detected.

44.4.3 Employees who have been overexposed

If an employee's annual whole-body dose exceeds 15 mSv, the RPA must notify the Health and Safety Executive (HSE) who will conduct an investigation to see if the working practices involved are in keeping with the ALARA (*as low as reasonably achievable*) principle (or whether improvements may be made which would lead to a reduction in the dose).

44.5 LOCAL RULES

Under IRR 1999, the employer has a legal responsibility to ensure that written local rules are produced for all departments (or areas) where employees are involved in work with ionizing radiation. These rules must be brought to the attention of all employees working in these departments. In practice, the RPA advises the employer on the formulation of these rules and it is the task of the RPS to ensure that the rules are known and put into practice by colleagues in their respective departments.

The local rules for a department should be displayed in a prominent position, or positions, within the department concerned, and should contain the following information:

- The names and contact details of the RPA and RPS for the department (or area).

- A description of each designated area in the department (see Sect. 44.5.1).
- Details of restrictions of access to such areas.
- Written systems of work detailing the procedures and protocols for the department.
- Details of any contingency plans.

44.5.1 Designated areas

There are two types of designated area (see Table 44.3): controlled and supervised areas. All designated areas must be delineated by physical boundaries, i.e. walls. However, in the case of radiography involving the use of mobile X-ray units, this requirement is dropped, provided that an area of at least 1.5 metres from the ray tube is under the continual supervision of the operator at all times. Warning signs must be posted at all entrances to the areas, preferably at eye level, and include a warning light to indicate if an X-ray unit is activated or an exposure is being made.

44.5.1.1 Design of designated areas

The function of the X-ray room is to provide an enclosure for the X-ray examination or treatment unit and limit access to the radiation area. It should also provide adequate shielding to the rest of the environment from the radiation produced, so that individuals outside the room do not receive a radiation dose that would exceed the annual effective dose limit to a member of the public. In diagnostic radiography, provision is made for a barrier inside the room behind which staff may be

protected from the radiation while they operate the unit, while viewing the patient through a protective window. If there is more than one X-ray tube operating from the generator in a diagnostic room, there must be a visual indication (usually a warning light) to indicate which tube is in circuit and capable of producing radiation if energized. With radiotherapy treatment rooms, due to the much higher radiation energies used, the equipment is operated from outside the treatment room and the patient viewed through a closed-circuit TV system. Entry to the treatment area is through a maze and the entry of an individual into the maze during treatment automatically terminates the treatment.

The level of radiation protection given by barriers and walls is usually stated in terms of their *lead-equivalent*.

> **Definition**
>
> The lead-equivalent of an absorbing material is the thickness of lead which would absorb the same amount of radiation as the given material when exposed to radiation of the same type and quality.

The lead-equivalent gives a basis for comparing one barrier with another at a given beam energy.

In the diagnostic range of beam energies (up to 150 keV), the photoelectric absorption within lead is significant owing to its high atomic number ($Z = 82$). For

Table 44.3 Description of designated areas

TYPE OF DESIGNATION	REQUIREMENTS FOR DESIGNATION	PERMITTED ACCESS
Controlled area	An area where any person is likely to receive an effective dose greater than 6 μSv per year or three-tenths of any relevant dose limit	A. Classified radiation workers B. Radiation workers who follow a written system of work, designed to restrict significant radiation exposure in that area C. Patients undergoing medical diagnostic or therapeutic exposures
Supervised area	A. An area where any person is likely to receive an effective dose greater than 1 mSv per year or one-tenth of any relevant dose limit B. An area under review for upgrading to a controlled area *Note:* a supervised area cannot be situated inside of a controlled area	Persons whose presence is necessary during a radiation exposure

this reason, many barriers (e.g. doors) in the diagnostic X-ray room incorporate a few millimetres of lead laminated with wood to give adequate radiation protection. Lead-glass windows are often fitted to such barriers to enable a visual contact to be maintained. The protection afforded by such a window must be at least the same amount as the protective barrier itself and there must be no gaps where the radiation is able to penetrate. The siting of such a barrier to protect staff must be such that the radiation must be scattered at least twice (greatly reducing its intensity) before reaching the opening in the barrier.

Wall thicknesses between X-ray rooms and adjacent areas must be such that any transmitted radiation will not produce a dose in excess of 1 mSv per year, which is the maximum dose for the general public. This figure must be calculated for all walls, floors, ceilings and windows of the X-ray rooms and is calculated by applying a *use factor*. The use factor is an estimation of the time when the radiation beam will be pointing towards that area. As a result of this calculation, the maximum dose received by a person sited on the far side of the barrier may be estimated and it must not exceed 1 mSv per year. In previous legislation, there was also an *occupancy factor*, which looked at the fraction of time a person was likely to spend in this area, but this factor has now been discontinued.

The materials used in the construction of the walls and floor of the X-ray room may contain lead sheeting or there may be sufficient thickness of other materials, such as concrete, to provide adequate absorption of the primary and scatter radiation produced in the room. The lead-equivalent of a concrete wall 15 cm thick is approximately 1.5 mm within the diagnostic energy range – this reflects the superior absorption of lead compared with concrete in this energy range. The lead-equivalent of such walls may be increased by the use of *barium sulphate plaster* as a thin coating on the walls. This is because of the high atomic number of barium ($Z = 56$).

As the beam energy increases, the advantage of lead over concrete diminishes, as there is a gradual shift from the predominance of photoelectric absorption to the predominance of Compton scattering. Thus the lead-equivalent of a barrier will increase with an increase in the photon energy – a greater thickness of lead will be required to give the same level of protection as the barrier. In the region of 1 MeV, the Compton scattering process predominates and lead has no real advantage over concrete since all materials have similar mass attenuation coefficients due to the Compton process. For this reason, many of the barriers used in radiotherapy departments are made of large thicknesses of concrete.

In conclusion, the design of a room, its wall thickness and the barriers must be such that the radiation dose received by patients, staff and members of the public is kept to a minimum in accordance with the ALARA principle. Further details of the design of diagnostic and therapy rooms will be found in specialized publications on this topic.

44.6 THE ROLE OF THE PRACTITIONER

The role of the practitioner is the *justification* of the request for the procedure. Practitioners are usually medically qualified individuals, although this role can be delegated to other radiographic professionals for some procedures, with the employer's approval.

Before justification can commence, the practitioner must check that the referrer has supplied sufficient data of the procedure requested. This includes the following:

- The patient's identification (and, if a female of childbearing age, the date of the patient's last menstrual period).
- Sufficient relevant medical data to permit the practitioner to decide if there is sufficient net benefit to the patient to allow justification of the procedure and, if the patient is to undergo a procedure where radionuclides are administered, if the patient is breastfeeding an infant.

The logical suggestion is that no unnecessary radiation dose should be received by any person, but where there is a net benefit for the patient the request would be justified.

For instance, the mammography screening programme has increased the early detection rate of breast cancer, and this in turn increased the survival rate from this condition. In the case of other cancers, the risk of death to the patient is considerably higher if a course of radiotherapy treatment is not given. An undetected aneurysm may burst causing the patient's death or other serious medical complications.

Another possibility is that the same information about the patient's condition can be gained without using ionizing radiation (e.g. ultrasound or MRI) and, in these cases, the practitioner should suggest this change of imaging modality to the referrer.

If the patient is a female of reproductive capacity (i.e. between the ages of 12 and 40), the practitioner must consider the possibility that the patient is or may be pregnant. The operator is also responsible for checking this at the time of examination.

44.6.1 Radiological examinations of women of reproductive capacity

The current rules concerning radiological examinations of women of reproductive capacity are as follow:

- Any woman who has an overdue or missed period should be treated as though she were pregnant.
- If the woman cannot answer 'no' to the question 'are you, or might you be, pregnant?' then she should be treated as though she were pregnant.

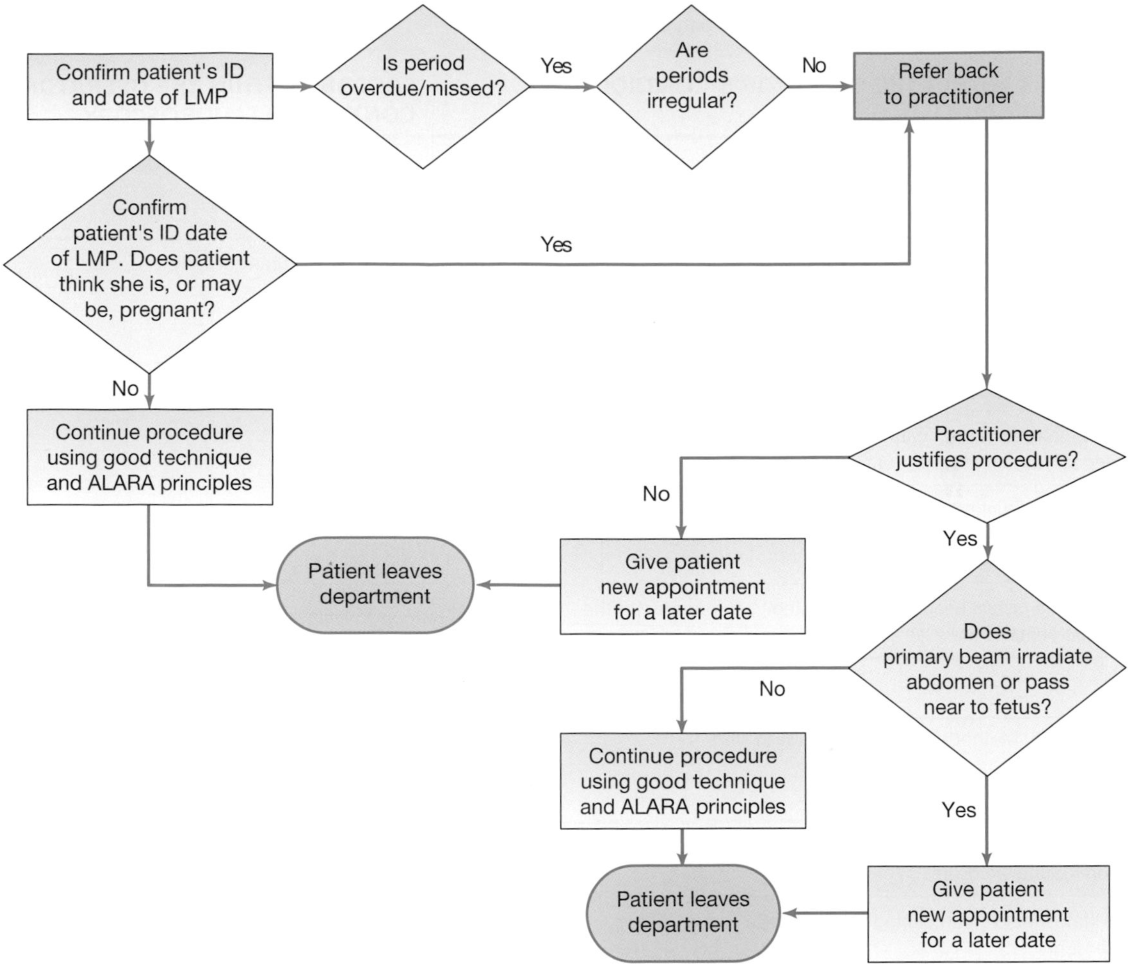

Figure 44.2 Flowchart of the scanning process carried out by an operator on women of reproductive capacity presenting for a radiographic examination.

- If the clinical indications are that an exposure should be made where the primary beam irradiates the fetus, then great care must be taken to minimize the number of views and the absorbed dose per view, but without jeopardizing the diagnostic value of the investigation.
- Provided good collimation is used, and equipment is properly shielded, radiographs of areas remote from the fetus (e.g. chest, skull, hand) may be done safely at any time during the pregnancy.

These recommendations do not reduce the care that should be taken in limiting the potential radiation dose to the fetus. The change in emphasis of the recommendations is that special precautions need only be taken if the woman is, or may be, pregnant – where 'pregnant' is defined as beginning when a menstrual period is overdue.

Other than this, there is no need for special limitations of exposures during a menstrual cycle, except for the normal requirements to keep all absorbed radiation doses as low as reasonably practicable. Good radiographic techniques should thus be used at all times to minimize radiation doses for all exposures.

A flow chart showing the progress of a woman of reproductive capacity presenting for a radiographic examination is given in Figure 44.2.

44.7 THE ROLE OF THE OPERATOR

The regulations define the operator as the individual (radiologist, radiographer or radiographic assistant) who is responsible for physically directing the X-ray exposure. They are the final link in the chain of radiation protection as they have a dual responsibility:

1. To keep the radiation dose to the patient, themselves and other staff and as low as reasonably practicable

Table 44.4 Methods of dose reduction to the patient

FACTORS WITHIN THE OPERATOR'S CONTROL IN RADIOGRAPHY	FACTORS WITHIN THE OPERATOR'S CONTROL IN FLUOROSCOPY
Selection of exposure factors, preferably using an anatomically programmed timer, so that the exposure is within the diagnostic reference level produced by the employer for the examination	Use of pulsed fluorography and image storage systems
Use of the highest practicable kVp	Use of digital fluorography
Making use of secondary radiation grids to reduce scatter reaching the image receptor	
Use of tissue displacement techniques with obese patients	
Use of immobilization with patients who cannot remain in position or keep still during the exposure	
Limitation of field size by use of collimation	
Utilizing gonad shields	
Use of the fastest image receptor system, consistent with the requirements of the examination	

Table 44.5 Methods of dose reduction to staff

RADIOGRAPHY	FLUOROGRAPHY
Only those whose presence is required should be in the room during exposures	All staff must wear adequate protective clothing, as specified in the written systems of work
All staff should stand behind the protective barrier during exposure	Use of automatic collimation
The X-ray tube must have adequate shielding	Staff should stand as far as possible from the primary beam
Operators should not expose themselves to the direct beam	Protective shielding should be incorporated in the generator to reduce dose from scattered radiation
Restless patients should be supported by immobilization devices	
Operators should not support restless patients	

but consistent with the clinical requirements of the examination. This includes:

- checking the patient's identity and that the practitioner has justified the procedure
- if the procedure has not been justified, referring the request back to the practitioner
- if the patient is a female of reproductive age, assessing the risk of pregnancy. If a risk of pregnancy is present, referring the request back to the practitioner for approval to proceed.

2. Once these checks have been completed, the procedure can commence. The operator should bear the points listed in Tables 44.4 and 44.5 in mind while carrying out the procedure.

Note: Many of the methods that reduce dose to the patient will also produce a reduction of dose to staff. Fluoroscopy results in higher radiation doses than conventional radiography and therefore good technique is even more essential to keep radiation doses to a minimum. The use of a modern fluoroscopic unit with pulsed fluoroscopy, image storage, automatic collimation and digitization of the image will result in a reduction of the radiation doses to patients and staff.

44.7.1 Reporting overexposure of patients

In the case of a known or suspected overexposure to a patient, the operator must inform the RPA. They will then report this to the Healthcare Commission, who will conduct an investigation into the incident and make recommendations to prevent the reoccurrence of similar incidents.

Summary

In this chapter, you should have learnt the following:
- The purpose and scope of radiation protection (see Sect. 44.2).
- An outline of the regulations affecting radiation protection (see Sect. 44.3).
- The organization of radiation safety in a hospital trust (see Sect 44.3.1).
- The responsibilities of the manufacturer (see Sect. 44.3.2).
- Dose-equivalent limits in radiation protection (see Sect. 44.4).
- The requirements for the designation of radiation workers (see Sect. 44.4.1).
- Methods of personnel monitoring (see Sect. 44.4.2).
- Procedure followed if an employee has been overexposed to radiation (see Sect. 44.4.3).
- Local rules (see Sect. 44.5).
- Designation of work areas in radiation protection (see Sect. 44.5.1).
- The design of designated areas in radiography and radiotherapy (see Sect. 44.5.1.1).
- The role of the practitioner (see Sect. 44.6).
- Special precautions in the radiological examination of women of reproductive capacity (see Sect. 44.6.1).
- The role of the operator and practical methods of radiation protection (see Sect. 44.7).
- Reporting of overexposure to a patient (see Sect. 44.7.1).

FURTHER READING

Allisy-Roberts, P., 2002. Medical and Dental Guidance Notes – A Good Practice Guide on All Aspects of Ionising Radiation Protection in the Clinical Environment. Institute of Physics and Engineering in Medicine, York, UK.

Ball, J.L., Moore, A.D., Turner, S., 2008. Ball and Moore's Essential Physics for Radiographers, fourth ed. Blackwell Scientific, London (Chapter 21).

Bushong, S.C., 2004. Radiologic Science for Technologists: Physics, Biology and Protection. Mosby, New York (Chapters 33–40).

HMSO., 1999. 1999/3232 The Ionising Radiation Regulations. HMSO, London.

HMSO., 2000. Statutory Instrument 2000/1059. The Ionising Radiation (Medical Exposure) Regulations. HMSO, London.

HSE., 2000. Working with Ionising Radiation – Ionising Radiation Regulations 1999. Approved code of Practice and Guidance. HSE Books, Sudbury.

Webb, S. (Ed.), 2000. The Physics of Medical Imaging, second ed. Institute of Physics, Bristol. (Chapter 2).

Part | 10 |

Appendices and tables

Appendix A

Mathematics for radiography

This appendix on the revision of mathematics is directed primarily at those whose mathematics is a little weak. However, many of the worked examples shown are chosen from topics in radiography.

For those studying for examinations, the following remarks may be of help. Examiners frequently complain of cramped, untidy mathematics which is difficult to follow. What they are hoping to see in the answer is a clear statement of the problem and an easy-to-follow development of the mathematics used to obtain the solution. This may be more important (and hence gain more marks) than simply obtaining the correct numerical answer. In fact, the correct answer simply recorded on its own with little or no supporting mathematical reasoning will not achieve many marks – remember that the examiner cannot know how you achieved the final answer unless you tell him/her. In practice, you should use phrases and sentences to tell the examiner how you have progressed from one step of the problem to the next as you move towards the eventual solution. This should also help you to think more clearly about what you are doing and also to check the integrity of your final answer – this is probably even more important with the widespread use of pocket calculators. A study of the worked examples in this appendix should clarify these points.

A.1 ALGEBRAIC SYMBOLS

The letters of the English and Greek alphabet (see Table D following the appendices) are often used to represent the magnitude of an unknown quantity. For example, an electrical potential difference may be represented by V volts, an angle by θ (i.e. theta) degrees or radians and an energy by E joules. Such a practice enables the symbols to be used in place of the actual numerical values of the quantities, and is of great practical use in solving equations (see App. A.4).

A.1.1 Suffixes

Suffixes are used to denote a specific value of a particular quantity. If we use the symbol I to denote the intensity of radiation from a particular source, then I will depend upon the distance from the source at which the intensity is measured (see Ch. 26). We may call a particular distance x, say, and denote the intensity of this distance by Ix – meaning *the intensity at x*. For another distance y, the corresponding value of intensity is Iy.

Similarly, if a quantity, N, changes with time, t, the value of N at any given time may be denoted by Nt.

Suffixes are used, then, to avoid ambiguity and are used as such in many chapters of this book.

A.2 FRACTIONS AND PERCENTAGES

Although fractions are not commonly used in radiographic calculations since they have been largely replaced with decimals, nevertheless a knowledge of how to manipulate fractions mathematically is useful in calculations involving Ohm's law (see Ch. 7) and capacitors (see Ch. 13). For this reason, a section on fractions and percentages is still included in this appendix.

A.2.1 Percentages

If a quantity increases in value by 50 per cent (%), then this means that it has become greater by one-half of its previous value. Thus, if the electric current passing through an X-ray tube was 200 mA, then an increase of 50% would bring this to 300 mA. Alternatively, it may be said that the new value is 150% of the original value.

In general terms, if a is the original value of a quantity and b is its new value, then:

the *percentage change* $= 100 \times \dfrac{b - a}{a}$

$\dfrac{100b}{a} =$ the *percentage* of b compared to a

$y\%$ of a is just $\dfrac{y}{100} \times a$

Examples

a. Original value $= 60$; new value $= 80$

The percentage change is then $100 \times \dfrac{20}{60} = 33\frac{1}{3}\%$

and the new value is $100 \times \dfrac{80}{60} = 133\frac{1}{3}\%$ of the original.

---

b. A quantity has reduced by 25%. What is the new value if it was 600 originally?

25% of 600 is just $\dfrac{25}{100} \times 600 = 150$

so the new value is $600 - 150 = 450$.

A percentage is a special case of a fraction, where one number is divided by another. The following sections describe how fractions may be added together and multiplied.

A.2.2 Addition of fractions

Suppose we have the fraction a/b, where a and b represent general numbers. Now the addition or subtraction of a/b to another fraction c/d rests on the fact that we can take any fraction and multiply top and bottom by the same factor (k, say) *without* altering its value:

i.e. $\dfrac{a}{b} = \dfrac{ka}{kb}$ (because the ks cancel)

It is the appropriate selection of k for each fraction which makes for the easy addition of fractions. For example, suppose we have:

$$\frac{2}{3} + \frac{5}{6}$$

If we multiply 2/3 by 2 (top and bottom), we shall have a fraction expressed in sixths, just like the second fraction:

$$\frac{2}{3} + \frac{5}{6} = \frac{2 \times 2}{2 \times 3} + \frac{5}{6} = \frac{4}{6} + \frac{5}{6} = \frac{9}{6} = 1\frac{1}{2}$$

Notice that we multiplied only the first fraction – we need not do the same thing to the second. This method is often very quick, particularly when only two or three simple fractions are involved, and is in fact entirely equivalent to the more general method of using the lowest common denominator (LCD), as illustrated in the following example:

$$\frac{2}{3} + \frac{3}{4} - \frac{5}{6} = \frac{(4 \times 2 + 3 \times 3 - 2 \times 5)}{12}$$
$$= \frac{(8 + 9 - 10)}{12} = \frac{7}{12}$$

Here, the LCD of the denominators 3, 4 and 6 is 12 and is therefore used as the overall denominator on the right-hand side. The individual denominators are then divided into 12, the result being multiplied by the respective numerator and summed (observing the correct signs) as shown in the example.

A.3 MULTIPLYING AND DIVIDING

A.3.1 Positive and negative numbers

It is obvious that $1 \times 8 = 8$, but what are -1×8, -1×-8 and 8×-1?

To avoid having to work out such problems from first principles every time, a simple rule has been developed which we may call Rule 1.

Rule 1
When multiplying or dividing two numbers together:
  Two (+)s make a (+).
  Two (−)s make a (+).
  A (+) and a (−) make a (−).

i.e. only when the signs are dissimilar is the result negative.

Examples

a. $-3 \times 4 = -12$
b. $14 \div -7 = -2$

c. $\dfrac{-40}{-4} = 10$

d. $-2 \times -4 \times -3 = 8 \times -3 = -24$

Exercise A.2

a. $28 \div 7$

b. $\dfrac{-36}{6}$

c. $\dfrac{144}{-4}$

d. -13×-3

e. $-7 \times \dfrac{-8}{-2}$

A.3.2 Fractions

The *multiplication* of two or more fractions is just a matter of simplification by cancellation (where possible) and then multiplying all the numerators together to form the new numerator, and all the denominators together to form the new denominator.

Examples

a. $\dfrac{2}{3} \times \dfrac{7}{5} = \dfrac{14}{15}$ (no cancellation possible)

b. $\dfrac{2}{3} \times \dfrac{9}{4} = \dfrac{\cancel{2}^1}{\cancel{3}_1} \times \dfrac{\cancel{9}^3}{\cancel{4}_2} = \dfrac{3}{2}$

The *division* of two fractions is straightforward provided that the following rule is obeyed.

Rule 2
When dividing by one or more fractions, turn those in the denominator upside down and multiply.

Let us say, by way of illustration, that we wish to divide 4 by ½:

$$\text{i.e. } \dfrac{4}{\dfrac{1}{2}}$$

Applying Rule 2, we turn ½ upside down and multiply:

$$\dfrac{4}{\dfrac{1}{2}} = 4 \times \dfrac{2}{1} = 8$$

Is this the answer we would expect intuitively? Well, the problem may be expressed as 'how many halves are there in 4?', and then it is obvious that the answer is 8. Some more examples to clarify the method:

a. $7 \div \dfrac{14}{9} = 7 \times \dfrac{9}{14} = \dfrac{9}{2}$

b. $\dfrac{\frac{3}{8}}{\frac{7}{11}} = \dfrac{3}{8} \times \dfrac{11}{7} = \dfrac{33}{56}$

c. $\dfrac{\frac{4}{9}}{\frac{-8}{27}} = \dfrac{4}{9} \times \dfrac{-27}{8} = \dfrac{-3}{2}$

d. $\dfrac{\frac{2}{3}}{\frac{4}{7} \times \frac{3}{5}} = \dfrac{2}{3} \times \dfrac{7}{4} \times \dfrac{5}{3} = \dfrac{35}{18}$

Exercise A.3

a. $\dfrac{\frac{-4}{11}}{\frac{7}{22}}$

b. $\dfrac{\frac{2}{9}}{\frac{7}{3} \times \frac{-2}{11}}$

c. $\dfrac{\frac{1}{3} \times \frac{2}{9}}{\frac{9}{1} \times \frac{1}{2}}$

A.3.3 Brackets

A bracket links two or more quantities together such that the bracket and its contents may be treated mathematically as a single quantity. If we wish to *remove* the brackets, then care over the plus and minus signs must be taken (Rule 1).

Examples

a. $2 \times (a - b) = 2 \times a - 2 \times b = 2a - 2b$
   Thus, each term in the bracket is multiplied by the term outside the bracket, with due regard for the sign convention.

b. $-4(c - 2d) = -4c + 8d$
   Note that the multiplication sign, present in Example a, has been omitted, as is usually the case.

c. $-3\left(\dfrac{-2a}{3} + b - \dfrac{1c}{7} \right) = 2a - 3b + \dfrac{3c}{7}$

Multiplying two or more brackets together can become quite involved. However, it is rare for problems in radiography to require even the multiplication of two brackets, but the method is outlined below for the sake of completeness.

Assume we wish to calculate:

$$(a + b)(c + d)$$
i.e. $(a + b)$ multiplied by $(c + d)$

To perform this calculation, we take the first term of the first bracket, a, and multiply it by $(c + d)$. Then we add the result to the multiplication of the second term, b, by $(c + d)$:

i.e. $(a + b)(c + d) = a(c + d) + b(c + d)$
$$= ac + ad + bc + bd$$

Again, we must be careful of the sign convention (Rule 1), as the following two worked examples show.

Examples

a. $(7 + c)(d - 8) = 7(d - 8) + c(d - 8) = 7d - 56 + cd - 8c$
b. $(4 - a)(3 - b + 2c) = 4(3 - b + 2c) - a(3 - b + 2c) = 12 - 4b + 8c - 3a + ab - 2ac$

Exercise A.4

a. $7a - 4(a - 2)$
b. $-6(-x + y - 3)$
c. $2(3a - 4) - 3(-a + 6)$

A.4 SOLVING EQUATIONS

Many of the types of equations encountered in problems associated with radiography are those in which a single 'unknown' (whose numerical value we wish to calculate) is 'mixed up' with several other numbers which may occur on both sides of the equation. (The solution of several equations involving several unknowns, i.e. simultaneous equations, is not normally required, and so will not be discussed here.) Our task, then, in the equations encountered, is to 'unscramble' the unknown so as to leave it on one side of the equation and all the numbers on the other side – the equation is then said to be 'solved'. This process is straightforward, provided that the following simple rule is obeyed:

Rule 3
Always perform the same operation to both sides of an equation.

This rule is intuitively obvious if it is imagined that the equals sign of the equation is the pivot of a pair of scales which is in exact balance. Whatever weight we now add to or subtract from one scale-pan must be added to or subtracted from the other or the scales will no longer be in balance. Similarly, if we double (say) the weight on one side we must do the same to the other – thus, provided we multiply by the same factor, balance is preserved and one side is equal to the other side. For example, consider the simple equation:

$$x - 2 = 3$$

If we add 2 to the left-hand side (LHS) of this equation the -2 will be cancelled, leaving x only. However, in accordance with Rule 3 above, we must add 2 to the right-hand side (RHS) in order to preserve equality:

$$\text{i.e. } x - 2 + 2 = 3 + 2 \text{ thus } x = 5$$

Putting $x = 5$ in the original equation, we have $5 - 2 = 3$, which is correct.

As another example, consider: $15 - y = 7$. Subtracting 15 from both sides so as to eliminate it from the LHS:

$$15 - y - 15 = 7 - 15 \quad \text{i.e. } -y = -8$$

Multiplying both sides by -1 in order to make both terms positive (Rule 1), we have:

$$-1 \cdot -y = -1 \cdot -8 \quad \text{i.e. } y = 8$$

(*Note:* The symbol '.' is often used, as above, to denote multiplication.)

Substituting our solution into the original equation to serve as a check, as in the previous example, we have:

$$15 - 8 = 7$$

thus verifying our answer.

It is apparent from these examples that a convenient way of picturing this type of mathematical operation is that of 'transferring a quantity from one side to the other and *changing its sign*'. Obviously, this only applies to the elimination of variables by addition or subtraction, *not* multiplication, which will be discussed in the next example.

Example

$$2 = 7 - \frac{5x}{2}$$

Proceeding as before,

$$\frac{5x}{2} = 7 - 2 = 5$$

$$\text{i.e. } \frac{5x}{2} = 5$$

We cannot now add or subtract anything to leave x on its own – we have to multiply by 2/5:

$$\text{i.e. } \frac{2}{5} \cdot \frac{5x}{2} = \frac{2}{5} \cdot 5$$

$$\text{i.e. } x = 2$$

This last step is known as *cross-multiplication* and may be pictured in the following manner:

    (cross-multiplication)

The double-ended arrows indicate that movement may be in either direction. Note that there is no change of sign.

One *incorrect* use of cross-multiplication occurs so frequently that it is worth a special mention here. Suppose we have the equation:

$$\frac{7x}{2} = \frac{3}{8} + \frac{x}{3}$$

if we cross-multiply in the following manner:

$$\frac{2}{7} \times \frac{7x}{2} = \frac{2}{7} \times \frac{3}{8} + \frac{x}{3} \text{ (incorrect)}$$

we obtain:

$$x = \frac{2 \cdot 3}{7 \cdot 8} + \frac{x}{3} \text{ (incorrect)}$$

The fault lies, of course, in the fact that Rule 3 has been disobeyed, i.e. the term $x/3$ remains unaltered although we were intending, by our cross-multiplication, to multiply both sides by 2/7. Hence, if we wished to cross-multiply at this stage, we should have obtained:

$$x = \frac{2 \cdot 3}{7 \cdot 8} + \frac{2 \cdot x}{7 \cdot 3} \text{ (correct)}$$

which may be further simplified to solve for x.

Exercise A.5

a. $\dfrac{2}{3}x = 4$

b. $\dfrac{7}{9}y - 1 = 13$

c. $q + \dfrac{3}{10} = \dfrac{5}{12}q$

d. $3\frac{3}{5}z - 12\frac{4}{5} = 1\frac{2}{5}z - \frac{7}{10}$

A.5 POWERS (INDICES)

An *index* is written at the top right of a quantity (the *base*) and refers to the number of times the quantity is multiplied by *itself*. For example, 5^3 means $5 \times 5 \times 5$ (i.e. 125). It is a convenient mathematical 'shorthand' to write powers of a number in this way. In this example, the index is a positive integer (i.e. 3), but this need not be the case for it may be positive, negative, fractional or decimal, as described below.

A.5.1 Combining indices

Let us assume that we have two numbers, 2^3 and 2^2, which we wish to combine by addition, multiplication and division in order to elicit general rules for the handling of indices.

A.5.1.1 Addition

Using the definition of an index as described above:

$$2^3 + 2^2 = 2 \cdot 2 \cdot 2 + 2 \cdot 2 = 8 + 4 = 12$$

Thus, when adding such numbers, each term is calculated separately prior to addition (or subtraction).

A.5.1.2 Multiplication

Again, from first principles, we have:

$$2^3 \cdot 2^2 = (2^3) \cdot (2^2) = 2^5 = 2^{(3+2)}$$

Hence, when multiplying two or more such numbers together, the rule is to *add* the indices.

A.5.1.3 Division

$$\frac{2^3}{2^2} = \frac{2 \cdot 2 \cdot 2}{2 \cdot 2} = 2 = 2^{(3-2)}$$

Thus, when dividing such numbers, the rule is to *subtract* the indices.

A.5.2 Negative indices

Suppose that we wish to divide 4^2 by 4^4. From first principles (Sect. A.5), we have:

Equation A.1

$$\frac{4^2}{4^4} = \frac{(4 \cdot 4)}{(4 \cdot 4 \cdot 4 \cdot 4)} = \frac{1}{4^2}$$

Also, by the rule on division as described above, we may subtract indices:

Equation A.2

$$\frac{4^2}{4^4} = 4^{(2-4)} = 4^{-2}$$

Since equations (A.1) and (A.2) are equal:

$$4^{-2} = \frac{1}{4^2}$$

In general, therefore:

Equation A.3

$$x^{-n} = \frac{1}{x^n}$$

i.e. to change a negative index to a positive index, just take the reciprocal, as shown in Equation A.3.

Examples

a. $10^{-2} = \dfrac{1}{10^2} = \dfrac{1}{100}$

b. $\dfrac{1}{10^{-6}} = \dfrac{1}{\frac{1}{10^6}} = 1 \times \dfrac{10^6}{1} = 10^6$

c. $\dfrac{420 \times 10^2}{2 \times 10^4} = 210 \times 10^{-2} = \dfrac{210}{10^2} = \dfrac{210}{100} = 2.1$

A.5.3 Fractional indices

What is meant by, say, $x^{1/2}$?

Now,

$$x^{1/2} \cdot x^{1/2} = x^{1/2 + 1/2} = x^1 = x$$

Also,

$$\sqrt{x} \cdot \sqrt{x} = x$$

from the definition of a square root.

Thus, from inspection of these two equations:

$$x^{1/2} = \sqrt{x}$$

i.e. $x^{1/2}$ is just the square root of x.
Similarly, $y^{1/3}$ is the cube root of y, etc.

Examples
a. $9^{1/2} = \sqrt{9} = \pm 3$
b. $9^{3/2} = (9^{1/2})^3 = (\pm 3)^3 = \pm 27$
c. $64^{1/3} = \sqrt[3]{64} = 4$

A.5.4 The zero index – x^0

A general number x raised to a power m is x^m. If we divide x^m by itself, the answer will obviously be 1. But $x^m \div x^m$ is x^{m-m} by the rules discussed above. Thus $1 = x^{m-m} = x^0$. Since we took any general number, this result is also general (except for 0^0, which is indeterminate).

Thus any number raised to the power zero is *unity*.

A.5.5 Indices to different bases

A problem on the inverse square law (see Ch. 26) frequently involves calculation of the form:

$$\frac{a \cdot b^2}{c^2}$$

Here a, b and c represent numbers whose values are known, having been specified by the problem. We wish to determine the best way of obtaining the final result, since b and c are frequently large numbers, whose squares are therefore even larger. This means that the probability of making an arithmetical error can be quite high if a laborious method of calculation is undertaken. However, a great simplification is possible if we remember that:

Equation A.4

$$\frac{b^2}{c^2} = \left(\frac{b}{c}\right)^2$$

Example
If $b = 90$ cm and $c = 60$ cm then b^2/c^2 the 'hard' way is:
$$\frac{b^2}{c^2} = \frac{90^2}{60^2} = \frac{8100}{3600} = \frac{81}{36}$$

which may be cancelled to give 2.25 – this exercise being left to the reader. The 'easy' way is to use Equation A.4, i.e.:

$$\frac{b^2}{c^2} = \left(\frac{b}{c}\right)^2 = \left(\frac{90}{60}\right)^2 = \left(\frac{3}{2}\right)^2 = 1.5^2 = 2.25$$

Note that the answers are the same, as we should expect, but that the second method involves cancelling of smaller numbers so that there is less likelihood of an arithmetical error.

Table A.1 Names of powers of 10

PREFIX	SYMBOL	POWER OF 10	EXAMPLE
mega	M	10^6	$1\,MW = 10^6$ watt
kilo	k	10^3	$1\,kV = 10^3$ volt
milli	m	10^{-3}	$1\,mA = 10^{-3}$ ampere
micro	μ	10^{-6}	$1\,\mu F = 10^{-6}$ farad
nano	n	10^{-9}	$1\,nm = 10^{-9}$ metre
pico	p	10^{-12}	$1\,pF = 10^{-12}$ farad

A.6 POWERS OF 10

When 10 is used as a base for indices, all the findings of the previous section apply. In addition, powers of 10 are very useful when measuring very large or very small quantities of a given unit, as shown in Table A.1.

Other names not shown in the table exist (see Table A after the appendices), but these are all that we shall need. It is advisable for the student to memorize these terms as they are in very common usage in radiography. The following exercise is included for this purpose.

Exercise A.6

a. An X-ray tube has a current of 0.05 amperes passing through it. How many milliamperes (mA) does this correspond to?
b. If the X-ray tube has a peak potential difference of 125 000 volts across it, what is the value in kilovolts (kVp)?
c. Express a capacitance of 0.000 065 farads in microfarads (μF).
d. A photon of light has a wavelength of 550 nanometres (nm). What is this in metres?

A.7 PROPORTIONALITY

A.7.1 Direct proportion

If a car is travelling at constant speed such that the petrol consumption is a steady 60 km.l^{-1}, then:

0.5 litre has been used after 30 km
1.0 litre has been used after 60 km
1.5 litres have been used after 75 km, etc.

Thus, the amount of petrol consumed is in *direct proportion* to the number of miles travelled, and we may write:

$$\text{litres} \propto \text{mileage}$$

where the sign '$\propto$' means 'is proportional to'. Alternatively, we may write:

$$\text{litres} = \left(\frac{1}{60}\right) \times \text{mileage}$$

In general, therefore, if two quantities y and x are directly proportional to each other, then:

$$y \propto x \text{ or } y = kx$$

where k is called the 'constant of proportionality'. Some examples of direct proportionality which are discussed in the main text include the following:

- The electric current (I) through a metallic conductor is proportional to the potential difference (V) across it, i.e. $I \propto V$ (Ohm's law; Ch. 7).
- Intensity of an X-ray beam $\propto$ tube current (mA) (Ch. 22).
- Intensity of an X-ray beam $\propto$ kilovoltage squared, i.e. intensity $\propto$ kV^2 (Ch. 22).

A.7.2 Inverse proportion

Suppose that we have many rectangles of equal area, k, but of differing heights (h) and widths (w). However, in each case the area is the same, so that:

$$h \times w = \text{constant } (k)$$

Then, since k is constant, we may write:

$$h = \frac{1}{w}$$

In this case, therefore, h and w are in *inverse* proportion, since w is halved if h is doubled, and vice versa. This is opposite to *direct* proportion, of course, where doubling (say) one quantity also doubles the other.

Examples of inverse proportion discussed in the main text include:

- The capacity (C) of a parallel-plate capacitor is inversely proportional to the separation (d) between its plates, i.e. $C \propto 1/d$ (Ch. 13).

- The intensity (I) from a point source of electromagnetic radiation is inversely proportional to the square of the distance (x) from the source, i.e. $I \propto 1/x^2$ (Ch. 26).
- The electrical resistant (R) of a given length of wire varies inversely as the area of cross-section (A), i.e. $R \propto 1/A$ (Ch. 7).

A.8 GRAPHS

A.8.1 Drawing and interpretation

A good understanding of the construction and interpretation of graphs is of great value in radiography, radiotherapy and nuclear medicine. The following simple but effective rules are offered in the drawing of good graphs:

- Each graph should take at least one-third of a page – use as large a scale as practicable so that you can make accurate readings.
- Each graph should have a clear, appropriate title.
- The axes, which should be drawn with a ruler, should be of approximately equal length.
- Both axes must be clearly labelled to show what is being measured and should contain units (cm, s, kg, etc.) where appropriate.
- The *independent* variable is normally on the x-axis, and the *dependent* variable on the y-axis, i.e. the variable which is being measured is plotted on the y-axis while the variable causing the change in y is plotted on the x-axis. If we consider plotting the radioactivity from a sample over a period of time, then the independent variable is time (plotted on the x-axis) while the dependent variable is the radioactivity (plotted on the y-axis).

The following examples have been chosen to illustrate both the drawing and the interpretation of graphs.

Example 1 – Direct proportion

As described in the last section, two quantities, x and y, are directly proportional to each other if $y = kx$, where k is a constant. Figure A.1 shows $y = kx$ in graphical form. The following points should be noted:

- The graph passes through the origin, since when $x = 0$, y is also equal to zero.
- The slope (or gradient) of the straight line produced is a measure of how steep it is and is defined as *the change in* y *divided by the corresponding change in* x. Since the graph passes through the origin, this is a convenient place from which to measure the changes. From this it can be seen that the slope is y/x. But from

---

the equation $y = kx$ it can be seen that $y/x = k$. Thus the slope increases as k increases.

- The general equation for a straight line will be in the form $y = mx + c$ where m is the gradient of the line and c is the intersection of the line with the y-axis – the value of x when $y = 0$.

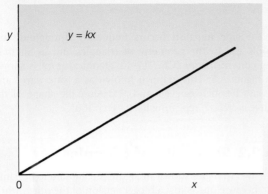

Figure A.1 Graph of $y = kx$, illustrating direct proportion.

Example 2 – Inverse proportion

Figure A.2 shows a graph of the inverse relationship between the capacitance, C, of a parallel-plate capacitor and the distance of separation of its plates, d, where $C \propto 1/d$ or $C = k/d$ for a specific capacitor.

From the graph it can be seen that as the distance between the plates increases, so the capacitance of the capacitor decreases.

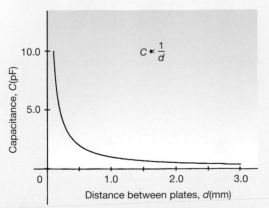

Figure A.2 Graph of $C \propto 1/d$, illustrating inverse proportion.

Example 3 – Rating graphs

Rating charts are supplied by the manufacturers of X-ray tubes, and contain a lot of information in graphical form which is an essential guide to the radiographer in the selection of 'safe' exposure factors, i.e. the combination of focal-spot size, kVp, mA and exposure time which will not cause damage to the X-ray tube.

An example of a rating chart is given by Figure A.3, where a family of curves represent the maximum permissible exposure factors for different settings of kVp. The use of rating graphs is discussed in detail in Chapter 31 and we only need to make the point here that points below a particular curve for one kVp setting are 'safe', while points above it lead to tube damage by overheating the anode.

Note the non-linear (logarithmic) scale on the x-axis. Logarithmic scales are discussed in Chapter 20.

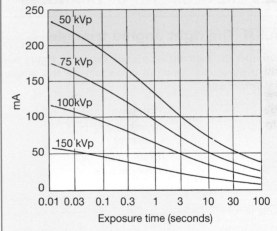

Figure A.3 Rating graph for an X-ray tube. Note the non-linear (logarithmic) scale on the x-axis.

A.8.2 Interpolation and extrapolation

It is often the case that a graph is drawn using a relatively small number of points, and that these points are joined together with a curve or straight line passing through them. The smooth curve or line makes it possible to 'read off' values from the graph, even when such values lie between the original points used to construct the graph. This procedure is known as *interpolation* and is one of the advantages of the graphical method.

If it is desired to determine the value of one of the plotted variables when it lies outside the range of the points used to plot the graph, the curve may be extended, or *extrapolated*, to reach this region. However, such an extrapolation can lead to large inaccuracies, since several different curves may seem equally suitable and there may be no way of knowing which one is correct!

Exercise A.7

a. Draw a graph of $y = 0.2x$, choosing values of x from 1 to 10 in steps of 1. Hence read from the graph the value of y when x is (i) 1.5, (ii) 9.5, (iii) 12, (iv) 0.5. Verify your answers by substitution into the original equation.
b. Repeat the same procedure for the equation $y = 0.2x^2$. (Note the increased uncertainty in obtaining the extrapolated value of y when $x = 12$.)

A.9 THE GEOMETRY OF TRIANGLES

A.9.1 The right-angled triangle

Consider the right-angled triangle shown in Figure A.4. The trigonometric functions of sine, cosine and tangent are defined as:

$$\sin A = \frac{\text{opposite}}{\text{hypotenuse}} = \frac{a}{b}$$

$$\cos A = \frac{\text{adjacent}}{\text{hypotenuse}} = \frac{c}{b}$$

$$\tan A = \frac{\text{opposite}}{\text{adjacent}} = \frac{a}{c}$$

Note that:

$$\frac{\sin A}{\cos A} = \frac{\dfrac{a}{b}}{\dfrac{c}{b}} = \frac{a}{b} \times \frac{b}{c} \text{ (by Rule 2)}$$

i.e. $\dfrac{\sin A}{\cos A} = \dfrac{a}{c} = \tan A$

Exercise A.8

a. Write down expressions for sin C, cos C and tan C from Figure A.4.
b. What is the value of $\sin^2 A + \cos^2 A$?

The sine function occurs frequently throughout this book, e.g. in the geometry of triangles and in alternating current theory (Ch. 11). Its graphical form is shown in Figure A.5. This graph is known as a 'sine wave', and always lies between +1 and −1. Also, the shape of the curve is *cyclical*, repeating itself every 360°.

A.9.2 Similarity of triangles

The two triangles shown in Figure A.6 are said to be 'similar' because one is just a bigger version of the other, while retaining the same *shape*. Thus, the corresponding angles of the two triangles are equal, but the lengths of the corresponding sides need not necessarily be so. However, if one side has a length which is double (say) that of the corresponding side of the other triangle, than *all* the sides

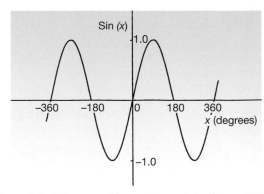

Figure A.5 A sine wave. The curve repeats itself every 360°.

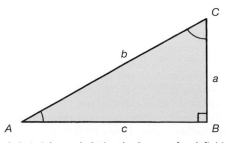

Figure A.4 A right-angled triangle. See text for definition of sine, cosine and tangent of an angle.

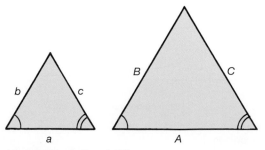

Figure A.6 Two similar triangles.

will be doubled compared to the other triangle. Generally, then, we may write:

Equation A.5

$$\frac{A}{a} = \frac{B}{b} = \frac{C}{c}$$

In many practical examples in radiography, however, the similar triangles look more like those shown in Figure A.7.

A.10 POCKET CALCULATORS AND CALCULATIONS IN EXAMINATIONS

Because the price of pocket calculators now puts them within the range of even the most impoverished student, the purchase of such a calculator is strongly recommended. 'Scientific' pocket calculators have the advantage that they can perform calculations which involve trigonometrical and logarithmic functions and so will be found especially useful. Many such calculators are also 'programmable' which means that formulae may be inserted into the calculator memory to allow it to perform certain calculations by simply inserting the appropriate data – a formula for Ohm's law could be inserted so that when the program is invoked the calculator will automatically calculate the resistance from the value of the potential and the current.

If you are to use a pocket calculator in examinations or if you are about to buy one, here are some suggestions which you might find helpful:

- Consider the types of calculations which you require from the calculator and do not buy one with lots of unnecessary functions – these simply increase your chance of error.
- Try out a calculator before you buy it (if possible) and, if you are about to use one in an examination, make sure you are familiar with its layout and functions.
- Find out the policy regarding the use of calculators in examinations at your university. Some universities will issue calculators for the purpose of examinations while others have specific regulations regarding programmable calculators.

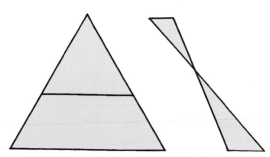

Figure A.7 Further examples of similar triangles.

- Remember that the calculator will only give the correct answer if the correct information is keyed into it. It is important to remember indices and also try to get some 'feel' for the magnitude of the correct answer.

A.11 LOGARITHMS

Although few students would now undertake calculations using logarithms as the chosen method – thanks to the ease of use of the pocket calculator – it is nevertheless helpful to have a basic grasp of the theory of logarithms to explain certain functions in radiography, e.g. it may be easier to understand the exponential equations (see Ch. 20) in their logarithmic form.

Definition
The *logarithm* of a number to a given *base* is the *power* by which the base must be raised to give the number.

Thus, the logarithm of 100 to the base 10 is 2 as $10^2 = 100$. This would normally be written as $\log_{10} 100 = 2$.

The base can be any number but, in practice, logarithms are usually to the base 10 or to the base e where e is the exponential number and is approximately equal to 2.7183.

Consider a situation where we wish to multiply two numbers a and b. If $a = 10^x$ and $b = 10^y$ then:

$$a \times b = 10^x \times 10^y = 10^{(x+y)}$$

Thus, from our initial definition of logarithms we can say:

$$\log_{10}(a \times b) = \log_{10} a + \log_{10} b$$

By a similar argument it can be shown that:

$$\log_{10}\left(\frac{a}{b}\right) = \log_{10} a - \log_{10} b$$

The main use of logarithms in radiography is to allow the simplification of complex formulae – if we consider the intensity of a beam of radiation which has travelled a distance x through a medium, this is given by the equation:

$$I_x = I_0 e^{-\mu x}$$

where I_x is the intensity of the radiation after a thickness x, I_0 is the initial intensity of the radiation, e is the exponential number and μ is the linear attenuation coefficient – these are all explained in Chapter 20. This equation is quite complicated to use in the above form but is much easier to use in its logarithmic form:

$$\log_e I_x = \log_e I_0 - \mu x$$

A.12 VECTOR QUANTITIES

In vector quantities, the quantity concerned has direction as well as dimension. Thus, in vector addition we need to take both these factors into account. This is probably best illustrated by two simple examples:

1. A man walks 30 metres in an easterly direction and then walks 20 metres in a northerly direction. How far must he walk in a straight line to get back to where he started? The situation may be visualized using Figure A.8. By applying Pythagoras' theorem to this we can calculate that the distance from C to A is 36 metres.

2. Forces $F_1 = 1$ newton, $F_2 = 4$ newtons and $F_3 = 2$ newtons are applied to a point source as shown in Figure A.9. What is the resultant force and what is its direction? As F_1 and F_3 are in opposite directions, the resultant force is the difference between F_1 and F_3 and is in the direction of F_3 as this is the larger of the two forces. We can now do vector addition (see Fig. A.10), where AB represents force F_2 and BD represents ($F_3 - F_1$). The resultant force is represented by AD. By

application of Pythagoras' theorem, the length of this line is 4.12 newtons. Tan A is BD/AB and thus A can be calculated as approximately 14°. Thus we can say that the resultant force measures 4.12 newtons and is in a direction 14° below the horizontal.

Appendix summary

- If we multiply or divide two +s or two −s, we get a +.
- If we multiply or divide a + and a − sign, we get a −.
- When dividing by a fraction, we can get the same result if we multiply by the fraction inverted (the fraction turned upside down).
- The following mathematical relationships have been established:

$$x^a \times x^b = x^{(a+b)}$$

$$\frac{x^a}{x^b} = x^{(a-b)}$$

$$x^{-a} = \frac{1}{x^a}$$

$$x^{\frac{1}{2}} = \sqrt{x}$$

$$\frac{x^a}{y^a} = \left(\frac{x}{y}\right)^a$$

- In direct proportion, $y \propto x$ or $y = kx$ while in inverse proportion, $y \propto 1/x$ or $y = c/x$ where k and c are constants of proportionality.
- Sin θ = opposite/hypotenuse; cos θ = adjacent/hypotenuse and tan θ = opposite/adjacent.
- Sine and cosine functions are cyclical, repeating themselves every 360°.
- When drawing graphs, use a manageable scale, use a ruler, label both axes and use a title.
- Similar triangles have the ratio of their corresponding sides equal.
- There are certain factors to consider when purchasing or using a pocket calculator.
- The basic theory of logarithms tells us that if $y = x^n$ then $\log_x y = n$.
- $\log_{10}(x \times y) = \log_{10}x + \log_{10}y$.
- $\log_{10}(x/y) = \log_{10}x - \log_{10}y$.
- In vector addition, we can get the resultant vector by joining the vectors end to end. The resultant vector is from the origin to the tip of the last vector.

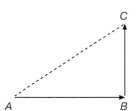

Figure A.8 Distances walked for calculation.

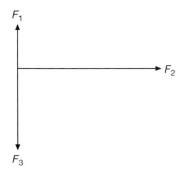

Figure A.9 Forces acting on a point.

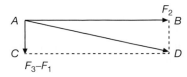

Figure A.10 Vector addition of forces.

ANSWERS TO EXERCISES

Exercise A.1

a. $\dfrac{11}{12} - \dfrac{5}{6} = \dfrac{11 - 10}{12} = \dfrac{1}{12}$

b. $\dfrac{7}{9} + \dfrac{2}{3} = \dfrac{7+6}{9} = \dfrac{13}{9} = 1\dfrac{4}{9}$

c. 20% of $50 = \dfrac{20}{100} \times 50 = 10$

d. $\dfrac{2}{3} - \dfrac{1}{4} + \dfrac{3}{5} = \dfrac{40 - 15 + 36}{60} = \dfrac{61}{60} = 1\dfrac{1}{60}$

e. $\dfrac{7}{11} + \dfrac{2}{9} - \dfrac{2}{3} = \dfrac{63 + 22 - 66}{99} = \dfrac{19}{99}$

f. Percentage change $= 100 \times \dfrac{(90 - 80)}{80}$

$= 100 \times \dfrac{10}{80} = 12.5\%$

Exercise A.2

a. $28 \div 7 = 4$

b. $\dfrac{-36}{6} = -6$

c. $\dfrac{144}{-4} = -36$

d. $-13 \times -3 = 39$

e. $-7 \times \dfrac{-8}{-2} = -7 \times 4 = -28$

Exercise A.3

a. $\dfrac{\frac{-4}{11}}{\frac{7}{22}} = \dfrac{-4}{11} \times \dfrac{22}{7} = \dfrac{-8}{7} = -1\dfrac{1}{7}$

b. $\dfrac{\frac{2}{9}}{\frac{7}{3} \times \frac{-2}{11}} = \dfrac{2}{9} \times \dfrac{3}{7} \times \dfrac{11}{-2} = \dfrac{-11}{21}$

c. $\dfrac{\frac{1}{3} \times \frac{2}{9}}{\frac{9}{1} \times \frac{1}{2}} = \dfrac{\frac{2}{27}}{\frac{9}{2}} = \dfrac{2}{27} \times \dfrac{2}{9} = \dfrac{4}{243}$

Exercise A.4

a. $7a - 4(a - 2) = 7a - 4a + 8 = 3a + a$

b. $-6(-x + y - 3) = 6x - 6y + 18$

c. $2(3a - 4) - 3(-a + 6) = 6a - 8 + 3a - 18 = 9a - 26$

Exercise A.5

a. $\dfrac{2}{3}x = 4$
$2x = 12$
$x = 6$

b. $\dfrac{7}{9}y - 1 = 13$
$7y - 9 = 117$
$7y = 126$
$y = 18$

c. $q + \dfrac{3}{10} = \dfrac{5}{12}q$
$12q + \dfrac{36}{10} = 5q$
$12q - 5q = \dfrac{-36}{10}$
$7q = \dfrac{-36}{10}$
$q = \dfrac{-36}{70}$
$= \dfrac{-18}{35}$

d. $3\dfrac{3}{5}z - 12\dfrac{4}{5} = 1\dfrac{5}{5}z - \dfrac{7}{10}$
$3\dfrac{3}{5}z - 1\dfrac{2}{5}z = 12\dfrac{4}{5} - \dfrac{7}{10}$
$2\dfrac{1}{5}z = 12\dfrac{1}{10}$
$\dfrac{11}{5}z = \dfrac{121}{10}$
$110z = 605$
$z = \dfrac{605}{110}$
$= 5\frac{1}{2}$

Exercise A.6

a. 50 mA
b. 125 kVp
c. 65 μF
d. 0.00000055 m

Exercise A.7

a. From the graph you should obtain the following readings:
  (i)   When $x = 1.5$, $y = 0.3$
  (ii) When $x = 9.5$, $y = 1.9$
  (iii) When $x = 12$, $y = 2.4$
  (iv) When $x = 0.5$, $y = 0.1$.

b. From the graph you should obtain the following readings:
   (i) When $x = 1.5$, $y = 0.45$
   (ii) When $x = 9.5$, $y = 18.05$
   (iii) When $x = 12$, $y = 28.8$
   (iv) When $x = 0.5$, $y = 0.05$.

Exercise A.8

a. From Figure A.4:
$$\sin C = c/b$$
$$\cos C = a/b$$
$$\tan C = c/a$$

b. From Figure A.4:
$$\sin^2 A + \cos^2 A = (a/b)^2 + (c/b)^2$$
$$= \frac{a^2 + c^2}{b^2}$$

But $a^2 + c^2 = b^2$ by Pythagoras' theorem.
Thus, $\sin^2 A + \cos^2 A = 1$.

Appendix | **B** |

Modulation transfer function

Modulation transfer function (MTF) is a mathematical method of assessing the resolving power of an imaging system, whether it be optical, radiographic or radioactive. The use of the MTF for this purpose was pioneered in the field of optics when it was discovered that a lens which was excellent at imaging the structure of very fine objects was not necessarily as good as another lens of lower resolving power when imaging coarser (i.e. larger) objects.

Definition

The MTF of an image is a numerical value determined by the division of the modulation (m_i) of the recorded image by the modulation of the stimulus (m_0):

Equation B.1

$$\text{MTF}(v) = m_i / m_0$$

B.1 MODULATION AND SPATIAL FREQUENCIES

As can be seen from the definition, the process of modulation is inherent in any description of the MTF and will therefore be considered first. Modulation is linked to spatial frequency. Consider the sine wave shown in Figure B.1,

which has a wavelength of X. The spatial frequency of this waveform is the number of cycles per unit length (say v cycles per cm), and is therefore given by $1/X$. The *modulation* of the object, m_0, is defined as:

Equation B.2

$$m_0 = \frac{(a - b)}{(a + b)}$$

where a and b are the height of the peaks and the troughs of the waveform respectively.

The units in which amplitude of the sine wave is recorded will differ with the application. e.g. X-ray intensity in radiography, light intensity for optical lenses, level of activity for gamma cameras or optical density for photographic film.

If it is supposed that an absorber is placed in the path of an X-ray beam such that it would produce a sinusoidal variation of intensity of the transmitted beam, then a perfect imaging system would produce a sine wave of the *same* modulation.

The *image modulation* would then be the same as the *object modulation*. However, in practice, the relative amplitude of the image modulation is reduced by the finite size of the focal spot; in addition, the recorded image is also affected by the characteristics of the image receptor. This tends to spread the image onto a larger area than theoretically desirable. Thus, the 'peaks' of the sinusoidal exposure tend to contribute to the 'troughs', so that an overall reduction in amplitude (and therefore modulation) is experienced.

This effect of a reduction in image modulation is small when the sinusoidal object has a long wavelength (low spatial frequency), but is of increasing importance as the wavelength is reduced to about 1 mm or less (spatial frequencies of 10 per cm or more). The image modulation therefore depends upon the spatial frequency of the object, and this forms the basis of the MTF, described below.

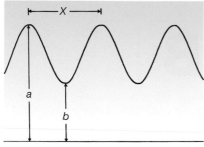

Figure B.1 The definition of modulation (see text).

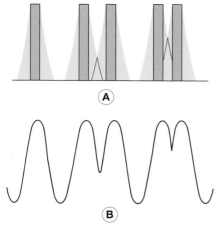

Figure B.2 The effect of increasing line-pairs per centimetre on spatial frequency. (A) Increasing geometric distortion as line-pair per millimetre increases; (B) the sine wave plot of the densities produced by (A).

B.2 MTF AND SPATIAL FREQUENCY

As seen, the MTF (Equation B.1) is defined as:

$$\text{MTF}(v) = m_i/m_0$$

In a perfect imaging system, the image is an exact copy of the object and so has the same modulation at all spatial frequencies. The MTF is therefore always unity for such a system. However, as the spatial frequency increases, it is to be expected that the imaging of fine detail (high spatial frequencies) would be worse (because of geometric distortion (Fig. B.2A)) and the image modulation is reduced (Fig. B.2B).

The graph shown in Figure B.3 shows three examples: an 'ideal' imaging system, where the MTF is 1 and is independent of the spatial frequency; a curve where the MTF is reduced at the higher frequencies due to geometric unsharpness (U_g) only and, lastly, a curve obtained when using a film/screen recording medium (U_g + screens).

The MTF is particularly useful in separating the individual causes of image degradation. MTFs due to each

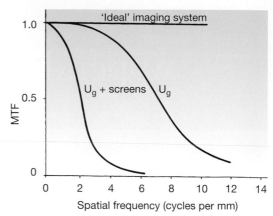

Figure B.3 The variation of the modulation transfer function (MTF) with spacial frequency for an ideal system, that due to geometric unsharpness (U_g), and that due to geometric unsharpness and screens (U_g + screens).

cause may be measured separately (MTF_1, etc.) and may be combined to produce the overall MTF of the system:

Equation B.3

$$\text{MTF} = \text{MTF}_1 \times \text{MTF}_2 \ldots$$

It thus becomes possible to predict the response of the overall system with various combinations of focal spot size, film/screen combinations, etc. if the MTF of each is known.

B.3 OBJECTS AS SPATIAL FREQUENCIES

A 'sinusoidal' object does not bear much similarity to the objects which are normally radiographed. However, it may be shown that the shape of any object may be obtained from the summation of sine and cosine waves of different amplitudes and frequencies (Fourier's theorem). Thus, if the MTF of the X-ray unit is known at each frequency, the overall response to the object may be determined.

As an example of the summation of amplitudes of different frequencies forming a shape, consider the flat-topped object shown by the dashed lines in Figure B.4A. The height of the object may be considered to represent the degree of absorption of the X-rays by the object, and its width as the physical size of the object. It may be shown that such a shape may be obtained by adding an infinite series of cosine waves (which are just sine waves displaced by 90°) of increasing frequency (f), where the amplitudes are given by:

Equation B.4

$$g = \frac{\sin(\pi f d)}{(2\pi f)}$$

The sum of the first 500 terms of such amplitudes is shown in Figure B.4A. The effect of including 2500 terms

344

Summation of all amplitudes

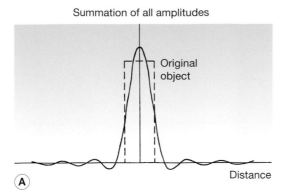

(A)

Distance

Summation of all amplitudes

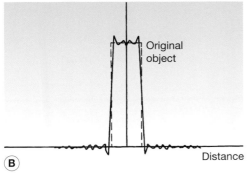

(B)

Distance

Figure B.4 The representation of a 'square' object (dashed lines) by the summation of frequencies of different amplitudes: (A) 500 terms; (B) 2500 terms. An infinite number of terms reproduces the object exactly.

(i.e. containing higher frequencies) is shown in Figure B.4B, where a closer approximation to the square shape is obtained. The agreement is exact when an infinite number of terms is included. However, the higher spatial frequencies present in the object are poorly reproduced in the image, because the MTF is low at high frequencies. Since the high frequencies are responsible for the 'square-ness' of the corners for objects such as shown in Figure B.3, sharp objects will be shown as being slightly blurred or out of focus. This is in accordance with the concept of *unsharpness*, as discussed earlier, and the two approaches are just two ways of looking at the same thing. The MTF is more mathematically rigorous as a complete descrip-tion of the imaging properties of the X-ray unit, but even this does not consider other problems such as statistical 'noise' within the image, known as '*quantum mottle*'.

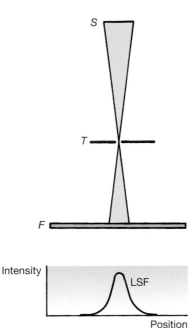

Figure B.5 The line spread function (LSF). *F*, image recording medium; *S*, source of X-rays; *T*, test object with narrow slit.

B.4 MEASUREMENT OF MTF

In practice it is difficult to manufacture sinusoidal objects in the numbers and wavelengths required and it would also be very time consuming to measure the image mod-ulation for every combination of frequency, position of absorber and image receptor for every object recorded. Fortunately, there is no need to do this: an intensity curve can be obtained by 'shining' an X-ray beam through a very narrow slit (see Fig. B.5).

Since the width of the slot is known, the blur or line spread function (LSF) of these images can be calculated, after taking into consideration all other factors affecting the 'blur' produced. These calculations are carried out by complex computer programs, the explanation of which is beyond the scope of this book. Once the LSF is known, it can in turn be used to calculate the MFT of the recorded image.

Appendix |C|

SI base units

SI base units were discussed in Chapter 4. Below are the precise definitions of these units.

C.1 MASS

The unit of mass is the *kilogram*. The mass of one kilogram is equal to the mass of the international platinum–iridium prototype of the kilogram.

C.2 LENGTH

The unit of length is the *metre*. The metre is the length equal to $1\,650\,763.73$ wavelengths in a vacuum of the radiation corresponding to the transition between the levels $2p_{10}$ and $5d_5$ of the krypton-86 atom.

C.3 TIME

The unit of time is the *second*. The second is the duration of $9\,192\,631\,770$ periods of the radiation corresponding to the transition between the two hyperfine levels of the ground state of the caesium-133 atom.

C.4 ELECTRIC CURRENT

The unit of electric current is the *ampere*. The ampere is the constant current which, if maintained in two straight parallel conductors of infinite length, of negligible circular cross-section and placed 1 metre apart in a vacuum, would produce between these conductors a force equal to 2×10^{-7} newton per metre of length.

C.5 TEMPERATURE

The unit of temperature is the *kelvin*. The kelvin is the fraction $1/273.16$ of the thermodynamic temperature of the triple point of water.

C.6 LUMINOUS INTENSITY

The unit of luminous intensity is the *candela*. The candela is the luminous intensity, in the perpendicular direction, of the surface of $1/600\,000$ square metre of a black body at the temperature of freezing platinum under a pressure of $101\,325$ newtons per square metre.

C.7 AMOUNT OF SUBSTANCE

The unit of amount of substance is the *mole*. The mole is the amount of substance of a system which contains as many elementary entities as there are atoms in $0.012\,kg$ of carbon-12.

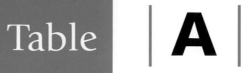

Table A Powers of 10

PREFIX	SYMBOL	FACTOR
exa	E	10^{18}
peta	P	10^{15}
tera	T	10^{12}
giga	G	10^{9}
mega	M	10^{6}
kilo	k	10^{3}
milli	m	10^{-3}
micro	μ	10^{-6}
nano	n	10^{-9}
pico	p	10^{-12}
femto	f	10^{-15}
atto	a	10^{-18}

Table B

Table B Physical constants

QUANTITY	VALUE
Avogadro's number, N_A	6.02×10^{23} mol^{-1}[a]
Velocity of light in a vacuum, c	3.00×10^{8} m.s^{-1}
Permittivity of a vacuum, ε_0	8.8×10^{-12} F.m^{-1}
Permeability of a vacuum, μ_0	1.26×10^{-6} Hm^{-1}
Electron rest mass, m_e	9.11×10^{-31} kg
Proton rest mass, m_p	1.672×10^{-27} kg
Neutron rest mass, m_n	1.675×10^{-27} kg
Planck's constant, h	6.63×10^{-34} J.s
Electronic charge, e	-1.60×10^{-19} C
[a] Or 6.02×10^{26} (kg.mol)$^{-1}$.	

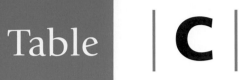

Table C Important conversion factors

QUANTITY	CONVERSION FACTOR
1 atomic mass unit (amu)	$= 1.66 \times 10^{-27}\,kg$
1 electron volt (eV)	$= 1.60 \times 10^{-19}\,J$
1 joule (J)	$= 6.24 \times 10^{18}\,eV$
Electron mass	$= 0.511\,MeV$
Proton mass	$= 938\,MeV$
Neutron mass	$= 940\,MeV$
1 angstrom (Å)	$0.1\,nm$

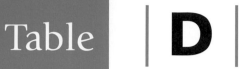

Table D Greek symbols and their common usage

NAME	SYMBOL		USAGE
	CAPITAL	LOWER CASE	
Alpha	A	α	α-Particle (He nucleus); also lower-case (α) is the flip angle in MRI
Beta	B	β	β-Particle (electron or positron)
Gamma	Γ	γ	γ-rays; also gyromagnetic ratio in MRI
Delta	Δ	δ	Δx or δx used to indicate change in x
Epsilon	E	ϵ	
Zeta	Z	ζ	
Eta	H	η	
Theta	Θ	θ	Used to represent angle
Iota	I	ι	
Kappa	K	κ	
Lambda	V	λ	(λ) Wavelength; radioactive decay constant
Mu	M	μ	(μ) Total linear attenuation coefficient
Nu	N	ν	(ν) Frequency of electromagnetic radiation
Xi	Ξ	ξ	
Omicron	O	o	
Pi	Π	π	(π) Linear attenuation coefficient for pair production
Rho	P	ρ	(ρ) Density of matter: resistivity
Sigma	Σ	σ	(σ) Linear attenuation coefficient for the Compton effect
Tau	T	τ	(τ) Linear attenuation coefficient for photoelectric absorption
Upsilon	Y	υ	
Phi	Φ	φ	Used to represent angle
Chi	X	χ	
Psi	Ψ	ψ	
Omega	Ω	ω	(Ω) Symbol used for resistance or impedance in ohm; (ω) used for precession frequency in MRI

MRI, magnetic resonance imaging.

Table D Greek symbols and their common usage

Table |E|

Table E The periodic table of elements

GROUP	1	2	3	4	5	6	7	8	9	10	11	12	13	14	15	16	17	18
PERIOD																		
1	1 H																	2 He
2	3 Li	4 Be											5 B	6 C	7 N	8 O	9 F	10 Ne
3	11 Na	12 Mg											12 Al	14 Si	15 P	16 S	17 Cl	18 Ar
4	19 K	20 Ca	21 Sc	22 Ti	23 V	24 Cr	25 Mn	26 Fe	27 Co	28 Ni	29 Cu	30 Zn	31 Ga	32 Ge	33 As	34 Se	35 Br	36 Kr
5	37 Rb	38 Sr	39 Y	40 Zr	41 Nb	42 Mo	43 Tc	44 Ru	45 Rh	46 Pd	47 Ag	48 Cd	49 In	50 Sn	51 Sb	52 Te	53 I	54 Xe
6	55 Cs	56 Ba	*	71 Lu	72 Hf	73 Ta	74 W	75 Re	76 Os	77 Ir	78 Pt	79 Au	80 Hg	81 Tl	82 Pb	83 Bi	84 Po	85 At	86 Rn
7	87 Fr	88 Ra	**	103 Lr	104 Rf	105 Db	106 Sg	107 Bh	108 Hs	109 Mt	110 Ds	111 Rg	112 Cn	113 Uut	114 Uuq	115 Uup	116 Uuh	117 Uus	118 Uuo
*Lanthanoids			57 La	58 Ce	59 Pr	60 Nd	61 Pn	62 Sm	63 Eu	64 Gd	65 Tb	66 Dy	67 Ho	68 Er	69 Tm	70 Yb		
**Actinoids			89 Ac	90 Th	91 Pa	92 U	93 Np	94 Pu	95 Am	96 Cm	97 Bk	98 Cf	99 Es	100 Fm	101 Md	102 No		

Table |F|

Table F Electron configuration of the elements

| ELEMENT | ATOMIC NO. | SYMBOL | NUMBER OF ELECTRONS IN SHELL | | | | | | |
			K	*L*	*M*	*N*	*O*	*P*	*Q*
Hydrogen	1	H	1						
Helium	2	He	2						
Lithium	3	Li	2	1					
Beryllium	4	Be	2	2					
Boron	5	B	2	3					
Carbon	6	C	2	4					
Nitrogen	7	N	2	5					
Oxygen	8	O	2	6					
Fluorine	9	F	2	7					
Neon	10	Ne	2	8					
Sodium	11	Na	2	8	1				
Magnesium	12	Mg	2	8	2				
Aluminium	13	Al	2	8	3				
Silicon	14	Si	2	8	4				
Phosphorus	15	P	2	8	5				
Sulphur	16	S	2	8	6				
Chlorine	17	Cl	2	8	7				
Argon	18	Ar	2	8	8				
Potassium	19	K	2	8	8	1			
Calcium	20	Ca	2	8	8	2			
Scandium	21	Sc	2	8	9	2			

(*Continued*)

359

ELEMENT	ATOMIC NO.	SYMBOL	NUMBER OF ELECTRONS IN SHELL						
			K	L	M	N	O	P	Q
Titanium	22	Ti	2	8	10	2			
Vanadium	23	V	2	8	11	2			
Chromium	24	Cr	2	8	13	1			
Manganese	25	Mn	2	8	13	2			
Iron	26	Fe	2	8	14	2			
Cobalt	27	Co	2	8	15	2			
Nickel	28	Ni	2	8	16	2			
Copper	29	Cu	2	8	18	1			
Zinc	30	Zn	2	8	18	2			
Gallium	31	Ga	2	8	18	3			
Germanium	32	Ge	2	8	18	4			
Arsenic	33	As	2	8	18	5			
Selenium	34	Se	2	8	18	6			
Bromine	35	Br	2	8	18	7			
Krypton	36	Kr	2	8	18	8			
Rubidium	37	Rb	2	8	18	8	1		
Strontium	38	Sr	2	8	18	8	2		
Yttrium	39	Yt	2	8	18	9	2		
Zirconium	40	Zr	2	8	18	10	2		
Niobium	41	Nb	2	8	18	12	1		
Molybdenum	42	Mo	2	8	18	13	1		
Technetium	43	Tc	2	8	18	14	1		
Ruthenium	44	Ru	2	8	18	15	1		
Rhodium	45	Rh	2	8	18	16	1		
Palladium	46	Pd	2	8	18	18			
Silver	47	Ag	2	8	18	18	1		
Cadmium	48	Cd	2	8	18	18	2		
Indium	49	In	2	8	18	18	3		
Tin	50	Sn	2	8	18	18	4		
Antimony	51	Sb	2	8	18	18	5		

ELEMENT	ATOMIC NO.	SYMBOL	NUMBER OF ELECTRONS IN SHELL						
			K	L	M	N	O	P	Q
Tellurium	52	Te	2	8	18	18	6		
Iodine	53	I	2	8	18	18	7		
Xenon	54	Xe	2	8	18	18	8		
Caesium	55	Cs	2	8	18	18	8	1	
Barium	56	Ba	2	8	18	18	8	2	
Lanthanum	57	La	2	8	18	18	9	2	
Cerium	58	Ce	2	8	18	20	8	2	
Praseodymium	59	Pr	2	8	18	21	8	2	
Neodymium	60	Nd	2	8	18	22	8	2	
Promethium	61	Pm	2	8	18	23	8	2	
Samarium	62	Sm	2	8	18	24	8	2	
Europium	63	Eu	2	8	18	25	8	2	
Gadolinium	64	Gd	2	8	18	25	9	2	
Terbium	65	Tb	2	8	18	26	9	2	
Dysprosium	66	Dy	2	8	18	28	8	2	
Holmium	67	Ho	2	8	18	29	8	2	
Erbium	68	Er	2	8	18	30	8	2	
Thulium	69	Tm	2	8	18	31	8	2	
Ytterbium	70	Yb	2	8	18	32	8	2	
Lutetium	71	Lu	2	8	18	32	9	2	
Hafnium	72	Hf	2	8	18	32	10	2	
Tantalum	73	Ta	2	8	18	32	11	2	
Tungsten	74	Wo	2	8	18	32	12	2	
Rhenium	75	Re	2	8	18	32	13	2	
Osmium	76	Os	2	8	18	32	14	2	
Iridium	77	Ir	2	8	18	32	15	2	
Platinum	78	Pt	2	8	18	32	17	1	
Gold	79	Au	2	8	18	32	18	1	
Mercury	80	Hg	2	8	18	32	18	2	
Thallium	81	Tl	2	8	18	32	18	3	

(Continued)

			NUMBER OF ELECTRONS IN SHELL						
ELEMENT	ATOMIC NO.	SYMBOL	K	L	M	N	O	P	Q
Lead	82	Pb	2	8	18	32	18	4	
Bismuth	83	Bi	2	8	18	32	18	5	
Polonium	84	Po	2	8	18	32	18	6	
Astatine	85	At	2	8	18	32	18	7	
Radon	86	Rn	2	8	18	32	18	8	
Francium	87	Fr	2	8	18	32	18	8	1
Radium	88	Ra	2	8	18	32	18	8	2
Actinium	89	Ac	2	8	18	32	18	9	2
Thorium	90	Th	2	8	18	32	18	10	2
Protactinium	91	Pa	2	8	18	32	20	9	2
Uranium	92	U	2	8	18	32	21	9	2
Neptunium	93	Np	2	8	18	32	23	8	2
Plutonium	94	Pu	2	8	18	32	24	8	2
Americium	95	Am	2	8	18	32	25	8	2
Curium	96	Cm	2	8	18	32	25	9	2
Berkelium	97	Bk	2	8	18	32	27	8	2
Californium	98	Cf	2	8	18	32	28	8	2
Einsteinium	99	Es	2	8	18	32	29	8	2
Fermium	100	Fm	2	8	18	32	30	8	2
Mendelevium	101	Md	2	8	18	32	31	8	2
Nobelium	102	No	2	8	18	32	32	8	2
Lawrencium	103	Lw	2	8	18	32	32	9	2
Rutherfordium	104	Rf	2	8	18	32	32	10	2
Dudnium	105	Dd	2	8	18	32	32	11	2
Saeborgium	106	Sg	2	8	18	32	32	12	2
Bohrium	107	Bh	2	8	18	32	32	13	2
Hassium	108	Hs	2	8	18	32	32	14	2
Meiterium	109	Mt	2	8	18	32	32	15	2
Darnstatium	110	Ds	2	8	18	32	32	17	1
Roentgenium	111	Rg	2	8	18	32	32	18	1

ELEMENT	ATOMIC NO.	SYMBOL	NUMBER OF ELECTRONS IN SHELL						
			K	L	M	N	O	P	Q
Copernicium	112	Cn	2	8	18	32	32	18	2
Ununtrium	113	Uut	2	8	18	32	32	18	3
Ununquadium	114	Uuq	2	8	18	32	32	18	4
Ununpentium	115	Uup	2	8	18	32	32	18	5
Ununquadium	116	Uuh	2	8	18	32	32	18	6
Ununseptium	117	Uus	2	8	18	32	32	18	7
Ununoctium	118	Uuo	2	8	18	32	32	18	8

Index